ADVANCES IN CLINICAL TRIAL BIOSTATISTICS

Biostatistics: A Series of References and Textbooks

1. *Design and Analysis of Animal Studies in Pharmaceutical Development*, edited by Shein-Chung Chow and Jen-pei Liu
2. *Basic Statistics and Pharmaceutical Statistical Applications*, James E. De Muth
3. *Design and Analysis of Bioavailability and Bioequivalence Studies, Second Edition, Revised and Expanded*, Shein-Chung Chow and Jen-pei Liu
4. *Meta-Analysis in Medicine and Health Policy*, edited by Dalene K. Stangl and Donald A. Berry
5. *Generalized Linear Models: A Bayesian Perspective*, edited by Dipak K. Dey, Sujit K. Ghosh, and Bani K. Mallick
6. *Difference Equations with Public Health Applications*, Lemuel A. Moyé and Asha Seth Kapadia
7. *Medical Biostatistics*, Abhaya Indrayan and Sanjeev B. Sarmukaddam
8. *Statistical Methods for Clinical Trials*, Mark X. Norleans
9. *Causal Analysis in Biomedicine and Epidemiology: Based on Minimal Sufficient Causation*, Mikel Aickin
10. *Statistics in Drug Research: Methodologies and Recent Developments*, Shein-Chung Chow and Jun Shao
11. *Sample Size Calculations in Clinical Research,* Shein-Chung Chow, Jun Shao, and Hansheng Wang
12. *Applied Statistical Designs for the Researcher*, Daryl S. Paulson
13. *Advances in Clinical Trial Biostatistics*, Nancy L. Geller

ADDITIONAL VOLUMES IN PREPARATION

ADVANCES IN CLINICAL TRIAL BIOSTATISTICS

edited by
NANCY L. GELLER
National Heart, Lung, and Blood Institute
National Institutes of Health
Bethesda, Maryland, U.S.A.

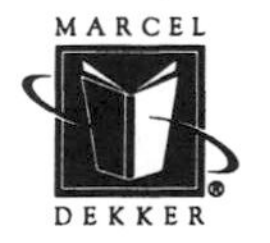

MARCEL DEKKER, INC. NEW YORK • BASEL

This book was edited by Nancy L. Geller in her private capacity. The views expressed do not necessarily represent the views of NIH, DHHS, or the United States.

Library of Congress Cataloging-in-Publication Data
A catalog record for this book is available from the Library of Congress.

ISBN: 0-8247-9032-4

This book is printed on acid-free paper.

Headquarters
Marcel Dekker, Inc., 270 Madison Avenue, New York, NY 10016, U.S.A.
tel: 212-696-9000; fax: 212-685-4540

Distribution and Customer Service
Marcel Dekker, Inc., Cimarron Road, Monticello, New York 12701, U.S.A.
tel: 800-228-1160; fax: 845-796-1772

Eastern Hemisphere Distribution
Marcel Dekker AG, Hutgasse 4, Postfach 812, CH-4001 Basel, Switzerland
tel: 41-61-260-6300; fax: 41-61-260-6333

World Wide Web
http://www.dekker.com

The publisher offers discounts on this book when ordered in bulk quantities. For more information, write to Special Sales/Professional Marketing at the headquarters address above.

Current printing (last digit):

10 9 8 7 6 5 4 3 2 1

PRINTED IN THE UNITED STATES OF AMERICA

Series Introduction

The primary objectives of the Biostatistics series are to provide useful reference books for researchers and scientists in academia, industry, and government, and also to offer textbooks for undergraduate and/or graduate courses in the area of biostatistics. The series provides comprehensive and unified presentations of statistical designs and analyses of important applications in biostatistics, such as those in biopharmaceuticals. A well-balanced summary is given of current and recently developed statistical methods and interpretations for both statisticians and researchers/scientists with minimal statistical knowledge who are engaged in the field of applied biostatistics. The series is committed to presenting easy-to-understand, state-of-the-art references and textbooks. In each volume, statistical concepts and methodologies are illustrated through real-world examples whenever possible.

Clinical research is a lengthy and costly process that involves drug discovery, formulation, laboratory development, animal studies, clinical development, and regulatory submission. This lengthy process is necessary not only for understanding the target disease but also for providing substantial evidence regarding efficacy and safety of the pharmaceutical compound under investigation prior to regulatory approval. In addition, it provides assurance that the drug products under investigation will possess good characteristics such as identity, strength, quality, purity, and stability after regulatory approval. For this purpose, biostatistics plays an important role in clinical research not only to provide a valid and fair assessment of the drug product under investigation prior to regulatory approval but also to ensure that the drug product possesses good characteristics with the desired accuracy and reliability.

This volume provides a comprehensive summarization of recent developments regarding methodologies in design and analysis of studies conducted in clinical research. It covers important topics in early-phase clinical development such as Bayesian methods for phase I cancer clinical trials and late-phase clinical development such as design and analysis of therapeutic equivalence trials, adaptive two-stage clinical trials, and cluster randomization trials. The book also provides useful approaches to critical statistical issues that are commonly encountered in clinical research such as multiplicity, subgroup analysis, interaction, and analysis of longitudinal data with missing values. It will be beneficial to biostatisticians, medical researchers, and pharmaceutical scientists who are engaged in the areas of clinical research and development.

Shein-Chung Chow

Preface

As the medical sciences rapidly advance, clinical trials biostatisticians and graduate students preparing for careers in clinical trials need to maintain knowledge of current methodology. Because the literature is so vast and journals are published so frequently, it is difficult to keep up with the relevant literature. The goal of this book is to summarize recent methodology for design and analysis of clinical trials arranged in standalone chapters.

The book surveys a number of aspects of contemporary clinical trials, ranging from early trials to complex modeling problems. Each chapter contains enough references to allow those interested to delve more deeply into an area. A basic knowledge of clinical trials is assumed, along with a good background in classical biostatistics. The chapters are at the level of journal articles in *Biometrics* or *Statistics in Medicine* and are meant to be read by second- or third-year biostatistics graduate students, as well as by practicing biostatisticians.

The book is arranged in three parts. The first consists of two chapters on the first trials undertaken in humans in the course of drug development (Phase I and II trials). The second and largest part is on randomized clinical trials, covering a variety of design and analysis topics. These include design of equivalence trials, adaptive schemes to change sample size during the course of a trial, design of clustered randomized trials, design and analysis of trials with multiple primary endpoints, a new method for survival analysis, and how to report a Bayesian randomized trial. The third section deals with more complex problems: including compliance in the assessment of treatment effects, the analysis of longitudinal data with missingness, and the particular problems that have arisen in AIDS clinical trials. Several of the chapters incorporate Bayesian methods, reflecting the recognition that these have become acceptable in what used to be a frequentist discipline.

The 20 authors of this volume represent five countries and 10 institutions. Many of the authors are well known internationally for their methodological contributions and have extensive experience in clinical trials practice as well as being methodologists. Each chapter gives real and relevant examples from the authors' personal experiences, making use of a wide range of both treatment and prevention trials. The examples reflect work in a variety of fields of medicine, such as cardiovascular diseases, neurological diseases, cancer, and AIDS. While it was often the clinical trial itself that gave rise to a question that required new methodology to answer, it is likely that the methods will find applications in other medical fields. In this sense, the contributions are examples of "ideal" biostatistics, transcending the boundary between statistical theory and clinical trials practice.

I wish to express my deep appreciation to all the authors for their patience and collegiality and for their fine contributions and outstanding expositions. I also thank my husband for his constant encouragement and Marcel Dekker, Inc., for their continuing interest in this project.

Nancy L. Geller

Contents

Contributors

Paul S. Albert, Ph.D. Mathematical Statistician, Biometrics Research Branch, Division of Cancer Treatment and Diagnosis, National Cancer Institute, National Institutes of Health, Bethesda, Maryland, U.S.A.

James S. Babb, Ph.D. Department of Biostatistics, Fox Chase Cancer Center, Philadelphia, Pennsylvania, U.S.A.

Abdel G. Babiker, Ph.D. Head, Division of HIV and Infections, and Professor of Medical Statistics and Epidemiology, Medical Research Council Clinical Trials Unit, London, England

Shelly L. Carter, Sc.D. Senior Biostatistician, The Emmes Corporation, Rockville, Maryland, U.S.A.

Michael P. Fay, Ph.D. Mathematical Statistician, Statistical Research and Applications, National Cancer Institute, National Institutes of Health, Bethesda, Maryland, U.S.A.

Dean Follmann, Ph.D. Chief, Biostatistics Research Branch, National Institute of Allergy and Infectious Diseases, National Institutes of Health, Bethesda, Maryland, U.S.A.

Laurence S. Freedman, M.A., Dip.Stat., Ph.D. Professor, Departments of Mathematics and Statistics, Bar-Ilan University, Ramat Gan, Israel

Nancy L. Geller, Ph.D. Director, Office of Biostatistics Research, National Heart, Lung, and Blood Institute, National Institutes of Health, Bethesda, Maryland, U.S.A.

Els Goetghebeur, Ph.D. Professor, Department of Applied Mathematics and Computer Science, University of Ghent, Ghent, Belgium

Eric S. Leifer, Ph.D. Mathematical Statistician, Office of Biostatistics Research, National Heart, Lung, and Blood Institute, National Institutes of Health, Bethesda, Maryland, U.S.A.

Juni Palmgren, Ph.D. Professor, Department of Mathematical Statistics and Department of Medical Epidemiology and Biostatistics, Stockholm University and Karolinska Institutet, Stockholm, Sweden

Mahesh Parmar, D.Phil., M.Sc., B.Sc. Professor of Medical Statistics and Epidemiology, Cancer Division, Medical Research Council Clinical Trials Unit, London, England

Michael A. Proschan, Ph.D. Mathematical Statistician, Office of Biostatistical Research, National Heart, Lung, and Blood Institute, National Institutes of Health, Bethesda, Maryland, U.S.A.

André Rogatko, Ph.D. Department of Biostatistics, Fox Chase Cancer Center, Philadelphia, Pennsylvania, U.S.A.

Joanna H. Shih, Ph.D. Mathematical Statistician, Biometric Research Branch, Division of Cancer Treatment and Diagnosis, National Cancer Institute, National Institutes of Health, Bethesda, Maryland, U.S.A.

Richard M. Simon, D.Sc. Chief, Biometric Research Branch, Division of Cancer Treatment and Diagnosis, National Cancer Institute, National Institutes of Health, Bethesda, Maryland, U.S.A.

Ann Sarah Walker, Ph.D., M.Sc. Medical Research Council Clinical Trials Unit, London, England

Simon Weeden, M.Sc. Senior Medical Statistician, Cancer Division, Medical Research Council Clinical Trials Unit, London, England

Margaret C. Wu, Ph.D.* Mathematical Statistician, Office of Biostatistics Research, National Heart, Lung, and Blood Institute, National Institutes of Health, Bethesda, Maryland, U.S.A.

David M. Zucker, Ph.D. Associate Professor, Department of Statistics, Hebrew University, Jerusalem, Israel

---

* Retired.

ADVANCES IN CLINICAL TRIAL BIOSTATISTICS

1
Bayesian Methods for Cancer Phase I Clinical Trials

James S. Babb and André Rogatko
Fox Chase Cancer Center, Philadelphia, Pennsylvania, U.S.A.

1. INTRODUCTION

1.1. Goal and Definitions

The primary statistical objective of a cancer phase I clinical trial is to determine the optimal dose of a new treatment for subsequent clinical evaluation of efficacy. The dose sought is typically referred to as the *maximum tolerated dose* (MTD), and its definition depends on the severity and manageability of treatment side effects as well as on clinical attributes of the target patient population. For most anticancer regimens, evidence of treatment benefit, usually expressed as a reduction in tumor size or an increase in survival, requires months (if not years) of observation and is therefore unlikely to occur during the relatively short time course of a phase I trial (O'Quigley et al., 1990; Whitehead, 1997). Consequently, the phase I target dose is usually defined in terms of the prevalence of treatment side effects without direct regard for treatment efficacy. For the majority of cytotoxic agents, toxicity is considered a prerequisite for optimal antitumor activity (Wooley and Schein, 1979) and the probability of treatment benefit is assumed to monotonically increase with dose, at least over the range of doses under consideration in the phase I trial. Consequently, the MTD of a cytotoxic agent typically corresponds to the highest dose associated with a tolerable level of toxicity. More precisely, the MTD is defined as the dose expected to produce some degree of medically unacceptable, dose limiting toxicity (DLT) in a specified proportion θ of patients (Storer, 1989; Gatsonis and Greenhouse, 1992). Hence we have

$$\text{Prob}\{\text{DLT} \mid \text{Dose} = \text{MTD}\} = \theta \tag{1}$$

where the value chosen for the target probability θ would depend on the nature of the dose limiting toxicity; it would be set relatively high when the DLT is a transient, correctable, or nonfatal condition, and low when it is lethal or life threatening (O'Quigley et al., 1990). Participants in cancer phase I trials are usually late stage patients for whom most or all alternative therapies have failed. For such patients, toxicity may be severe before it is considered an intolerable burden (Whitehead, 1997). Thus, in cancer phase I trials, dose limiting toxicity is often severe or potentially life threatening and the target probability of toxic response is correspondingly low, generally less than or equal to 1/3. As an example, in a phase I trial evaluating 5-fluorouracil (5-FU) in combination with leucovorin and topotecan (see Sec. 1.4.1), dose limiting toxicity was defined as any treatment attributable occurrence of: (1) a nonhematologic toxicity (e.g., neurotoxicity) whose severity according to the Common Toxicity Criteria* of the National Cancer Institute (1993) is grade 3 or higher; (2) a grade 4 hematologic toxicity (e.g., thrombocytopenia or myelosuppression) persisting at least 7 days; or (3) a 1 week or longer interruption of the treatment schedule. The MTD was then defined as the dose of 5-FU that is expected to induce such dose limiting toxicity in one-third of the patients in the target population. As illustrated with this example, the definition of DLT should be broad enough to capture all anticipated forms of toxic response as well as many that are not necessarily anticipated, but may nonetheless occur. This will reduce the likelihood that the definition of DLT will need to be altered or clarified upon observation of unanticipated, treatment-attributable adverse events—a process generally requiring a formal amendment to the trial protocol and concomitant interruption of patient accrual and treatment.

It is important to note that there is currently no consensus regarding the definition of the MTD. When the phase I trial is designed

* The Common Toxicity Criteria can be found on the Internet at http://ctep.info.nih.gov/CTC3/default.htm.

according to traditional, non-Bayesian methods (e.g., the up-and-down schemes described in Storer, 1989), an empiric, data-based definition is most often employed. Thus, the MTD is frequently taken to be the highest dose utilized in the trial such that the percentage of patients manifesting DLT is equal to a specified level such as 33%. For example, patients are often treated in cohorts, usually consisting of three patients, with all patients in a cohort receiving the same dose. The dose is changed between successive cohorts according to a predetermined schedule typically based on a so-called modified Fibonacci sequence (Von Hoff et al., 1984). The trial is terminated the first time at least some number of patients (generally 2 out of 6) treated at the same dose exhibit DLT. This dose level constitutes the MTD. The dose level recommended for phase II evaluation of efficacy is then taken to be either the MTD or one dose level below the MTD (Kramar et al., 1999). Although this serves as an adequate working definition of the MTD for trials of nonparametric design, such an empiric formulation is not appropriate for use with most Bayesian and other parametric phase I trial design methodologies. Consequently, it will be assumed throughout the remainder of this chapter that the MTD is defined according to Eq. (1) for some suitable definition of DLT and choice of target probability θ.

The fundamental conflict underlying the design of cancer phase I clinical trials is that the desire to increase the dose slowly to avoid unacceptable toxic events must be tempered by an acknowledgment that escalation proceeding too slowly may cause many patients to be treated at suboptimal or nontherapeutic doses (O'Quigley et al., 1990). Thus, from a therapeutic perspective, one should design cancer Phase I trials to minimize both the number of patients treated at low, nontherapeutic doses as well as the number given severely toxic overdoses.

1.2. Definition of Dose

Bayesian procedures for designing phase I clinical trials require the specification of a model for the relationship between dose level and treatment related toxic response. Depending on the agent under investigation and the route and schedule of its administration, the model may relate toxicity to the physical amount of agent given each patient, or to some target drug exposure such as the area under the time vs. plasma concentration curve (AUC) or peak plasma concentration. The choice of formulation is dependent on previous experience and medical theory and is beyond the scope of the present chapter. Consequently, it will be assumed that the appropriate representation of dose level has been determined prior to specification of the dose-toxicity model.

1.3. Choice of Starting Dose

In cancer therapy, the phase I trial often represents the first time a particular treatment regimen is being administered to humans. Due to consequent safety considerations, the starting dose in a cancer phase I trial is traditionally a low dose at which no significant toxicity is anticipated. For example, the initial dose is frequently selected on the basis of preclinical investigation to be one-tenth of the murine equivalent LD_{10} (the dose that produces 10% mortality in mice) or one-third the toxic dose low (first toxic dose) in dogs (Geller, 1984; Penta et al., 1992). Conversely, several authors (e.g., O'Quigley et al., 1990) suggest that the starting dose should correspond to the experimenter's best prior estimate of the MTD, which may not be a conservative initial level. This may be appropriate since starting the trial at a dose level significantly below the MTD may unduly increase the time and number of patients required to complete the trial and since retrospective studies (Penta et al., 1992; Arbuck, 1996) suggest that the traditional choice of starting dose often results in numerous patients being treated at biologically inactive dose levels. In the sequel, it will be assumed that the starting dose is predetermined; its choice based solely on information available prior to the onset of the trial.

1.4. Examples

Selected aspects of the Bayesian approach to phase I trial design will be illustrated using examples based on two phase I clinical trials conducted at the Fox Chase Cancer Center.

5-FU Trial

In this trial a total of 12 patients with malignant solid tumors were treated with a combination of 5-fluorouracil (5-FU), leucovorin, and topotecan. The goal was to determine the MTD of 5-FU, defined as the dose that, when administered in combination with 20 mg/m^2 leucovorin and 0.5 mg/m^2 topotecan, results in a probability $\theta = 1/3$ that a DLT will be manifest within 2 weeks. The relevant data obtained from this trial are given in Table 1.

Table 1 Dose Level of 5-FU (mg/m^2) and Binary Assessment of Treatment-Induced Toxic Response for the 12 Patients in the 5-FU Phase I Trial

Patient[a]	5-FU Dose	Response
1	140	No DLT
2	210	No DLT
3	250	No DLT
4	273	No DLT
5	291	No DLT
6	306	No DLT
7	318	No DLT
8	328	No DLT
9	337	No DLT
10	345	No DLT
11	352	DLT
12	338	DLT

[a] Patients are listed in chronological order according to date of accrual.

PNU Trial

The incorporation of patient-specific covariate information into a Bayesian design scheme will be exemplified through a phase I study of PNU-214565 (PNU) involving patients with advanced adenocarcinomas of gastrointestinal origin (Babb and Rogatko, 2001). Previous clinical and preclinical studies demonstrated that the action of PNU is moderated by the neutralizing capacity of anti-SEA antibodies. Based on this, the MTD of PNU was defined as a function of the pretreatment concentration of circulating anti-SEA antibodies. Specifically, the MTD was defined as the dose level expected to induce DLT in a proportion $\theta = .1$ of the patients with a given pretreatment anti-SEA concentration.

2. GENERAL BAYESIAN METHODOLOGY

The design and conduct of phase I clinical trials would benefit from statistical methods that can incorporate information from preclinical studies and sources outside the trial. Furthermore, both the investigator and patient might benefit if updated assessments of the risk of toxicity were available during the trial. Both of these needs can be addressed within a Bayesian framework. In Sections 2.1 through 2.5 we present a description of selected Bayesian procedures developed for the specific case where toxicity is assessed on a binary scale (presence or absence of DLT), only a single agent is under investigation (the levels of any other agents being fixed) and no relevant pretreatment covariate information is available to tailor the dosing scheme to individual patient needs. We discuss extensions and modifications of the selected methods in Section 3.

2.1. Formulation of the Problem

Dose level will be represented by the random variable X whose realization is denoted by x. For notational compactness, the same variable will be used for any formulation of dosage deemed appropriate. Thus, for example, X may represent some target drug exposure (e.g., AUC), the physical amount of agent in appropriate units (e.g., mg/m^2), or the amount of agent expressed as a multiple of the starting dose, and might be expressed on a logarithmic or other suitable scale. It will be assumed throughout that the MTD is expressed in a manner consistent with X.

The data observed for k patients will be denoted $D_k = \{(x_i, y_i); i = 1, \ldots, k\}$, where x_i is the dose administered patient i, and y_i is an indicator for dose limiting toxicity assuming the value $y_i = 1$ if the ith patient manifests DLT and the value $y_i = 0$, otherwise. The MTD is denoted by γ and corresponds to the dose level expected to induce dose limiting toxicity in a proportion θ of patients.

In the ensuing sections, a general Bayesian paradigm for the design of cancer phase I trials will be described in terms of three components:

1. A *model* for the dose-toxicity relationship. The model specifies the probability of dose limiting toxicity at each dose level as a function of one or more unknown parameters.
2. A *prior distribution* for the vector $\boldsymbol{\nu}$ containing the unknown parameters of the dose-toxicity model. The prior will be represented by a probability density function h defined on the parametric space Θ specified for $\boldsymbol{\nu}$. It is chosen so that $H(I) = \int_I h(\mathbf{u})\, d\mathbf{u}$ is an assessment of the probability that $\boldsymbol{\nu}$ is contained in $I \subseteq \Theta$ based solely on the information available prior to the onset of the phase I trial.

3. A *loss function* quantifying the total cost associated with the administration of any permissible dose level. The loss will be expressed through a function L defined on $S \times \Theta$, where S is the set of dose levels available for use in the trial. Hence, $L(x, \boldsymbol{\nu})$ denotes the loss incurred by treating a patient at dose level $x \in S$ when $\boldsymbol{\nu} \in \Theta$ obtains.

Through an application of Bayes' theorem the dose-toxicity model and prior distribution can be used to derive the posterior distribution of $\boldsymbol{\nu}$ given D_k. Hence, we obtain a function Π_k defined on the parametric space Θ such that $\int_I \Pi_k(\mathbf{u})d\mathbf{u}$ is the conditional probability that $\boldsymbol{\nu}$ is contained in $I \subseteq \Theta$ given the data available after k patients have been observed. We can then compute

$$EL_k(x) = \int_\Theta L(x, \mathbf{u})\Pi_k(\mathbf{u})\,d\mathbf{u}$$

representing the posterior expected loss associated with dose $x \in S$ after observation of k patients. When a phase I trial is designed according to strict Bayesian decision-theoretic principles, dose escalation proceeds by selecting for each patient the dose level $x \in S$ minimizing the posterior expected loss given the prevailing data. Thus, after the responses of k patients have been observed, the next patient (or cohort of patients) would be administered the dose x_{k+1} satisfying

$$EL_k(x_{k+1}) = \min\{EL_k(x) : x \in S\}$$

or, equivalently,

$$x_{k+1} = \arg\min_{x \in S}\{EL_k(x)\}.$$

As an alternative, several authors (e.g., O'Quigley et al., 1990; Gasparini and Eisele, 2000) consider Bayesian designs wherein dose levels are chosen to minimize $L(x, \hat{\boldsymbol{\nu}}_k)$, where $\hat{\boldsymbol{\nu}}_k$ is an estimate of $\hat{\boldsymbol{\nu}}$ based on the data available after k patients have been observed. Typically, $\hat{\boldsymbol{\nu}}_k$ corresponds to the mean, median or mode of the posterior distribution Π_k.

The vast majority of cancer phase I clinical trial designs are sequential in nature. That is, subsequent to one or more patients being treated at a prespecified initial dose, dose levels are selected one at a time on the basis of the data available from all previously treated patients. However, nonsequential designs (e.g., Tsutakawa, 1972, 1975; Flournoy, 1993) have also been proposed wherein the design vector $\mathbf{x}$, representing the entire collection of dose levels to be used in the trial, is chosen prior to the onset of the trial. In such circumstances, $\mathbf{x}$ is chosen to minimize the expected loss with respect to the prior distribution h and patients (or cohorts of patients) are then randomly assigned to the dose levels so obtained. In the ensuing formulations only sequential designs will be explicitly discussed. In other words, we consider designs that select doses on the basis of the information conveyed by the posterior distribution Π_k rather than the prior distribution h.

2.2. Dose-Toxicity Model

A mathematical model is specified for the relationship between dose level and the probability of dose limiting toxicity. The choice of model is based on previous experience with the treatment regimen under investigation, preclinical toxicology studies, medical theory, and computational tractability. We note that the dose to be administered to the first patient or cohort of patients is typically chosen on the basis of prior information alone. Thus, its selection does not in general depend on the model for the dose-toxicity relationship. Consequently, it may be advantageous to delay the specification of the model until after a pharmacologic and statistical evaluation of the data from the cohort of patients treated at the preselected starting dose.

The models most frequently used in cancer phase I clinical trials are of the form

$$\text{Prob}\{\text{DLT}|\text{Dose} = x\} = F(\beta_0 + \beta_1 x)^{\delta} \tag{2}$$

where F is a cumulative distribution function (CDF) referred to as the tolerance distribution, δ and β_1 are both assumed to be positive so that the probability of dose limiting toxicity is a strictly increasing function of dose, and one or more of δ, β_0 and β_1 may be assumed known. Most applications based on this formulation use either a logit or probit model with typical examples including the two-parameter logistic (Gatsonis and Greenhouse, 1992; Babb et al., 1998)

$$\text{Prob}\{\text{DLT}|\text{Dose} = x\} = \frac{\exp(\beta_0 + \beta_1 x)}{1 + \exp(\beta_0 + \beta_1 x)} \tag{3}$$

(with $\delta = 1$ assumed known) and the one-parameter hyperbolic tangent (O'Quigley et al., 1990).

$$\text{Prob}\{\text{DLT}|\text{Dose} = x\} = \left[\frac{\tanh(x) + 1}{2}\right]^{\delta}. \tag{4}$$

To facilitate comparisons between these two models, the hyperbolic tangent model can be rewritten as

$$\text{Prob}\{\text{DLT}\,|\,\text{Dose} = x\} = \left[\frac{\exp(2x)}{1 + \exp(2x)}\right]^{\delta}$$

which is consistent with the form given in Eq. (2) with $\beta_0 = 0$ and $\beta_1 = 2$ assumed known. For exposition we consider the two-parameter logistic model given in (3). With this model the MTD is

$$\gamma = \frac{\ln(\theta) - \ln(1 - \theta) - \beta_0}{\beta_1}.$$

An illustration of the model is shown in Figure 1 and properties of the model are given in (Johnson et al., 1995).

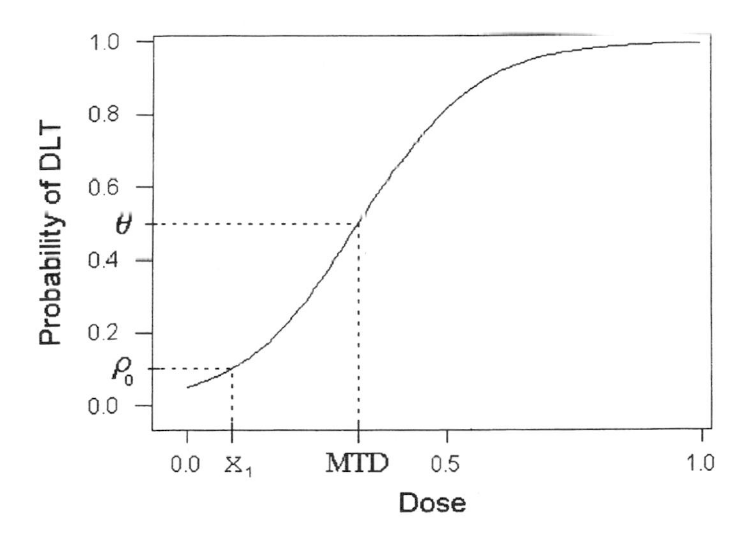

Figure 1 Example of the logistic tolerance distribution used as a model for the dose-toxicity relationship. In this representation dosage has been standardized so that the range of permissible doses is contained in the unit interval (i.e., $S = [0, 1]$). For illustration, the starting dose is taken to be $x_1 = 0.1$ and the probability of DLT at x_1 is denoted by ρ_0. The MTD has arbitrarily been defined as the (standardized) dose for which the probability of dose limiting toxicity is equal to $\theta = 0.5$.

An alternative formulation describes the dose-toxicity relationship as it applies to the set $S = \{x_1, x_2, \ldots, x_k\}$ of prespecified dose levels available for use in the trial. For example, Gasparini and Eisele (2000) present a curve-free Bayesian phase I design discussed the possibility of using one prior distribution (the design prior) to determine dose assignments during the phase I trial and a separate prior (the inference prior) to estimate the MTD upon trial completion. Although the use of separate priors for design and inference may appear inconsistent, its usefulness is defended by arguing that analysis occurs later than design (Tsutakawa, 1972). Consequently, our beliefs regarding the unknown parameters of the dose-toxicity model may change during the time from design to inference in ways not entirely accounted for by a sequential application of Bayes' theorem.

Since estimation of the MTD is the primary statistical aim of a phase I clinical trial, our subsequent attention will be focused on dose-toxicity models parameterized in terms of $\boldsymbol{\nu} = [\gamma \quad \omega]$ for some choice of (possibly null) vector ω of nuisance parameters. To facilitate elicitation of prior information, the nuisance vector ω should consist of parameters that the investigators can readily interpret.

As discussed above, the starting dose of a phase I trial is frequently selected on the basis of preclinical investigation. Consequently, prior information is often available about the risk of toxicity at the initial dose. To exploit this, Gatsonis and Greenhouse (1992) and Babb et al., (1998) considered the logistic model given by (3) parameterized in terms of the MTD

$$\gamma = \frac{\ln(\theta) - \ln(1-\theta) - \beta_0}{\beta_1}$$

and

$$\rho_0 = \frac{\exp(\beta_0 + \beta_1 x_1)}{1 + \exp(\beta_0 + \beta_1 x_1)}$$

the probability of DLT at the starting dose. Due to safety considerations, the dose for the first patient (or patient cohort) is typically chosen so that it is believed a priori to be safe for use with humans. Consequently, it is generally assumed that $\rho_0 \leq \theta$. This information about the initial dose can be expressed through a marginal prior distribution for ρ_0 whose mass is concentrated on $[0, \theta]$. Examples include the truncated beta (Gatsonis and Greenhouse, 1992) and uniform distributions (Babb et al., 1998) defined on the interval $(0, a)$ for some known value $a \leq \theta$. Prior information about the MTD is frequently more ambiguous. Such prior ignorance can be reflected through the use of vague or non-informative priors. Thus, for example, the marginal prior distribution of the MTD might scheme in which the toxicity probabilities are modeled directly as an unknown k-dimensional parameter vector. That is, the dose-toxicity model is given by

$$\text{Prob}\{\text{DLT}|\text{Dose} = x_i\} = \theta_i \quad i = 1, 2, \ldots, k \tag{5}$$

with $\boldsymbol{\nu} = [\theta_1 \quad \theta_2 \quad \ldots, \quad \theta_k]$ unknown. The authors maintain that by removing the assumption that the dose-toxicity relationship follows a specific parametric curve, such as the logistic model in (3), this model permits a more efficient use of prior information. A similar approach is based on what has variously been referred to as an empiric discrete model (Chevret, 1993), a power function (Kramar et al., 1999; Gasparini and Eisele, 2000) or a power model (Heyd and Carlin, 1999). The model is given by

$$\text{Prob}\{\text{DLT}|\text{Dose} - x_i\} = \hat{\theta}_i^{\delta} \tag{6}$$

where $\delta > 0$ is unknown and $\hat{\theta}_i$ ($i = 1, 2, \ldots, k$) is an estimate of the probability of DLT at dose level x_i based solely on information available prior to the onset of the phase I trial. With this model the toxicity probabilities can be increased or decreased through the parameter $\boldsymbol{\nu} = \delta$ as accumulating data suggests that the regimen is more or less toxic than was suggested by prior opinion. As noted by Gasparini and Eisele (2000), the empiric discrete model of Eq. (6) is equivalent to the hyperbolic tangent model of Eq. (4) provided one uses as prior estimates

$$\hat{\theta}_i = \frac{\tanh(x_i) + 1}{2} \quad i = 1, 2, \ldots, k\,.$$

2.3. Prior Distribution

The Bayesian formulation requires the specification of a prior probability distribution for the vector $\mathbf{v}$ containing the unknown parameters of the dose-toxicity model. The prior distribution is subjective; i.e., it conveys the opinions of the investigators prior to the onset of the trial. It is through the prior that information from previous trials, clinical and preclinical experience, and medical theory are incorporated into the analysis. The prior distribution should be concentrated in some meaningful way around a prior guess $\hat{\nu}_0$ (provided by the clinicians), yet it should also be sufficiently diffuse as to allow for dose escalation in the absence of dose limiting toxicity (Gasparini and Eisele, 2000). We note that several authors (e.g., Tsutakawa, 1972, 1975) have be taken to be a uniform distribution on a suitably defined interval (Babb et al., 1998) or a normal distribution with appropriately large variance (Gatsonis and Greenhouse, 1992).

Example: 5-FU Trial (continued)

The statistical goal of the trial was to determine the MTD of 5-FU when administered in conjunction with 20 mg/m^2 leucovorin and 0.5 mg/m^2 topotecan. The dose-toxicity model used to design the trial was that given by Eq. (3), reparameterized in terms of $\nu = [\gamma \quad \rho_0]$. Preliminary studies indicated that 140 mg/m^2 of 5-FU was well tolerated when given concurrently with up to 0.5 mg/m^2 topotecan. Consequently, this level was selected as the starting dose for the trial and was believed a priori to be less than the MTD. Furthermore, previous trials involving 5-FU alone estimated the MTD of 5-FU as a single agent to be 425 mg/m^2. Since 5-FU has been observed to be more toxic when in combination with topotecan than when administered alone, the MTD of 5-FU in combination with leucovorin and topotecan was assumed to be less than 425 mg/m^2. Overall, previous experience with 5-FU led to the assumption that $\gamma \in [140, 425]$ and $\rho_0 < 1/3$ with prior probability one. Based on this, the joint prior probability density function of $\boldsymbol{\nu}$ was taken to be

$$h(\boldsymbol{\nu}) = 57^{-1} I_{\Theta}(\gamma, \rho_0) \qquad \Theta = [140, 425] \times [0, 0.2] \tag{7}$$

where, for example, I_S denotes the indicator function for the set S [i.e., $I_S(x) = 1$ or 0 according as x does or does not belong to S]. It follows from (7) that the MTD and ρ_0 were assumed to be independently and marginally distributed as uniform random variables. In the example above, there was a suitable choice for an upper bound on the range of dose levels to be searched for the MTD. That is, prior experience with

5-FU suggested that, when given in combination with topotecan, the MTD of 5-FU was a priori believed to be less than 425 mg/m^2. In consequence, the support of the prior for the MTD was finite. In many contexts, there will not be sufficient information available prior to the onset of the phase I trial to unambiguously determine a suitable upper bound for the MTD (and hence for the range of dose levels to be searched). In this case, one might introduce a hyperparameter X_{max} and specify a joint prior distribution for the MTD and X_{max} as

$$h(\gamma, X_{max}) = f_1(\gamma \mid X_{max}) f_0(X_{max})$$

with, to continue the 5-FU example, $f_1(\gamma|X_{max})$ denoting the probability density function (pdf) of a uniform random variable on [140, 425] and f_0 (X_{max}) a monotone decreasing pdf defined on [425, ∞), such as a truncated normal with mean 425 and suitable standard deviation.

Flournoy (1993) considered the two-parameter logistic model in Eq. (3) reparameterized in terms of the MTD and the nuisance parameter $\omega = \beta^2$. The parameters γ and ω were assumed to be independent a priori with γ having a normal and ω having a gamma distribution. Thus, the joint prior distribution of $\mathbf{v} = [\gamma \quad \beta^2]$ was defined on $\Theta = \Re \times (0, \infty)$ by

$$h(\boldsymbol{\nu}) = [\Gamma(a)b^a\sigma\sqrt{2\pi}]^{-1}\beta^{2(a-1)}\exp\left(\frac{-(\gamma-\mu)^2}{2\sigma^2} - \frac{\beta^2}{b}\right).$$

As rationale for the choice of prior distribution for ω, it was noted that ω^{-1} is proportional to the variance of the logistic tolerance distribution and that the gamma distribution is frequently used to model the inverse of a variance component. In order to determine values for the hyperparameters a, b, μ, and σ, physicians were asked to graph curves corresponding to a prior 95% confidence band for the true dose-toxicity relationship. Values were then chosen for the hyperparameters so that the 95% confidence intervals at selected doses, as determined by the upper and lower hand drawn graphs at each dose, agreed with the corresponding confidence intervals implied by the prior.

Various authors (e.g., Chevret, 1993; Faries, 1994; Moller, 1995; Goodman et al., 1995) studying the continual reassessment method (O'Quigley et al., 1990) have considered monoparametric dose-toxicity models such as the hyperbolic tangent model of Eq. (4) and the empiric discrete model given by (6). Prior distributions used for the unknown parameter δ include the exponential

$$g(\delta) = \exp(-\delta) \qquad \delta \in (0, \infty) \tag{8}$$

and the uniform

$$g(\delta) = 1/3 \qquad \delta \in (0, 3) \tag{9}$$

corresponding to priors observed to work well in computer simulation studies (O'Quigley et al., 1990; Chevret, 1993). Since the hyperbolic tangent model implies that

$$\gamma = \frac{\ln \theta^{1/\delta}}{1 - \theta^{1/\delta}}$$

the priors induced for the MTD by the choice of (8) and (9) as the prior distribution for δ are

$$h(\gamma) = |J| \exp\left[\frac{\ln(\theta)}{\ln(1 + e^{2\gamma}) - 2\gamma}\right] \quad \gamma \in (-\infty, \infty)$$

and

$$h(\gamma) = \frac{|J|}{3} \quad \gamma \in \left(-\infty, \ln\frac{\theta^{1/3}}{1 - \theta^{1/3}}\right)$$

respectively, where the Jacobian is given by

$$J = \frac{-2\ln(\theta)}{(1 + e^{2\gamma})[\ln(1 + e^{2\gamma}) - 2\gamma]^2}$$

and $|J|$ is the absolute value of the determinant of J. Chevret (1993) conducted a simulation study to compare the relative utility of using exponential, gamma, log-normal, uniform, and Weibull distributions as priors for the lone unknown parameter in the dose-toxicity models given by Eqs. (4) and (6) or in the two-parameter logistic model with known intercept parameter. The results suggested that estimation of the MTD was not significantly affected by the choice of prior distribution and that no one prior distribution performed consistently better than the others under a broad range of circumstances.

An alternative formulation of the prior distribution, suggested by Tsutakawa (1975) and discussed by Patterson et al. (1999) and Whitehead (1997), is based on a prior assessment of the probability of DLT at selected dose levels. As a simple example, consider two prespecified dose levels z_1 and z_2. These dose levels need not be available for use in the phase I trial, but often represent doses used in previous clinical investigations. For $i = 1, 2$, positive constants $t(i)$ and $n(i)$ are chosen so that $t(i)/n(i)$ corresponds to a prior estimate of the probability of DLT at the dose z_i. The prior for $\boldsymbol{\nu}$ is then specified as

$$h(\boldsymbol{\nu}) = \kappa \prod_{i=1}^{2} p(z_i \mid \boldsymbol{\nu})^{t(i)} [1 - p(z_i \mid \boldsymbol{\nu})]^{n(i)-t(i)}$$

where κ is the standardizing constant rendering h a proper probability density function and $p(\cdot|\boldsymbol{\nu})$ is the model for the dose-toxicity relationship parameterized in terms of $\boldsymbol{\nu}$. In this formulation the prior is proportional to the likelihood function for $\boldsymbol{\nu}$ given a data set in which, for $i = 1, 2$, $n(i)$ patients were treated at dose z_i with exactly $t(i)$ manifesting DLT. Consequently, this type of prior is typically referred to as a "pseudodata" prior. As noted by Whitehead (1997), the pseudodata might include observations from previous studies at one or both of z_1 and z_2. Such data might be downweighted to reflect any disparity between previous and present clinical circumstances by choosing values for the $n(i)$ that are smaller than the actual number of previous patients observed.

The curve-free method of Gasparini and Eisele (2000) is based on the dose-toxicity model given by (5). Hence, the dose-toxicity relationship is modeled directly in terms of $\boldsymbol{\nu} = [\theta_1 \quad \theta_2 \quad \ldots \quad \theta_k]$, the vector of toxicity probabilities for the k dose levels selected for use in the trial. The prior selected for ν is referred to as the product-of-beta prior and can be described as follows. Let $\psi_1 = 1 - p_1$ and for $i = 2, 3, \ldots, k$, let $\psi_i = (1 - p_i)/(1 - p_{i-1})$. The product-of-beta prior is the distribution induced for $\boldsymbol{\nu}$ by the assumption that the ψ_i $(i = 1, 2, \ldots, k)$ are independent with ψ_i distributed as a beta with parameters a_i and b_i. The authors provide a method for determining the hyperparameters a_i and b_i so that the marginal prior distribution of θ_i is concentrated near $\hat{\theta}_i$, corresponding to the clinicians' prior guess for θ_i, and yet disperse enough to permit dose escalation in the absence of toxicity. They also discuss why alternative priors, such as the ordered Dirichlet distribution, may not be appropriate for use in cancer phase I trials designed according to the curve-free method.

2.4. Posterior Distribution

Perceptions concerning the unknown model parameters change as the trial progresses and data accumulate. The appropriate adjustment of subjective opinions can be made by transforming the prior distribution h through an application of Bayes' theorem. Thus, we obtain the posterior distribution Π_k which reflects our beliefs about $\boldsymbol{\nu}$ based on a combination of prior knowledge and the data available after k patients have been observed.

The transformation from prior to posterior distribution is accomplished through the likelihood function. If we denote the dose-toxicity model parameterized in terms of $\boldsymbol{\nu}$ as

$$p(x|\boldsymbol{\nu}) = \text{Prob}\{\text{DLT}\,|\,\text{Dose} = x\}$$

then the likelihood function for $\nu = [\gamma \quad \omega]$ given the data D_k is

$$L(\boldsymbol{\nu}|D_k) = \prod_{i=1}^{k} p(x_i|\boldsymbol{\nu})^{y_i}\{1 - p(x_i|\boldsymbol{\nu})\}^{1-y_i}.$$

Bayes' theorem then implies that the joint posterior distribution of (γ, ω) given the data D_k is

$$\Pi_k(\gamma, \omega|D_k) = \frac{L(\gamma, \omega|D_k)h(\gamma, \omega)}{\int L(\mathbf{u}|D_k)h(\mathbf{u})d\mathbf{u}}$$

where the integral is over Θ. To facilitate exposition, it will hereafter be assumed that the prior distribution h is defined on some set $\Gamma \times \Omega$ containing the parameter space Θ such that $\gamma \in \Gamma$ and $\omega \in \Omega$ with prior probability 1. Whenever necessary, this will entail extending h from Θ to $\Gamma \times \Omega$ by defining h to be identically equal to zero on the difference $(\Gamma \times \Omega)\backslash\Theta$. This convention will simplify ensuing formulations without a loss of generality. For example, the marginal posterior distribution of the MTD given the data from k patients can then be simply expressed as

$$P_k(\gamma) = \int_{\Omega} \Pi_k(\gamma, \mathbf{u} \mid D_k) d\mathbf{u}$$

irrespective of whether or not γ and ω were assumed to be independent a priori.

Example: 5-FU Trial (continued)

The dose-toxicity relationship was modeled according to the logistic tolerance distribution given by (3) reparameterized in terms of $\boldsymbol{\nu} = [\gamma\ \rho_0]$, where ρ_0 is the probability of DLT at the starting dose $x_1 = 140$. As shown by Eq. (7), the prior distribution for ν was taken to be the uniform on $\Gamma \times \Omega = [140, 425] \times [0, .2]$. It follows that the marginal posterior probability density function of the MTD given the data D_k is

$$P_k(\gamma) = \int_0^{0.2} \Pi_{i=1}^k \frac{(\exp\{y_i f(\gamma, u|x_i)\}}{[1 + \exp\{f(\gamma, u|x_i)\})} du \quad \gamma \in [140, 425]$$

where

$$f(\gamma, u|x_i) = \frac{(\gamma - x_i)\ln\{u/(1-u)\} + (x_i - 140)\ln\{\theta/(1-\theta)\}}{\gamma - 140}.$$

The marginal posterior distribution P_k represents a probabilistic summary of all the information about the MTD that is available after the observation of k patients. Figure 2 shows the marginal posterior distribution of the MTD given the data shown in Table 1.

2.5. Loss Function

As each patient is accrued to the trial, a decision must be made regarding the dose level that the patient is to receive. In a strict Bayesian setting, the decisions are made by minimizing the posterior expected loss associated with each permissible choice of dose level. To accomplish this, the set S of all permissible dose levels is specified and a loss function is chosen to quantify the cost or loss arising from the administration of each permissible dose under each possible value of $\boldsymbol{\nu}$. The loss may be expressed in financial terms, in terms of patient well-being, or in terms

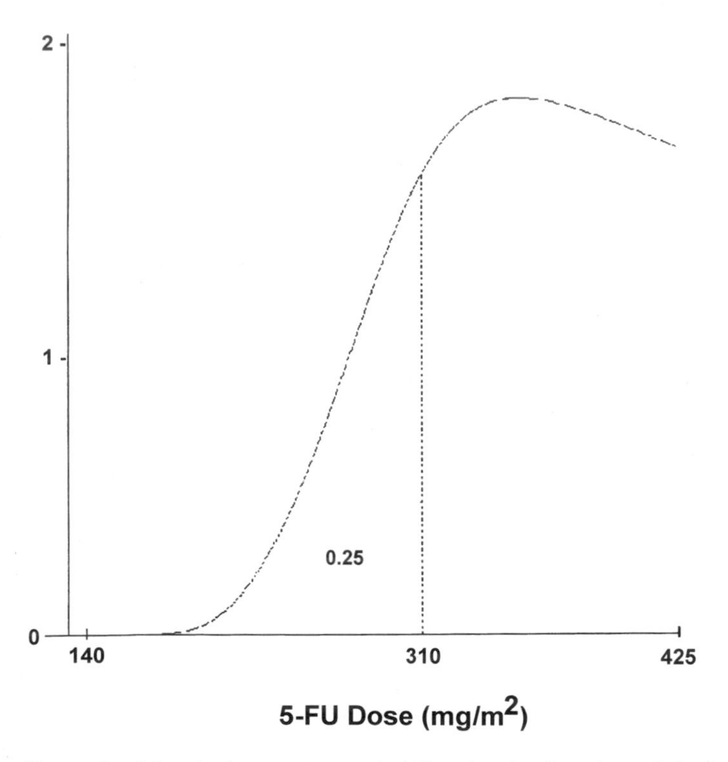

Figure 2 Marginal posterior probability density function of the MTD of 5-FU given the data from all 12 patients treated in the 5-FU phase I trial.

of the gain in scientific knowledge (Whitehead, 1997). Uncertainty about ν is reflected through the posterior distribution and the expected loss associated with each permissible dose x is determined by averaging the loss attributed to x over the parameter space $\Gamma \times \Omega$ according to the posterior distribution Π_k. Thus, after k patients have been observed, the posterior expected loss associated with dose $x \in S$ is

$$EL_k(x) = \int_{\Theta} L(x, \mathbf{u}) \, \Pi_k(\mathbf{u}) d\mathbf{u}$$

and the next patient would receive the dose

$$x_{k+1} = \arg \min_{x \in S} \{EL_k(x)\}.$$

For example, the dose for each patient might be chosen to minimize the posterior expected loss with respect to the loss function $L(x, \nu) = d\{\theta, p(x, \nu)\}$ or $L(x, \nu) = m(x, \gamma)$ for some choice of metrics d and m defined on the unit square and $S \times \Gamma$, respectively. Thus, patients might be treated at the mean, median, or mode of the marginal posterior distribution of the MTD, corresponding to the respective choices of loss function $L(x, \nu) = (x - \gamma)^2$, $L(x, \nu) = |x - \gamma|$, and $L(x, \nu) = I_{(0,\varepsilon)}(|x - \gamma|)$, for some arbitrarily small positive constant ε.

Instead of minimizing the posterior expected loss, dose levels can be chosen so as to minimize the loss function after substituting an estimate for ν. Consequently, given the data from k patients, one might estimate ν as $\hat{\nu}_k$ and administer to the next patient the dose

$$x_{k+1} = \arg \min_{x \epsilon S} \{L(x, \hat{\nu}_k)\}.$$

In the remainder of this section we describe various loss functions that have been discussed in the literature concerning cancer phase I clinical trials.

Since the primary statistical aim of a phase I clinical trial is to determine the MTD, designs have been presented which seek to maximize the efficiency with which the MTD is estimated. As an example, Tsutakawa (1972, 1975) considered the following design which, for simplicity, we describe in terms of a dose-toxicity model whose only unknown parameter is γ. Let $\mathbf{x}$ denote the vector of dose levels to be administered to the next cohort of patients accrued to the trial. Given $\gamma = \gamma_0$, the posterior variance of γ before observing the response at x is approximated by the loss function

$$L(\boldsymbol{x}, \gamma_0) = \{B(h) + I(x, \gamma_0)\}^{-1}$$

where $B(h)$ is a nonnegative constant which may depend on the prior h chosen for γ and $I(x, \gamma_0)$ is the Fisher information contained in the sample when using $\mathbf{x}$ and γ_0 obtains. The constant term B is introduced so that $L(x, \gamma_0)$ is bounded above (when $B > 0$) and so that L becomes the exact posterior variance of γ under suitable conditions. The method is illustrated using the specific choice $B(h) \propto \tau^{-1}$, where τ is the variance of the prior distribution assumed for γ. After observing the responses of k patients, the doses to be used for the next cohort are given by the vector $\mathbf{x}$ minimizing

$$EL_k(x) = \int_\Gamma L(\mathbf{x}, \mathbf{u}) \, \Pi_k(\mathbf{u}) \, d\mathbf{u}$$

the expected loss with respect to the posterior distribution Π_k of $\nu = \gamma$. Methods to accomplish the minimization of G are discussed in Tsutakawa

(1972, 1975) and presented in (Chaloner and Larntz, 1989). Once x has been determined, random sampling without replacement can be used to determine the dose level contained in x that is to be administered each patient in the next cohort.

For cancer phase I trials, we typically seek to optimize the treatment of each individual patient. Attention might therefore focus on identifying a dose that all available evidence indicates to be the best estimate of the MTD. This is the basis for the continual reassessment method (CRM) proposed by O'Quigley et al. (1990). In the present context their original formulation can be described as follows. Let $p(\cdot|\boldsymbol{\nu})$ denote the model selected for the dose-toxicity relationship parameterized in terms of $\boldsymbol{\nu}$. Given the data from k patients, the probability of DLT at any permissible dose level $x \in S$ can be estimated as

$$\hat{\theta}_k(x) = \int_{\Theta} p(x|\mathbf{u})\,\Pi_k(\mathbf{u})d\mathbf{u}$$

or

$$\hat{\theta}_k(x) = p(x|\hat{\boldsymbol{\nu}}_k) \tag{10}$$

where $\hat{\boldsymbol{\nu}}_k$ denotes an estimate of $\boldsymbol{\nu}$. The next patient is then treated at the dose for which the estimated probability of DLT is as close as possible, in some predefined sense, to the target probability θ. Thus, for example, after observation of k patients, the next patient might receive the dose level x_{k+1} satisfying

$$|\hat{\theta}_k(x_{k+1}) - \theta| \leq |\hat{\theta}_k(x) - \theta| \quad \forall x \in S$$

In an effort to balance the ethical and statistical imperatives inherent to cancer phase I trials, methods have been proposed to construct dose sequences that, in an appropriate sense, converge to the MTD as fast as possible subject to a constraint on each patient's predicted risk of being administered an overdose (Eichhorn and Zacks, 1973, 1981; Babb et al., 1998) or of manifesting DLT (Robinson, 1978; Shih, 1989). Thus, for example, the Bayesian feasible methods first considered by Eichhorn and Zacks (1973) select dose levels for use in the trial so that the expected proportion of patients receiving a dose above the MTD does not exceed a specified value α, called the feasibility bound. This can be accomplished by administering to each patient the dose level corresponding to the α-fractile of the marginal posterior cumulative distribution function (CDF) of the

MTD. Specifically, after k patients have been observed, the dose for the next patient accrued to the trial is

$$x_{k+1} = F_k^{-1}(\alpha) \tag{11}$$

where

$$F_k(x) = \int_0^x \int_\Omega \prod_k(\gamma, \omega)\, d\omega\, d\gamma \tag{12}$$

is the marginal posterior CDF of the MTD given D_k. Thus, subsequent to the first cohort of patients, the dose selected for each patient corresponds to the dose having minimal posterior expected loss with respect to

$$L(x, \nu) = \begin{cases} \alpha(\mathrm{g} - x) & \text{if } x \leq \gamma \text{ (i.e., if } x \text{ is an underdose)} \\ (1-\alpha)(x-\gamma) & \text{if } x > \gamma \text{ (i.e., if } x \text{ is an overdose).} \end{cases}$$

The use of this loss function implies that for any $\delta > 0$ the loss incurred by treating a patient at δ units above the MTD is $(1-\alpha)/\alpha$ times greater than the loss associated with treating the patient at δ units below the MTD. This interpretation might provide a meaningful basis for the selection of the feasibility bound (Babb et al., 1998). The value selected for the feasibility bound will determine the rate of change in dose level between successive patients. Low values will result in a cautious escalation scheme with relatively small increments in dose, while high values would result in a more aggressive escalation. In a typical application the value of the feasibility bound is initially set at a small value ($\alpha = 0.25$, say) and then allowed to increase in a predetermined manner until $\alpha = 0.5$. The rationale behind this approach is that uncertainty about the MTD is highest at the onset of the trial and a small value of α affords protection against the possibility of administering dose levels much greater than the MTD. As the trial progresses, uncertainty about the MTD declines and the likelihood of selecting a dose level significantly above the MTD becomes smaller. Consequently, a relatively high probability of exceeding the MTD can be tolerated near the conclusion of the trial because the magnitude by which any dose exceeds the MTD is expected to be small.

As defined by Eichhorn and Zacks (1973), a dose sequence $\{x_j\}_{j=1}^{n}$ is *Bayesian feasible* of level $1 - \alpha$ if $F_j(x_{j+1}) \leq \alpha$, $\forall j = 1, \ldots, n-1$, where F_j the marginal posterior CDF of the MTD given D_j as defined in Eq. (12). Correspondingly, the design of a phase I clinical trial is said to be Bayesian feasible (of level $1 - \alpha$) if the posterior probability that each patient receives an overdose is no greater than the feasibility bound α. Zacks et al., (1998) showed that the dose sequence specified by Eq. (11) is consistent (i.e., under suitable conditions, the dose sequence converges in probability to the MTD) and is optimal among Bayesian feasible designs in the sense that it minimizes $\int_\Gamma \int_\Omega (\gamma - x_k) I_{(-\infty, x_k)}(\gamma) \Pi_k(\gamma, \omega)\, d\omega\, d\gamma$, the expected amount by which any given patient is underdosed. Consequently, the method defined by equation (11) is referred to as the optimal Bayesian feasible design.

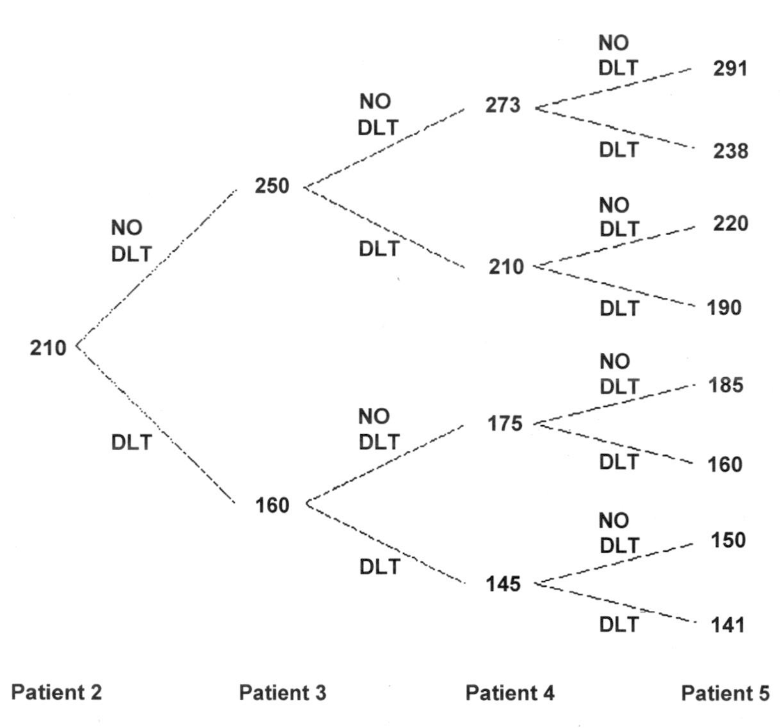

Figure 3 Dose levels for patients 2–5 of the 5-FU trial conditional on the treatment-attributable toxicities observed.

Example: 5-FU Trial (continued)

The 5-FU trial was designed according to the optimal Bayesian feasible dose escalation method known as EWOC (Babb et al., 1998). For this trial the feasibility bound was set equal to $\alpha = 0.25$, this value being a compromise between the therapeutic aim of the trial and the need to avoid treatment attributable toxicity. Consequently, escalation of 5-FU between successive patients was to the dose level determined to have posterior probability equal to 0.25 of being an overdose (i.e., greater than the MTD). The first patient accrued to the trial received the preselected dose 140 mg/m^2. Based on the EWOC algorithm, as implemented according to Rogatko and Babb (1998), the doses administered the next four patients were selected according to the schedule given in Figure 3.

In contrast to the Bayesian feasible methods, the prediction approaches of Robinson (1978) and Shih (1989) provide sequential search procedures which control the probability that a patient will exhibit DLT. Their formulation is non-Bayesian, being based on the coverage distribution (Shih, 1989) rather than the posterior distribution of ν.

3. MODIFICATIONS AND EXTENSIONS

3.1. Maximum Likelihood

In its original presentation CRM (O'Quigley et al., 1990) utilized Bayesian inference. Subsequently, to overcome certain difficulties associated with the Bayesian approach (see, for example, Gasparini and Eisele, 2000) a maximum likelihood based version of CRM (CRML) was introduced (O'Quigley and Shen, 1996). Essentially, the Bayesian and likelihood based approaches differ with respect to the method used to estimate the probability of DLT at each permissible dose level. Thus, for example, both CRM and CRML might utilize the estimates given by Eq. (10) with $\hat{\nu}_k$ respectively corresponding to either a Bayesian or maximum likelihood estimate of ν. Simulation studies (Kramar et al., 1999) comparing Bayesian CRM with CRML showed the methods to have similar operating characteristics. However, one key distinction between the Bayesian and likelihood approaches is that the latter requires a trial to be designed in stages. More specifically, the maximum likelihood estimate, $\hat{\theta}_k(x)$, of the probability of DLT at any dose x will be trivially equal to either zero or one, or perhaps even fail to exist, until at least one patient manifests DLT and one fails to exhibit DLT. Hence, the use of CRML must be preceded by an initial stage whose design does not require maximum likelihood estimation. This stage might be designed according to Bayesian principles (e.g., by original CRM) or by use of more traditional up-and-down schemes based on a modified Fibonacci sequence. Once at least one patient manifests and one patient is treated without DLT, the first stage can be terminated and subsequent dose escalations can be determined through the use of CRML. Since CRML is inherently non-Bayesian, it will not be discussed further in this chapter. Instead we refer interested readers to O'Quigley and Shen (1996) and Kramar et al. (1999) for details regarding the implementation of CRML.

3.2. Delayed Response

Since cancer patients often exhibit delayed response to treatment, the time required to definitively evaluate treatment response can be longer than the average time between successive patient accruals. Consequently, new patients frequently become available to the study before the responses of all previously treated patients have unambiguously been determined (O'Quigley et al., 1990). It is therefore important to note that Bayesian procedures do not require knowledge of the responses of all patients currently on study before a newly accrued patient can begin treatment. Instead, the dose for the new patient can be selected on the basis of whatever data are currently available (O'Quigley et al., 1990; Babb et al, 1998). Thus, it can be left to the discretion of the clinician to determine whether to treat a newly accrued patient at the dose recommended on the basis of all currently known responses, or to wait until the resolution of one or more unknown responses and then treat the new patient at an updated determination of dose.

3.3. Rapid Initial Escalation

Recently, ethical concerns have been raised regarding the large number of patients treated in cancer phase I trials at potentially biologically inactive dose levels (Hawkins, 1993; Dent and Eisenhauer, 1996). A summary (Decoster et al., 1990) of the antitumor activity and toxic deaths reported for 6639 phase I cancer patients revealed that only 0.3% ($n = 23$) exhibited a complete response, 4.2% (279) manifested a partial response and toxic deaths occurred in only 0.5% (31) of the patients. A similar review of 6447 patients found that only 4.2% achieved an objective response (3.5% partial response, 0.7% complete remission). As a result, the last several years have seen the production of numerous suggested modifications of the standard trial paradigm (ASCO, 1997). Such design alternatives, often referred to as accelerated titration designs (Simon et al., 1997), begin with an aggressive, rapid initial escalation of dose and mandate switching to a more conservative approach when some prespecified target is achieved. The switching rule is usually based on a defined incidence of some level of toxicity (e.g., the second hematologic toxicity of grade 2 or higher), or a pharmacologic endpoint such as 40% of the AUC at the mouse LD_{10}. In the context of Bayesian phase I designs, Moller (1995) and Goodman et al. (1995) proposed two-stage phase I dose escalation schemes wherein implementation of a Bayesian design was preceded by a rapid ad hoc dose escalation phase. There may be considerable advantage in adopting the two-stage trial design since the first stage may not only reduce the incidence of non-therapeutic dose assignments, but would also provide meaningful prior information on which to base the Bayesian design of the second stage.

3.4. Constrained Escalation

In their inception, Bayesian methods were not widely accepted in the context of cancer phase I clinical trials. The major criticism was that they might unduly increase the chance of administering overly toxic dose levels (Faries, 1994). Consequently, many recently proposed Bayesian design methods (e.g., Faries, 1994; Moller, 1995; Goodman et al., 1995) incorporate guidelines that limit the magnitude by which the dose level can be increased between successive patients. As an example, the protocol of the PNU trial prohibited escalation at any stage of the trial to a dose level greater than twice the highest dose previously administered without induction of dose limiting toxicity (Babb and Rogatko, 2001). Similarly, designs have been proposed (Faries, 1994) wherein each dose is selected from a small number of prespecified levels according to CRM, but with escalation between successive cohorts limited to one dose level. As an alternative, the trial might be designed to provide maximal statistical efficiency subject to some formal constraint reflecting patient safety. For example, the dose for each patient might be selected so as to minimize the posterior expected variance of the MTD (as in Tsutakawa, 1972, 1975; Flournoy, 1993) over the subset of permissible dose levels that are Bayesian feasible at some level $1 - \alpha$ (as in Eichhorn and Zacks, 1973; Babb et al., 1998).

3.5. Multinomial and Continuous Response Measures

Phase I trials frequently provide more information about toxicity than is exploited by the methods described in Section 2. For example, whereas the above methods use a binary assessment of toxic response, toxicity is often measured on a multinomial scale, graded according to NCI toxicity criteria, or through a variable that can be modeled as continuous (e.g., white blood cell count). This additional information can be incorporated into the trial design through an extension of the dose-toxicity model. To illustrate this in the multinomial setting, we consider a trinomial response measure Y that assumes the values 0, 1, and 2 according as each patient manifests "mild," "moderate," or dose limiting toxicity. The variable Y may represent a summary of all relevant adverse events by recording the highest level of toxicity observed for each patient. The dose-toxicity model can then be specified through the functions

$$\phi_i(x|\boldsymbol{\nu}) = \text{Prob}\{Y = i|\text{Dose} = x\} \quad i = 0, 1, 2$$

given by

$$\phi_2(x|\boldsymbol{\nu}) = F(\alpha_2 + \beta_2 x)$$

$$\phi_1(x|\boldsymbol{\nu}) = F(\alpha_1 + \beta_1 x) - \phi_2(x|\boldsymbol{\nu})$$

and

$$\phi_0(x|\boldsymbol{\nu}) = 1 - \phi_2(x|\boldsymbol{\nu}) - \phi_1(x|\boldsymbol{\nu})$$

where F is a tolerance distribution and the elements of $\boldsymbol{\nu} = [\alpha_1 \quad \alpha_2 \quad \beta_1 \quad \beta_2]$ satisfy $\alpha_1 \geq \alpha_2 > 0$ and $\beta_1 \geq \beta_2 > 0$. Examples include McCullagh's (1980) proportional odds regression model, as considered in the context of phase I and II clinical trials by Thall and Russell (1998).

Wang et al. (2000) propose an extension of CRM for the case where the definition of DLT includes multiple toxicity grades and/or different types of toxicity (e.g., a grade 4 hematologic and grade 3^+ nonhemetalogic toxicity) having potentially different clinical consequences. As a specific example, they consider the case where DLT is defined as either a grade 3 or grade 4 toxicity. The extension requires the specification of a probability θ^*, which is strictly less than the target probability θ used in the definition of the MTD. The authors propose the specific choice $\theta^* = \theta/w$ where the weight w reflects the relative seriousness of grade 3 and 4 toxicities. For example, if grade 4 is considered twice as serious or difficult to manage as grade 3, then $w = 2$. Treatment response is still recorded as the binary indicator for DLT and no changes are made to the dose-toxicity model or prior distribution underlying CRM. However, whereas CRM will always select the dose level having estimated probability of DLT closest to the target θ, the extended version recommends using the dose with estimated probability of DLT nearest θ^* after the observation of a grade 4 toxicity. Hence, whenever a grade 3 or lower toxicity is observed, the extended CRM selects the dose level with estimated DLT probability nearest θ, exactly as prescribed by standard CRM. Only upon observation of a grade 4 toxicity will the extended version select a dose different from (more precisely, less than or equal to) that recommended by CRM. As a result, use of the extended version of CRM will result in a more cautious escalation of dose level in the presence of severe toxicity.

When toxicity can be modeled as a continuous variable Y the MTD is defined in terms of a threshold τ representing a level of response deemed clinically unacceptable. For example, if it is desirable that Y not exceed τ, then dose limiting toxicity corresponds to the event $\{Y \geq \tau\}$ and the MTD is defined as the dose γ such that

$$\text{Prob}\{Y \geq \tau \mid \text{Dose} = \gamma\} = \theta.$$

The dose-toxicity model can be specified by assuming that the conditional distribution of Y given dose $= x$ has some continuous probability density function with mean

$$\mu_x = \beta_0 + \beta_1 x$$

and standard deviation

$$\sigma_x = g(x)\sigma$$

where g is a function defined on the permissible dose set S. For example, Eichhorn and Zacks (1973, 1981) consider the case where the conditional distribution of Y given dose is lognormal. Specifically, it is assumed that the logarithm of the measured physical response Y, given dose $= x$, is normally distributed with mean $\mu_x = \beta_0 + \beta_1 (x - x_0)$ and standard deviation equal to either $\sigma_x = (x - x_0)\sigma$ (case 1) or $\sigma_x = \sigma$ (case 2), where $\sigma > 0$ is known, β_0 and β_1 are unknown and x_0 is a predetermined dose level at which the probability of DLT is assumed negligible.

Upon specification of the dose-toxicity model, a Bayesian designed trial would proceed according to the steps outlined above: a prior is specified for the unknown parameters of the model, a loss function is defined on $S \times \Theta$, and dose levels are chosen so as to minimize the posterior expected loss.

3.6. Designs for Drug Combinations

In the development of a new cancer therapy, the treatment regimen under investigation will often consist of two or more agents whose levels are to be determined by phase I testing. In such contexts, a simple approach is to conduct the trial in stages with the level of only one agent escalated in each stage. The methods described above can then be implemented to design each stage. An example of this is given by the 5-FU trial.

Example: 5-FU Trial (continued)

The protocol of the 5-FU trial actually included two separate stages of dose escalation. In the first stage, outlined above, 12 patients were each administered a dose combination consisting of 20 mg/m^2 leucovorin, 0.5 mg/m^2 topotecan, and a dose of 5-FU determined by the EWOC algorithm. In the second stage, the level of 5-FU was held fixed at 310 mg/m^2, corresponding to the dose recommended for the next (i.e., thirteenth) patient had the first stage been allowed to continue. An additional 12 patients were accrued during the second stage with each patient receiving 310 mg/m^2 5-FU, 20 mg/m^2 leucovorin, and a dose of topotecan determined by EWOC. For these 12 patients the feasibility bound was initially set equal to 0.25 (as in the first stage) and then allowed to increase by 0.05 with each successive dose assignment until the value $\alpha = 0.5$ was attained. Hence, for example, the first two patients in stage 2 received respective doses of topotecan determined to have posterior probability 0.25 and 0.3 of exceeding the MTD. All stage 2 patients including and subsequent to the sixth patient received a dose of topotecan corresponding to the median of the marginal posterior distribution of the MTD given the prevailing data.

A single stage scheme was proposed by Flournoy (1993) as a method to determine the MTD of a combination of cyclophosphamide (denoted x) and busulfan (y). To define a unique MTD and implement design methods appropriate for single agent regimens, attention was restricted to a set S of dose combinations lying along the line segment delimited by the points $(x, y) = (40, 6)$ and $(x, y) = (180, 20)$. Since for any $(x, y) \in S$ the level of one agent is completely determined by the level of the other, the design methods described above for single agent trials can be used to select dose combinations in the multiple agent trial. As an example, Flournoy (1993) considered a design wherein k patients are to be treated at each of six equally spaced dose combinations to be selected from the set S defined above. The single agent design method of Tsutakawa (1980) was implemented to determine the optimal placement and spacing of the dose combinations and so define the set of dose combinations to be used in the trial. This approach can easily be generalized to accommodate either nonlinear search regions or combinations of more than two agents. For example, the set S of dose levels to be searched for an MTD could be chosen so that given any two distinct dose combinations in S, one will have the levels of all agents higher than the other. As a result, the combinations in S can be unambiguously ordered and the dose-toxicity relationship can be meaningfully modeled as an increasing function of the distance of each permissible dose combination from the "minimum" combination. Since this formulation represents each permissible dose combination by a single real number, the design methods described above for single agent trials can be used to select dose combinations in the multiple agent trial.

Since the curve-free method of Gasparini and Eisele (2000) is applicable whenever dose levels can be meaningfully ordered, it can be used to design a phase I study of treatment combinations. With this approach one must preselect k dose combinations $d_1, d_2, \ldots, d_k$ ordered so that, with prior probability one, $\text{Prob}\{\text{DLT}|\text{Dose} = d_i\} \leq \text{Prob}\{\text{DLT}|\text{Dose} = d_j\}$ for all $i < j$. The dose-toxicity relationship is then modeled according to Eq. (5) and a pseudodata prior is assumed for $\boldsymbol{\nu} = [\theta_1 \ \ \theta_2 \ \ \ldots \ \ \theta_k]$, where $\theta_i = \text{Prob}\{\text{DLT}|\text{Dose} = d_i\}$. It is important to note that by not requiring the specification of a parametric curve relating the toxicity probabilities of different dose combinations, this approach eliminates the need to model any synergism or interaction between the agents.

Kramar et al. (1999) describe the application of CRML in a phase I trial to determine the MTD of the combination of docetaxel and irinotecan. The method is based on the discrete empiric model given by Eq. (6). Use of this model requires a procedure for obtaining a prior estimate of the probability of DLT at each of the k dose combinations preselected for use in the trial. Kramar et al. (1999) describe how the estimates can be obtained prior to the onset of the phase I trial by using data from trials investigating each agent separately. Once these estimates have been obtained, the multiple agent trial can proceed according to CRML exactly as it applies to a single agent trial.

3.7. Incorporation of Covariate Information

As defined above, the MTD may well quantify the average response of a specific patient population to a particular treatment, but no allowance is made for individual differences in susceptibility to the treatment (Dillman and Koziol, 1992). Recent developments in our understanding of the genetics of drug-metabolizing enzymes and the importance of individual patient differences in pharmacokinetic and relevant clinical parameters is leading to the development of new treatment paradigms (ASCO, 1997). For example, the observation that impaired renal function can result in reduced clearance of carboplatin, led to the development of dosing formulas based on renal function that permit careful control over individual patient exposure (Newell, 1994). Consequently, methods are being presented for incorporating observable patient characteristics into the design of cancer phase I trials.

In cancer clinical trials, the target patient population can often be partitioned according to some categorical assessment of susceptibility to treatment. Separate phase I investigations can then be conducted to determine the appropriate dose for each patient sub-population. As an example, the NCI currently accounts for the contribution of prior therapy by establishing separate MTDs for heavily pretreated and minimally pretreated patients. In such contexts, independent phase I trials can be designed for each patient group according to the methods outlined above. Alternatively, a single trial might be conducted with relevant patient information directly incorporated into the trial design. Thus, the dose-toxicity relationship is modeled as a function of patient attributes represented by the vector c of covariate measurements. For exposition, we consider the case where a single covariate observation c is obtained for each patient. The relationship between dose and response might then be characterized as

$$p(x, c) = \frac{\exp(\alpha + \beta x + \delta c)}{1 + \exp(\alpha + \beta x + \delta c)} \tag{13}$$

where

$$p(x, c) \equiv \text{Prob}[\text{DLT}|\text{Dose} = x, \text{Covariate} = c].$$

The overall design of the trial will depend in part on whether or not the observation c can be obtained for each patient prior to the onset of treatment. For example, when the covariate assessment can be made before the initial course of treatment, the dose recommended for phase II testing can be tailored to individual patient needs. Specifically, the MTD for patients with covariate c is defined as the dose $\gamma(c)$ such that $p\{\gamma(c), c\} = \theta$. Thus, $\gamma(c)$ is the dose that is expected to induce DLT in a proportion θ of patients with pretreatment covariate observation c. When relevant covariate information can only be accumulated after or during the course of treatment (as would be true for most pharmacokinetic assessments), the information can be used to improve the efficiency with which the MTD is determined, but cannot form the basis for a tailored dosing regimen. In this case, a global MTD is defined representing the dose recommended for use by all patients in the target population.

Upon specification of a joint prior distribution for the unknown model parameters, the conduct of the trial would proceed along the lines given in Sections 2.4 and 2.5 (see, for example, Babb and Rogatko, 2001). Consequently, we conclude this section with an example illustrating the specification of the prior distribution in the PNU trial. Alternative formulations are given in Mick et al. (1994) and Piantadosi and Liu (1996).

Example: PNU Trial (continued)

Preliminary studies with PNU indicated that dose levels should be adjusted for baseline pretreatment concentrations of circulating anti-SEA antibodies. Consequently, the MTD $\gamma(c)$ was defined to be the dose level of PNU (ng/kg) that produces DLT in a proportion $\theta = 0.1$ of the patients with baseline anti-SEA equal to c, as assessed 3 days prior to the onset of treatment. The small value chosen for θ reflects the severity of the treatment induced toxicities (e.g., myelosuppression) observed in previous studies.

Prior to the recognition of the importance of anti-SEA, a total of 77 patients were treated at dose levels between 0.01 and 37 ng/kg. The results suggested that, irrespective of anti-SEA concentration, patients could be safely treated at 0.5 ng/kg and that patients with anti-SEA concentration equal to c (pmol/ml) could tolerate doses up to $M(c) = \min\{3.5, c/30\}$ ng/kg without significant toxicity. Hence,

$$x_1(c) = I_{(0,15]}(c) + (c/30)I_{(15,105]}(c) + 3.5I_{(105,\infty)}(c)$$

was chosen as both the starting dose and the minimum permissible dose for the trial. Due to the nature of the agent and as a precaution, it was decided not to consider doses above 1000 ng/kg and to never treat a patient at a dose above his/her pretreatment anti-SEA (in pmol/mL).

Consequently, the set of permissible doses levels for patients with pretreatment anti-SEA concentration equal to c is

$$S(c) = \{x : x_1(c) \leq x \leq \min(c, 1000)\}.$$

The model for the dose-toxicity relationship was taken to be the logistic model given in equation (13) with both dose and anti-SEA expressed on the natural log scale. To account for the fact that anti-SEA mitigates the toxic effects of PNU, it was assumed that $\delta < 0$. To elicit prior information it was necessary to reformulate the dose-toxicity model in terms of parameters the clinicians could readily interpret. Since the clinicians could easily understand the probability of DLT associated with selected combinations of dose and anti-SEA, the model was expressed in terms of $\gamma(c_2)$, $\rho_1 = \rho\{0.5, c_1\}$ and $\rho_2 = \rho\{0.5, c_2\}$ for values $c_1 = 0.01$ and $c_2 = 1800$ selected to span the range of anti-SEA concentrations expected in the trial. We note that ρ_1 and ρ_2 are the probabilities of DLT when the minimum allowable dose 0.5 ng/kg is administered to patients with pretreatment anti-SEA $c_1 = 0.05$ and $c_2 = 1800$, respectively. $\gamma(c_2)$ is the MTD associated with the maximum anticipated concentration of anti-SEA. Since the probability of DLT at a given dose is a decreasing function of anti-SEA, we have $\rho_2 < \rho_1$. Thus, the parameter space associated with $\omega = [\rho_1, \rho_2]$ was taken to be $\Omega = \{(x, y){:}\ 0 \leq x \leq \theta, 0 \leq y \leq x\}$. The prior distribution of $\boldsymbol{\nu} = [\gamma(c_2), \omega]$ was specified by assuming $\gamma(c_2)$ and ω to be independent a priori with ω distributed as a uniform on Ω and with $\ln\{\gamma(c_2)\}$ distributed as a uniform on $[\ln(3.5), \ln(1000)]$. Thus, the prior distribution was taken to be

$$h\{\gamma(c_2), \omega\} \propto \gamma(c_2)^{-1} I_{[3.5,1000]}\{\gamma(c_2)\} I_{\Omega}(\omega).$$

3.8. Monitoring Safety and Efficacy in Phase I and II Trials

Upon completion of the phase I trial a decision is made to either remove the treatment from further investigation or to progress to a phase II evaluation of treatment efficacy. In the phase II setting, patients are treated at an estimate of the MTD and the primary statistical focus is on the incidence of some threshold level of antitumor activity. Typically it is assumed that the agent is sufficiently safe at the recommended phase II dose. Consequently, safety considerations are rarely formally accounted for in the design of phase II trials (Thall et al., 1996). However, since the phase II dose is generally determined on the basis of data from a relatively small number (usually 20 or fewer) of phase I patients, the safety of the new agent at the recommended dose may not be well established (Conaway and Petroni, 1996). Consequently, designs for early phase clinical trial are being proposed (e.g., Conaway and Petroni, 1996; Thall et al., 1996; Thall and Russell, 1998, Thall et al., 1999) which permit the monitoring of both patient safety and treatment efficacy. Such designs are considered here since they represent what can be regarded as combination phase I/II trials (Thall and Russell, 1998).

For the combination phase I/II trial, both safety and efficacy are assessed as binary endpoints (Conaway and Petroni, 1996). For example, safety is represented by the indicator variable for dose limiting toxicity while efficacy is indicated by the presence or absence of a given level of antitumor activity (such as complete remission or a reduction of at least 50% in the largest tumor diameter). The method of Thall and Russell (1998) is based on a trinary assessment of overall treatment response. Thus, response is represented by a random variable Y such that: $Y = 0$ if neither DLT nor the desired efficacy outcome is manifest; $Y = 1$ if a patient exhibits positive response without DLT; and $Y = 2$ if DLT is manifest (either with or without positive response to treatment). The relationship between dose and overall response is modeled by assuming that the conditional distribution of Y given dose follows McCullagh's (1980) proportional odds regression model. Specifically, letting $\varphi_i(x) = \text{Prob}\{Y \geq i | \text{Dose} = x\}$, $i = 0, 1, 2$, and writing $\text{logit}(p) = \log[p/(1 - p)]$, the dose-toxicity model is given by

$$\text{logit}[\varphi_i(x)] = \mu_i + \beta x \quad i = 1, 2$$

and

$$\varphi_0(x) = 1 - \varphi_1(x)$$

with $\mu_1 > \mu_2$ and $\beta > 0$. As noted by Thall and Russell (1998), an important consequence of the model is that the probability of the desired outcome $Y = 1$ (i.e., positive response without DLT) is not necessarily a monotone function of dose, which is in accordance with clinical experience. The prior distribution is specified by assuming that μ_1, μ_2, and β are independently distributed as uniform random variables on their respective domains. The authors present a graphical method for determining appropriate domains for the model parameters. The design of the trial requires specification of probabilities θ_1 and θ_2 and thresholds τ_1 and τ_2 such that a given dose x is considered to be insufficiently efficacious if

$$\prod\nolimits_k^* \{p_1(x) < \theta_1\} > \tau_1 \tag{14}$$

and intolerably toxic if

$$\prod\nolimits_k^* \{p_2(x) > \theta_2\} > \tau_2 \tag{15}$$

where, for $i = 1, 2$, $p_i(x) = \text{Prob}\{Y = i|\text{Dose} = x\}$ and $\Pi_k^*(E)$ denotes the posterior probability of the event E given the data available after observation of k patients. A dose level x is said to be acceptable if it is deemed neither insufficiently efficacious nor intolerably toxic. The probabilities θ_1 and θ_2 are specified by the clinicians and represent standards defining acceptable rates of toxicity and positive response. The thresholds τ_1 and τ_2 are chosen on the basis of simulation studies so that the final design has adequate operating characteristics. Once these probabilities and thresholds have been chosen, the trial progresses as follows. A predetermined number N of patients are treated in cohorts of fixed size with each patient in a cohort receiving the same dose. The first cohort of patients is administered the lowest dose in the permissible dose set $S = \{x_1, x_2, \ldots, x_k\}$. Subsequently, if the last dose used is:

- Unacceptably toxic according to (15), then terminate the trial if the last dose is the lowest permissible dose x_1; or deescalate the dose one level.
- Acceptably toxic, but unacceptably active according to (14), then terminate the trial if the last dose is the highest permissible dose x_k; terminate the trial if the next higher dose is unacceptably toxic; or escalate the dose one level if the next higher dose has acceptable toxicity.
- Acceptable, then treat the next cohort at the acceptable dose x^* $\in S$ minimizing $\Pi_k^* \{p_1(x^*) < \theta_1\}$, subject to the constraint that the dose not be escalated by more than one level unless some patients have been treated at all intermediate dose levels.

4. STATISTICAL CONSIDERATIONS

Upon completion of the phase I trial the MTD can be estimated by minimizing the posterior expected loss with respect to some choice of loss function L. Thus, the dose that is recommended for use in a subsequent phase II trial is the level

$$\hat{\gamma} = \arg\min_{\gamma \in \Gamma} \left\{ \int_{\Omega} L(\gamma, \mathbf{u}) \prod_{n} (\gamma, \mathbf{u}) d\mathbf{u} \right\}$$

where n is the total number of patients accrued to the trial. Candidate estimators would include the mean, median, and mode of the marginal posterior distribution of the MTD. Consideration should be given to asymmetric loss functions since under- and overestimation of the MTD would have very different consequences. To reflect the often substantial difference in the characteristics of the phase I and II patient populations, estimation of the MTD can be based on a different prior distribution or loss function than was used to design the phase I trial (Tsutakawa, 1972, 1975). A further separation of the design and inferential aspects of the phase I trial has been suggested by authors (e.g., Watson and Pelli, 1983) who recommend the use of Bayesian methods to design the trial and the use of maximum likelihood to estimate the MTD.

As discussed in Gatsonis and Greenhouse (1992) and indicated by Eq. (10), Bayesian methods can also be used to derive an estimate $\hat{\theta}_k(x)$ of the probability of DLT at a specific dose x. Such information might be incorporated into the informed consent process and provide a basis for statistical stopping rules or for modifying other aspects of the study design.

In addition to being a means to design a phase I trial, Bayesian procedures provide a useful summary of all the information available at any time in the trial. For example, the precision with which the phase II dose has been determined can be reflected through the highest posterior density (HPD) credible interval for the MTD. The HPD credible interval is constructed so that it contains the most likely values for the target dose and so that the posterior probability that it contains the true MTD is equal to a specified credibility level δ. Since the length of a credible interval measures our uncertainty about the parameter under investigation, the HPD credible interval for the MTD would provide a suitable basis for determining when the phase II dose has been determined with sufficient precision that no further phase I testing is required. Similarly, Goodman et al. (1995) suggest a stopping rule based on the length of the 95% HPD credible interval for the unknown slope parameter in the two-parameter logistic dose-toxicity model of Eq. (3) with known intercept. Heyd and Carlin (1999) present simulation results for this stopping rule.

5. CONCLUDING REMARKS

One of the challenging aspects associated with cancer phase I clinical trials is the need to make accurate assessments of the dose levels to be given patients at the onset trial when only limited information is available. The Bayesian approach permits full utilization of the information available from preclinical studies generally conducted prior to the onset of the trial. Furthermore, since the Bayesian designs do not in general rely on asymptotic properties, they are suitable for use in the small sample setting typical of most cancer phase I trials. As result, many researchers are currently focused on improving the performance and generality of phase I design methodologies through the Bayesian perspective.

REFERENCES

Arbuck, S. G. (1996). Workshop on phase I study design. Annals of Oncology 7:567–573.

ASCO special report. Critical role of phase I clinical trials in cancer treatment. Journal of Clinical Oncology 15:853–859.

Babb, J., Rogatko, A., Zacks, S. (1998). Cancer phase I clinical trials: Efficient dose escalation with overdose control. Statistics in Medicine 17:1103–1120.

Babb, J. S., Rogatko, A. (2001). Patient specific dosing in a cancer phase I clinical trial. Statistics in Medicine 20:2079–2090.

Chaloner, K., Larntz, K. (1989). Optimal Bayesian design applied to logistic regression experiments. Journal of Planning and Inference 21:191–208.

Chevret, S. (1993). The continual reassessment method in cancer phase I clinical trials: A simulation study. Statistics in Medicine 12:1093–1108.

Conaway, M. R., Petroni, G. R. (1996). Designs for phase II trials allowing for a trade-off between response and toxicity. Biometrics 52:1375–1386.

Decoster, G., Stein, G., Holdener, E. E. (1990). Responses and toxic deaths in phase I clinical trials. Annals of Oncology 1:175–181.

Dent, S. F., Eisenhauer, E. A. (1996). Phase I trial design: Are new methodologies being put into practice? Annals of Oncology 6:561–566.

Dillman, R. O., Koziol, J. A. (1992). Phase I cancer trials: Limitations and implications. Molecular Biotherapy 4:117–121.

Eichhorn, B. H., Zacks, S. (1973). Sequential search of an optimal dosage I. Journal of American Statistical Association 68:594–598.

Eichhorn, B. H., Zacks, S. (1981). Bayes sequential search of an optimal dosage: Linear regression with both parameters unknown. Communications in Statistics-Theory and Methods 10:931–953.

Faries, D. (1994). Practical modifications of the continual reassessment method for phase I cancer clinical trials. Journal of Biopharm 4:147–164.

Flournoy, N. (1993). A clinical experiment in bone marrow transplantation: Estimating a precentage point of a quantal response curve. In: Gatsonis, C., Hodges, J. S., Kass, R. E., Singpurwalla, D., eds. Lecture Notes in Statistics. New York: Springer-Verlag, pp. 324–336.

Gasparini, M., Eisele, J. (2000). A curve-free method for phase I clinical trials. Biometrics 56:609–615.

Gatsonis, C., Greenhouse, J. B. (1992). Bayesian methods for phase I clinical trials. Statistics in Medicine 11:1377–1389.

Geller, N. L. (1984). Design of phase I and II clinical trials in cancer: a statistician's view. Cancer Investigation 2:483–491.

Goodman, S. N., Zahurak, M. L., Piantadosi, S. (1995). Some practical improvements in the continual reassessment method for phase I studies. Statistics in Medicine 5:1149–1161.

Hawkins, M. J. (1993). Early cancer clinical trials: Safety, numbers, and consent. Journal of the National Cancer Institute 85:1618–1619.

Heyd, J. M., Carlin, B. P. (1999). Adaptive design improvements in the Continual Reassessment Method for phase I studies. Statistics in Medicine 18: 1307–1321.

Johnson, N. L., Kotz, S., Balakrishnam, N. (1995). Continuous Univariate Distributions. New York: John Wiley.

Kramar, A., Lebecq, A., Candalh, E. (1999). Continual reassessment methods in phase I trials of the combination of two drugs in oncology. Statistics in Medicine 18:1849–1864.

McCullagh, P. (1980). Regression models for ordinal data (with discussion). Journal of the Royal Statistical Society 42:109–142.

Mick, R., Lane, N., Daugherty, C. (1994). Physician-determined patient risk of toxic effects: impact on enrollment and decision making in phase I cancer trials. Journal of the National Cancer Institute 86:1685–1693.

Moller, S. (1995). An extension of the continual reassessment methods using a preliminary up-and-down design in a dose finding study in cancer patients, in order to investigate a greater range of doses. Statistics in Medicine 14: 911–923.

National Cancer Institute (1993). Investigator's handbook: A manual for participants in clinical trials of investigational agents sponsored by the Division of Cancer Treatment, National Cancer Institute.

Newell, D. R. (1994). Pharmacologically based phase I trials in cancer chemotherapy. Hematology Oncology Clinics of North America 8:257–275.

O'Quigley, J., Pepe, M., Fisher, L. (1990). Continual reassessment method: A practical design for phase I clinical trials in cancer. Biometrics 46:33–48.

O'Quigley, J., Shen, L. (1996). Continual Reassessment Method: A likelihood approach. Biometrics 52:673–684.

Patterson, S., Francis, S., Ireson, M., Webber, D., Whitehead, J. (1999). A novel Bayesian decision procedure for early-phase dose-finding studies. Journal Biopharm Statistics 9:583–597.

Penta, J. S., Rosner, G. L., Trump, D. L. (1992). Choice of starting dose and escalation for phase I studies of antitumor agents. Cancer Chemotherapy and Pharmacology 31:247–250.

Piantadosi, S., Liu, G. (1996). Improved designs for dose escalation studies using pharmacokinetic measurements. Statistics in Medicine 15:1605–1618.

Rogatko, A., Babb, J. (1998). Escalation with overdose control. User's guide. Version 1. beta. The URL address is http://www.fccc.edu/users/rogatko/ewoc.html.

Robinson, J. A. (1978). Sequential choice of an optimal dose: A prediction intervals approach. Biometrika 65:75–78.

Shih, W. J. (1989). Prediction approaches to sequentially searching for an optimal dose. Biometrics 45:623–628.

Simon, R., Freidlin, B., Rubinstein, L., Arbuck, S. G., Collins, J., Christian, M. C. (1997). Accelerated titration designs for phase I clinical trials in oncology. Journal of the National Cancer Institute 89:1138–1147.

Storer, B. (1989). Design and analysis of phase I clinical trials. Biometrics 45:925–937.

Thall, P. F., Simon, R. M., Estey, E. H. (1996). New statistical strategy for monitoring safety and efficacy in single-arm clinical trials. Journal of Clinical Oncology 14:29.

Thall, P. F., Russell, K. E. (1998). A strategy for dose-finding and safety monitoring based on efficacy and adverse outcomes in phase I/II clinical trials. Biometrics 54:251–264.

Thall, P. F., Estey, E. H., Sung, H. G. (1999). A new statistical method for dose-finding based on efficacy and toxicity in early phase clinical trials. Investigational New Drugs 17:155–167.

Tsutakawa, R. K. (1972). Design of experiment for bioassay. Journal of American Statistical Association 67:584–590.

Tsutakawa, R. K. (1975). Bayesian inference for bioassay. Technical Report 5. Mathematical Sciences, University of Missouri: Columbia.

Tsutakawa, R. K. (1980). Selection of dose levels for estimating a percentage point of a logistic response curve. Journal of the Royal Statistical Society. Series C: Applied Statistics 29:25–33.

Von Hoff, D. D., Kuhn, J., Clark, G. (1984). Cancer Clinical Trials: Methods and Practice. Oxford University Press.

Wang, C., Chen, T. T., Tyan, I. (2000). Designs for phase I cancer clinical trials with differentiation of graded toxicity. Communications in Statistics—Theory and Methods 29:975–987.

Watson, A. B., Pelli, D. G. (1983). QUEST: A Bayesian adaptive psychometric method. Perception and Psychometrics 33:113–120.

Whitehead, J. (1997). Bayesian decision procedures with application to dose-finding studies. International Journal of Pharmaceutical Medicine 11:201–208.

Wooley, P. V., Schein, P. S. (1979). Methods of Cancer Research. New York: Academic Press.

Zacks, S., Rogatko, A., Babb, J. (1998). Optimal Bayesian-feasible dose escalation for cancer phase I clinical trials. Statistics and Probability Letters 38:215–220.

2

Design of Early Trials in Stem Cell Transplantation: A Hybrid Frequentist-Bayesian Approach*

Nancy L. Geller and Eric S. Leifer
National Heart, Lung, and Blood Institute, National Institutes of Health, Bethesda, Maryland, U.S.A.

Dean Follmann
National Institute of Allergy and Infectious Diseases, National Institutes of Health, Bethesda, Maryland, U.S.A.

Shelly L. Carter
The Emmes Corporation, Rockville, Maryland, U.S.A.

1. INTRODUCTION

Clinical trials in humans generally progress from dose finding trials (phase I) to first trials of efficacy (phase II) to definitive trials of efficacy (phase III). In the interest of making development of clinical therapy more efficient, we propose combining phase I and II trials so that once dose finding is completed, patients can continue entry at that dose, and the first assessment of efficacy can be made. The concept itself is simple,

* Nancy L. Geller, Dean Follmann, and Eric Leifer wrote this chapter in their private capacity. The views expressed in the chapter do not necessarily represent the views of NIH, DHHS, or the United States.

but has not found widespread application. While the phase I/II portion may use any of the designs in the literature, we have nested the phase I escalation portion into frequentist phase II designs with early stopping rules. In addition, in the phase II portion of the trial, we include Bayesian stopping rules for safety.

We have applied these designs in a series of allogeneic peripheral blood stem cell transplantation (PBSC) trials with HLA-identical siblings as donors. These trials differ from conventional bone marrow transplantation trials in that the preparative regimen is immunosuppressive, but not myeloablative. However, the sequella of PBSC transplantation are similar to those of bone marrow transplantation and much is known about bone marrow transplantation. We incorporate this prior knowledge into our designs.

There are many possibilities for a primary endpoint in transplantation trials. The earliest endpoint is engraftment, because for a patient to survive disease-free, the donor cells must first engraft and the engraftment must be sustained. The goal in transplantation is for the donor's immune system to replace the patient's; this is known as full donor chimerism. Thus full donor chimerism is a second early endpoint. If mixed donor chimerism (less than full donor chimerism) is not achieved by day 100, it is unlikely that full donor chimerism will ever occur. Thus mixed donor chimerism by day 100 is another early endpoint. Following a transplant, patients are at risk for acute graft versus host disease (aGVHD), usually defined as occurring prior to day 100. Thus, aGVHD of grade II or less by day 100 might be used as an endpoint. Failure in any of these endpoints might result in death. Another cause of early death is infection, which might occur because the patient is immune-suppressed. Thus transplant-related mortality, that is, death due to the transplant or its sequella by day 100 or 200, is another possible primary endpoint.

Aside from these early endpoints, other usual cancer disease endpoints may be considered, such as complete response (absence of disease) by a certain day, or survival to a certain day. When therapy is well developed and definitive trials are undertaken, it is commonplace to use disease-free survival or even overall survival as the trial endpoint.

The choice of the primary endpoint in a transplantation trial depends on the developmental stage of the therapy. Because our trials were among the first PBSC transplants, they were designed to select a preparative regimen that had high probability of achieving donor engraftment. As treatment became more successful, the primary endpoint of succeeding trials would focus on endpoints either further along in time or sustained for a longer period.

2. A PHASE I/II DESIGN FOR PBSC TRANSPLANTATION TRIALS

The initial trial was designed as a phase I/II study. The primary goal was to find the minimal dose of preparative regimen (of three considered) which would establish that the probability of engraftment by day 42 was greater than .80. If such a dose were found, we would assess efficacy by accruing a sufficient number of patients to estimate the proportion of response (complete or partial response for at least one month's duration) with a prespecified precision (e.g., to within $\pm .20$).

The null hypothesis H_0 that the proportion p of patients that engraft by day 42, was at most .80 was tested versus the alternative hypothesis H_A that the proportion of patients who engraft was at least .95:

$$H_0: p \leq .80 \qquad \text{versus} \qquad H_A: p \geq .95.$$

We chose a design with overall significance level .05 and power .80.

We used Simon's optimal two-stage design (1989). Simon's design is optimal in the sense that among all two-stage designs (of the prescribed size and power) that allow for acceptance (but not rejection) of H_0 after the first stage, it has the minimum expected sample size under the point-null hypothesis $p = .80$. The rationale is that it is often attractive to investigators to minimize sample size when the treatment is unsuccessful, but that sample size is less of concern when the treatment is successful.

Patients were to be entered in two stages, with the first (minimum) dose level of the preparative regimen stopped after the first stage if there were not a sufficient number of engraftments. If, among the first 9 patients treated, 7 or fewer engrafted, H_0 would be accepted and the trial would stop. Thus we could stop with as few as two failures, even if they were the first two patients entered into the trial. In that case, the preparative regimen would be escalated to the second dose level. However, if at least 8 patients engrafted at the first dose level, up to 20 additional patients would be enrolled at that dose. If there were three failures (even before all 20 additional patients were enrolled), we would stop using the first preparative regimen, in this case accepting H_0, and the dose of the preparative regimen would be escalated. In any case, a 95% confidence interval for the proportion of engraftment would be given which considered the two-stage design (Jennison and Turnbull, 1983).

If the initial preparative regimen were found to have a low proportion of engraftment (i.e., H_0 was accepted), we would proceed to the second preparative regimen dose level. We would then use the same design as described above to test the same hypotheses with the second preparative regimen. If the second preparative regimen were found to have a low proportion of engraftment (i.e., we accept H_0), the third preparative regimen would be used and the same hypotheses tested.

The first preparative regimen at which H_0 was not accepted in favor of H_A would be the recommended dose for further study. For such a regimen, a 95% confidence interval for response (conditional on engraftment) would be given. If the null hypothesis were accepted for any of the three preparative regimens, other preparative regimens would need to be considered in another trial. In addition, a 95% confidence interval for response to this preparative regimen (counting graft failures as treatment failures) may be given.

An attractive feature of this design is that it uses the same patients to undertake phase I and II activities, i.e., dose finding and hypothesis testing, all while using the optimality properties of Simon's design, which was developed for phase II designs. For the specific design described above, we note that for a particular dose under investigation, H_0 is accepted when either a second patient fails to engraft among the first nine patients tested at that dose, or a third patient fails in any case. In this way, the expected number of patients given an inadequate dose of the preparative regimen is minimized.

There are, of course, other ways in which phase I and II activities could be combined. Instead of Simon's design, we have sometimes used Fleming's (1982) design in the same fashion as described above. Fleming's (1982) design allows early stopping to either accept or reject the null hypothesis. Since Fleming's design is ultimately based on Wald's (1947) sequential probability ratio test, it approximately minimizes expected sample sizes under the point-null *and* point-alternative hypotheses. These designs are preferable in certain situations to Simon's designs which, as discussed above, only minimizes expected sample size under the point-null hypothesis.

Alternatively, doses could be escalated according to methods of O'Quigley, et al. (1990, 2001) or Stylianou and Flournoy (2002) or Rogatko and Babb (2003). Such escalation schemes were designed to undertake dose finding efficiently and if they are used in a phase I/II trial, it is likely that additional patients for the phase II portion of the trial will be required. The phase I/II trial proposed here does not require additional patients for phase II.

When there are a sufficient number of engraftments to accept a preparative regimen in the particular design we propose, we can estimate the response proportion (conditional on engraftment) in addition to performing hypothesis testing on the proportion of patients that engraft. If there were no responders in 19 engrafters, we could also conclude that the response proportion (conditional on engraftment) is .15 or less with 95% confidence. If there were no responders in 29 engrafters, we could conclude with 95% confidence that the response proportion (conditional on engraftment) is .10 or less.

3. BAYESIAN STOPPING RULE FOR SAFETY

The trial described in Section 2 was monitored by a data and safety monitoring board, which expressed a concern that engraftment by day 42 was not sufficient to assure the longer term safety of the patients who underwent this procedure. They requested a stopping rule for a longer term endpoint to monitor safety. We chose 100 day transplant-related mortality (TRM) as the safety endpoint. TRM encompasses multiple causes of death and so serves as a suitable safety endpoint. Thus patients who died because of failure to engraft, graft failure after engraftment, toxicity from the preparative regimen, graft versus host disease or infection would count as failures in the safety endpoint. Day 100 was chosen to include the early sequella of the transplant, but not later events, such as chronic graft versus host disease or recurrence. To monitor day 100 TRM, we adopted a Bayesian approach which formally incorporated "prior" expectations about the proportion of patients experiencing TRM.

Several authors have used Bayesian methods in other settings. Thall and Simon (1994) discuss Bayesian guidelines for phase II trials where comparison to a previously established standard will be made and the data are monitored continuously. Thall et al., (1995) discuss Bayesian sequential monitoring in phase II trials with multiple outcomes. Follmann and Albert (1999) discuss Bayesian monitoring with censored data. Thall and Russell (1998) use a Bayesian approach to assess dose and efficacy simultaneously by defining adverse, efficacious and neither as outcomes and using a cumulative odds model.

The proportion of patients experiencing TRM up through day 100 post-transplant, p_{TRM}, was assumed to follow a binomial distribution. For the prior distribution of p_{TRM}, we used the beta distribution. This was done for two reasons. First, it is a "natural" conjugate prior for the binomial distribution; that is, the likelihood functions for both the beta and the binomial distributions have the same functional form (Berger, 1985). Thus, the posterior distribution may be easily recalculated each time a patient is evaluated. Second, using a beta prior has the following attractive property: Suppose a beta prior distribution with parameters a and b is used, and so its mean is $a/(a + b)$ and variance is $ab/[(a + b)^2 (a + b + 1)]$. Further, suppose that among n patients enrolled, y have not engrafted (failure), and the remaining $n - y$ have engrafted (success). Then the posterior beta distribution has parameters $a + y$ and $b + (n - y)$ and mean $(a + y) / (n + a + b)$. This mean is the maximum likelihood estimate of p_{TRM} based on $a + y$ successes and $(n - y) + b$ failures. Thus the prior may be thought of as contributing a "imaginary" failures and b "imaginary" successes to the posterior distribution and so is "worth" $a + b$ "patients" compared to the n "real" patients that have been enrolled (Santner and Duffy, 1989).

This interpretation provides a simplified approach to specifying the prior distribution. We specify the prior mean at say r and take the worth of the prior to be a modest proportion of the total planned sample size, that is, $a + b$ is a modest proportion of n. This assures that the prior will be influential in the early stage of the study, but that later, the data will dominate the prior.

A stopping boundary would be reached if the proportion experiencing TRM exceeds the anticipated proportion with posterior probability at some threshold, say .90 or .95. From prior experience we anticipated the mean to be .20 and we take our prior to be "worth" six patients. Thus the parameters of the prior distribution were 1.2 and 4.8 which also implies that the variance of the prior distribution is .0229.

We took the threshold probability for stopping as .90. That is, we would recommend stopping if the number of patients patients experiencing TRM implied the posterior distribution had .90 of its probability mass exceeding the mean of the prior, .20. For the purpose of preserving power, we did not allow for stopping after every patient, but, instead, after groups of patients. The resulting stopping boundaries are given in Table 1.

In implementing this stopping rule, it is important to be even-handed in counting those alive and dead by 100 days. Strictly speaking, we should not tally a patient as having 100 day TRM or not until their

Table 1 Bayesian Stopping Rule for 100 Day TRM

No. patients	Stop if number of transplant-related deaths by day 100 reaches or exceeds
9	4
19	7
28	9

100 day enrollment anniversary has passed. However, if meeting the boundary is certain to occur, we can relax this restriction. For example, if the first four patients enroll simultaneously and all die within 10 days, there is no need to wait an additional 90 days to say the boundary has been crossed.

The stopping rule was assessed by simulation. Based on 10,000 repetitions, the probability of meeting the stopping boundary was .16 under the null hypothesis of $p_{TRM} = .80$ and .88 under the alternative hypothesis that $p_{TRM} = .40$. We concluded that the likelihood of stopping was satisfactory to protect patient safety for 100 day TRM. It is important to undertake simulations to evaluate the repeated sampling behavior of planned stopping rules in order to feel comfortable about their performance.

S+ programs for Bayesian stopping rules and their assessment are available from the authors.

4. A PHASE II TRIAL DESIGN WITH AN INTERMEDIATE ENDPOINT AND BAYESIAN STOPPING RULES FOR EARLY FAILURE

Several phase I/II PBSC transplantation clinical trials were designed for different diseases using the paradigm above. The new treatment method was considered successful, in that there was one preparative regimen that gave engraftment in a high proportion of cases in several different trials. Because of this progress, the next set of trials used a longer term primary endpoint, 200 day disease-free survival. A Bayesian stopping rule for earlier failure was also included.

Here is an example of a design to estimate the 200 day disease-free survival which was used in a PBSC transplant trial of patients with debilitating non-malignant hematological diseases. The expected 200 day disease-free survival for such patients was .30. Forty-five patients were to be enrolled. After all patients had been followed for 200 days, a 95% confidence interval for the 200 day survival was to be given based on the Kaplan–Meier (1958) estimate and Greenwood's formula (1926) for the variance. This sample size is the number of patients required (assuming that no early stopping was permitted) to estimate the true 200 day survival proportion to within approximately $\pm.13$ with 95% confidence if the Kaplan–Meier estimate of 200 day survival was in the range of .30–.40 (Simon and Lee, 1982).

In this trial, we also considered Bayesian stopping rules for early failure. We illustrate with a stopping rule for acute GVHD (grade 3 or higher up to day 100) based on a Bayesian formulation. Prior experience in transplantation has resulted in the proportion of patients with grade 3 or higher acute GVHD. $p_{a\mathrm{GVHD}}$, is most likely to be .20. Given that there would be 45 patients in the trial, we used a beta prior distribution with mean .20 and "worth" 18 patients, i.e., with parameters 4 and 16 (variance 0.0076). With this prior distribution, the probability of grade 3 or higher acute GVHD was unlikely to be less than .08 (prior probability .06) or greater than .40 (prior probability .02), also consistent with experience. Stopping would be recommended whenever the posterior distribution had .95 of its mass exceeding the mean of the prior distribution, .20. The stopping rule is shown in Table 2.

Table 2 Bayesian Stopping Rule for Acute GVHD

No. patients	No. cases to recommend stopping
5–6	5
7–10	6
11–13	7
14–17	8
18–21	9
22–25	10
26–29	11
30–33	12

This stopping rule was assessed by simulation. Based on 10,000 repetitions, the probability of stopping early for an excess of acute GVHD over the course of the trial was .04 when $p_{a\text{GVHD}} = .20$ and .76 when $p_{a\text{GHVD}} = .40$. This was deemed reasonable for protecting patient safety.

5. A PHASE II DESIGN WITH MULTIPLE PRIORITIZED ENDPOINTS

Other designs are feasible for the phase II portion of a phase I/II trial. Several authors have considered trials with multiple endpoints in the phase II setting. Conaway and Petroni (1995), Jennison and Turnbull (1993), and Thall et al. (1995) design trials which evaluate bivariate responses and such designs might be considered in the phase II portion of a phase I/II trial.

Below we present a method for a phase II portion of a phase I/II trial, where a priority among multiple endpoints can be specified. As an example, consider using mixed chimerism by day 100 and absence of disease at day 100 as joint endpoints. Suppose we are interested in testing if the proportion of those with mixed chimerism at day 100 is .75, but this is only of interest if the proportion of those with absence of disease at day 100 is at least .50.

1. Test

   $H_{01}: p$ (disease at day 100) $\leq .50$ versus

   $H_{A1}: p$ (disease at day 100) $> .50$

2. If H_{01} is rejected (at, say, $\alpha = .05$), test

   $H_{02}: p$ (mixed chimerism) $\leq .75$ versus

   $H_{A2}: p$ (mixed chimerism) $> .75$

   at the same level $\alpha = .05$.

Because the two hypotheses are prioritized and H_{02} is not tested unless H_{01} is rejected, the overall type I error of this procedure is .05, that is $P(\text{Reject } H_{01} \text{ or } H_{02} \mid H_{01} \text{ and/or } H_{02} \text{ is true}) = .05$. The procedure preserves α because the second hypothesis is tested only if the first is rejected, but not otherwise. Of course if H_{02} were tested regardless of whether H_{01} was rejected, then the overall type I error would be inflated to

$P(\text{Reject } H_{01} \mid H_{01} \text{ is true}) + P(\text{Reject } H_{02} \mid H_{02} \text{ is true})$; this quantity could be as large as .10.

Suppose we set sample size to have adequate power to test the first hypothesis. With two-sided $\alpha = .05$ and power .90, for example, a sample size of 65 can detect the alternative that the proportion of patients with disease at day 100 is .70. We might introduce some planned interim analyses, which would lower the power slightly. We recommend sample size be set based on the power to detect an alternative of interest on the endpoint with first priority, since the lower priority hypotheses may not be tested. One would also calculate the power to detect a difference of interest on the secondary hypothesis. If a larger sample size is needed for the secondary endpoint than the primary endpoint, it might seem natural to increase the difference of interest on the secondary hypothesis. However, we recommend reconsidering if the priority of the endpoints is correct, and, in particular, if this is the approach that is appropriate.

6. DISCUSSION

This chapter presents designs for phase I/II trials. Simon's designs, which were developed for the phase II frequentist setting, were used to establish stopping rules for finding a safe dose level in the phase I portion of our trial, as well as for hypothesis testing in the phase II portion, if a safe dose was found. When a safe dose was found, we also proposed an estimate of treatment efficacy at the safe dose level. In addition, we incorporate Bayesian stopping rules for safety.

What is the logical basis for combining frequentist and Bayesian approaches in early trials? For those who prefer a frequentist approach, the argument can be made that when there is prior knowledge about safety endpoints, a Bayesian approach is appropriate. The associated toxicities and the course of recovery for those undergoing PBSC transplantation are well known from bone marrow transplantation. The frequentist can use his or her preferred design for the primary endpoint, yet incorporate this wealth of experience into the secondary endpoints. For those who prefer Bayesian approaches altogether, one could undertake a phase I/II trial with both phases Bayesian.

For the frequentist, the safety stopping rules do not affect α, but lower the power of the trial. That is, the possibility of stopping for safety reasons makes it easier to miss a treatment effect of interest. However, if a trial is stopped early for safety reasons, the treatment effect is of limited interest. Both the number of stopping rules for safety and the possible stopping times should also be limited to avoid an excessive decrease in power and to reduce the chance of stopping unnecessarily.

The choice of primary endpoints in early trials is difficult and must rely on clinical judgment. The statistician can help the clinician keep in mind that new therapies should be assessed by early endpoints and it is only when treatment is better established that longer term endpoints should be primary. In designing early trials, recent designs, such as those that prioritize among multiple endpoints, should be considered. The frequentist approach to efficacy with a Bayesian approach for safety provides a paradigm for efficient design of these early studies.

REFERENCES

Berger, J. O. (1985). Statistical Decision Theory and Bayesian Analysis. 2d ed. New York: Springer-Verlag.

Conaway, M. R., Petroni, G. R. (1995). Bivariate sequential designs for phase II clinical trials. Biometrics 51:656–664.

Fleming, T. R. (1982). One-sample multiple testing procedure for phase II clinical trials. Biometrics 38:143–151.

Follmann, D. A., Albert, P. (1999). Bayesian monitoring of event rates with censored data. Biometrics 55:603–607.

Greenwood, M. (1926). A report on the natural duration of cancer. Reports on Public Health. Vol. 33. London: H.M. Stationery Office, pp. 1–26.

Jennison, C., Turnbull, B. (1983). Confidence intervals for a binomial parameter following a multistage test with application to MIL-STD 105D and medical trials. Technometrics 25:49–58.

Jennison, C., Turnbull, B. W. (1993). Group sequential tests for bivariate safety endpoints. Biometrics 49:741–752.

Kaplan, E. L., Meier, P. (1958). Nonparametric estimation from incomplete observations. Journal of the American Statistical Association 53:457–481.

O'Quigley, J., Hughes, M. D., Fenton, T. (2001). Dose-finding designs for HIV studies. Biometrics 57:1018–1029.

O'Quigley, J., Pepe, M., Fisher, L. (1990). Consistency of continual reassessment method in dose finding studies. Biometrika 83:395–406.

Rogatko, A., Babb, J. (2003). Bayesian methods in phase I clinical trials. In: Geller, N., ed. Contemporary Biostatistical Methods in Clinical Trials. New York: Marcel Dekker, pp. 1–40.

Santner, T. J., Duffy, D. E. (1989). The Statistical Analysis of Discrete Data. New York: Springer-Verlag, pp. 24–25.

Simon, R. (1989). Optimal two-stage designs for phase II clinical trials. Controlled Clinical Trials 10:1–10.

Simon, R., Lee, Y. J. (1982). Nonparametric confidence limits for survival probabilities and median survival time. Cancer Treatment Reports 66:37–42.

Stylianou, M., Flournoy, N. (2002). Dose finding using the biased coin up-and-down design and isotonic regression. Biometrics 58:171–177.

Thall, P. F., Russell, K. E. (1998). A strategy for dose-finding and safety monitoring based on efficacy and adverse outcomes in Phase I/II clinical trials. Biometrics 54:251–264.

Thall, P., Simon, R. (1994). Practical Bayesian guidelines for Phase IIB clinical trials. Biometrics 50:337–349.

Thall, P., Simon, R., Estey, E. (1995). Bayesian sequential monitoring designs for single-armed clinical trials with multiple outcomes. Statistics in Medicine 357–379.

3

Design and Analysis of Therapeutic Equivalence Trials

Richard M. Simon
National Cancer Institute, National Institutes of Health, Bethesda, Maryland, U.S.A.

1. INTRODUCTION

Active control clinical trials compare a new treatment to a treatment known to be active in the disease in question. Active control trials are sometimes called non inferiority trials or therapeutic equivalence trials and we will use the terms interchangeably. There are two common objectives to active control trials. The first is to demonstrate that the new treatment (E, experimental) is effective relative to no treatment or relative to a placebo. In the context of a serious or life-threatening disease, if there is an effective treatment (C, active control), it will not be justifiable to perform a randomized clinical trial comparing E to placebo or no treatment (P). Consequently, demonstration of the effectiveness of E is often attempted by comparing E to C. The hope is that if one can conclude that E is equivalent to C and if C is known to be effective, then E must be effective.

The second objective of an active control trial is to determine whether E is equivalent to C. For example, C may represent mastectomy for breast cancer and E lumpectomy with radiation treatment. Or C may be 12 months of adjuvant chemotherapy after surgery for colon cancer and E may be 6 months of chemotherapy. The goal of demonstrating therapeutic equivalence frequently occurs when E is a less debilitating or less toxic version of C. The goal of demonstrating that E is effective relative to P frequently occurs when E is a new drug for which one seeks regulatory approval.

Therapeutic equivalence trials should not be confused with bioequivalence trials. The goal of a bioequivalence trial is to compare the serum concentrations of a specified molecule as functions of time for two treatments. The treatments often represent two different routes or schedules of administration of a drug. Bioequivalence trials are often conducted as small two-period crossover studies. Because the endpoint permits the use of the crossover design to eliminate interpatient variability and because the endpoint can usually be measured precisely, the bioequivalence objective can usually be accomplished adequately with relatively few patients.

In contrast to bioequivalence trials, therapeutic equivalence or active control trials are problematic. There are two major problems. One is that we can never establish that E is equivalent to C. In statistical hypothesis testing we frequently express the null hypothesis that E is equivalent to C. It is a fallacy, however, to believe that failure to reject a null hypothesis represents demonstration of its truth. We will describe in the next section several statistical formulations of active control trials that attempt to deal with the problem that one can never establish the equivalence of two treatments.

The second major problem with the strategy of trying to establish effectiveness of E through a therapeutic equivalence trial is that C must be known to be effective. This means effective with regard to the endpoint used in the active control trial and that endpoint must be a measure of patient benefit. Many active control trials fail at this point. For example, in several types of advanced cancer, standard treatments are used for which there is little evidence of effectiveness. The treatments are known to be "active" in the sense that they cause partial shrinkage of a percentage of tumors, but that shrinkage is not direct evidence of effective palliation or patient benefit, particularly in light of the toxicities of the treatments. To know that C is effective, one should generally have randomized clinical trials of C versus P that establishes the effectiveness of C with regard to a medically meaningful endpoint that can be used in the active control trial. Even that is not enough because one must be able to conclude that C is effective for the patients to be studied in the active control trial. Hence there must be evidence that the patients to be included in the active control trial are very similar to those that were included in the randomized trials of C versus P that established the effectiveness of C.

In the following sections we will describe the statistical approaches that are commonly used for the design and analysis of active control trials. We will elaborate on the problems of establishing therapeutic equivalence or treatment effectiveness via active control trials and will critique the commonly used statistical formulations. We will also present a new Bayesian approach to the design and analysis of active control trials and will illustrate its application.

2. COMMONLY USED STATISTICAL FORMULATIONS

2.1. Testing the Null Hypothesis of Equivalence

Most clinical trials are designed to test the null hypothesis that the two treatments are equivalent with regard to the primary endpoint. For an active control trial, the null hypothesis can be represented as H_0: $F_E = F_C$, where F_E denotes the distribution function of the endpoint for treatment E and F_C is defined analogously. Let the probability of rejecting H_0 be no greater than α whenever H_0 is true. The usual approach is to define an alternative hypothesis H_A that represents the smallest difference between the treatments that is medically important. If the distribution functions F_E and F_C are normal with possibly different means but the same variances, then the distance between F_E and F_C can be represented by the difference in means $\Delta = \mu_C - \mu_E$. In order to have power $1-\beta$ for rejecting the null hypothesis when the alternative hypothesis $\Delta = \Delta^*$ is true, we require

$$\frac{\Delta^*}{\tau} = z_{1-\alpha} + z_{1-\beta} \tag{1}$$

where $\tau = \sqrt{2\sigma^2/n}$ is the standard error of the maximum likelihood estimate (MLE) of Δ, $z_{1-\alpha}$ and $z_{1-\beta}$ are percentiles of the standard normal distribution and n is the sample size per treatment arm. Equation (1) can be used for planning the sample size of the trial. When the endpoint is binary, a number of normal approximations are available for sample size planning, one of the most accurate being that of Casagrande et al. (1978). For time to event endpoints, the target number of events can be planned using the results of Rubenstein et al. (1981) when the alternative hypothesis is based on proportional hazards.

A major objection to the conventional statistical formulation of testing the null hypothesis for active control trials is that failure to reject the null hypothesis is often considered a basis for accepting the null hypothesis. In superiority trials, acceptance of the null hypothesis is equivalent to rejection of the experimental treatment E. If the clinical trial is inadequately small, it will have poor statistical power and will likely result in failure to reject the null hypothesis. Consequently, an inadequately tested new treatment will not be adopted. The decision structure is reversed, however, for active control trials. Acceptance of the null hypothesis is acceptance of therapeutic equivalence. This may lead to adoption of the experimental treatment E. Here an inadequately small trial will likely lead to failure to reject the null hypothesis and acceptance of therapeutic equivalence. There are other defects, in addition to inadequate sample size, that can impair the statistical power of an active control trial and lead to erroneous adoption of E. Having many patients lost to follow-up, many protocol violations or selecting patients who are unlikely to benefit from either treatment are but a few examples.

In using this formulation one must bear in mind that for active control trials the type 2 error β is at least as important as the type 1 error α because the decision structure is reversed from the formulation for superiority trials. Hence it is not unusual to use $\beta = .05$ and $\alpha = .10$ for active control trials. It is also noteworthy that the significance test is one-sided for active control trials.

The issue of sample size planning for active control trials is complex and will be dealt with more fully in Section 3.2. Most trials with the objective of demonstrating equivalence of a less debilitating or more convenient therapy for a life-threatening disease, however, must be very large. This is because the secondary endpoints of convenience or less debilitation are desirable only if one is assured that the decrease in efficacy for the primary endpoint is very small. Hence the trial must have high power for rejecting the null hypothesis for a very small value of Δ^*. This results in a large sample size.

2.2. Testing a Nonnull Hypothesis

Inadequately sized active control trials are sometimes taken as convincing demonstration of equivalence by a large portion of the medical audience. Many do not appreciate that failure to reject the null hypothesis is not a valid basis for concluding that the null hypothesis is true, particularly when the statistical power is low. In order to limit the potential for misinterpretation of active control trials, Blackwelder (1982) proposed that they be designed and analyzed by testing the alternative hypothesis H_A: $\mu_C - \mu_E = \Delta^*$. If the power for rejecting $\Delta = \Delta^*$ is low, then the conclusion will be that the treatments are not equivalent and hence E will not be accepted.

For the normal model with common variance, in order to test $\Delta = \Delta^*$ with one-sided significance level β and power $1-\alpha$ for rejecting $\Delta = \Delta^*$ when $\Delta = 0$, the resulting sample size is given by the same formula (1) as described above for the conventional formulation. For binary or time-to-event endpoints, the sample size formulas for the two formulations differ somewhat because the standard error of the maximum likelihood estimate of treatment difference is not the same under the null and alternative hypotheses. But the differences are not large. The main potential advantage of the approach of basing the analysis on testing the alternative hypothesis is to protect against erroneous acceptance of the null hypothesis when the statistical power is poor because of inadequate sample size.

2.3. Confidence Intervals

Many of the misinterpretations of the results of active control trials can be avoided by reporting confidence intervals for the treatment difference rather than significance tests (Simon, 1993). Unfortunately, confidence intervals are rarely reported. When they are, it is usually confidence intervals for each treatment mean rather than for the difference.

We do clinical trials to learn about the relative merits of two treatments. The relative merits are based on various types of outcomes. Sensible clinical decision making is based on weighing trade-offs among the differences between the treatments with regard to multiple endpoints. Clinical decisions are often based on the magnitudes of effects that can be expected; hence, estimation is crucial. The most common problem with significance tests is that they are misinterpreted as measures of the magnitude of effect. A "statistically significant" effect is considered an important effect and a nonstatistically significant effect is considered no effect. Although this is a problem with the interpretation and not with the tool itself, it indicates that investigators and clinicians want measures of effect in order to make their decisions. Significance tests are poor surrogates for binary indicators of clinical significance. This is because they are determined simultaneously by the magnitude of the effect and the precision by which it is measured. A major effect in a small study may not be statistically significant and a small effect in a large study may be statistically significant. There has been such an overreliance on significance tests that sometimes even point estimates of the magnitude of effect get buried. Confidence intervals are less easily mistaken for decision procedures and help focus attention on one component of the decision process, estimating the size of effects.

Many published clinical trials are noninformative rather than negative. That is, the confidence interval is consistent with both clinically significant and with null effects. One might argue that a statement of the statistical power of the study would have served equally well. This is not true, although the influential article by Freiman and Chalmers has led a generation of clinical trialists to believe that it is (Frieman et al., 1978). Statistical power does not utilize the results actually obtained. Hence, a study with limited power may reliably demonstrate that an experimental treatment is not better than control to a clinically significant degree if the observed difference favors control. This is illustrated in the results for 71 "negative" clinical trials published by Frieman et al. (1978). There were 50 clinical trials with less than 90% power for detecting a 50% reduction in the event rate. Of these 50, a 90% confidence interval excludes effects as large as a 50% reduction in 16 (32%) cases. Hence confidence intervals are more informative than power statements in the reporting of results. The paper by Simon describes for clinical investigators how to calculate such confidence intervals for treatment effects and why one should (Simon, 1986). That paper provides simple approximate methods for computing confidence intervals for treatment effects in common situations such as with binary or time to event endpoints. The confidence interval makes explicit the strengths and limitations of the trial for distinguishing between null and alternative hypotheses.

One can also plan the size of an active control trial based on a confidence interval analysis (Makuch and Simon, 1978; Durrleman and Simon, 1990). Suppose one plans to report a one-sided $1-\alpha$ level confidence interval for $\Delta = \mu_C - \mu_E$. This confidence interval can be written $\hat{\Delta} + z_{1-\alpha}\tau$, where $\hat{\Delta}$ is the maximum likelihood estimator of Δ and τ is its standard error. We may wish to conclude that E is not substantially inferior to C if the upper confidence limit is no greater than a specified Δ^*. If $\Delta = 0$, the probability that the upper confidence limit is less than Δ^* is $\Phi(\Delta^*/\tau - z_{1-\alpha})$ where Φ is the cumulative distribution function for the standard normal distribution. Requiring that this probability equals $1-\beta$ results in Eq. (1). A lower $1-\alpha$ level confidence limit for Δ is $\hat{\Delta} - z_{1-\alpha}\tau$. If this lower limit exceeds 0, then one may conclude that the treatments are not equivalent. If $\Delta = \Delta^*$, the probability that the lower limit exceeds zero is again $\Phi(\Delta^*/\tau - z_{1-\alpha})$. Hence, for the case of normal endpoints with equal variance, expression (1) provides for a probability of $1-\beta$ that the $1-\alpha$ one-sided upper confidence limit is less than Δ^* when $\Delta=0$ and a probability $1-\beta$ that the $1-\alpha$ one-sided lower confidence limit is greater than zero when $\Delta = \Delta^*$. Since both conditions are relevant, it seems appropriate to design the trial for use of a two-sided $1-2\alpha$ confidence interval. In many cases, it may be reasonable to use $2\alpha = 0.1$ and $1-\beta = 0.9$. A more stringent condition for planning is to require that the width of the confidence interval be Δ^*. This ensures that in all cases either $\Delta \geq \Delta^*$ is excluded or $\Delta \leq 0$ is excluded. It requires a substantially greater number of patients however. For sample size planning with time to event data one can use expression (1) with the approximation that $\sigma^2 = \text{total events}/4$.

2.4. Specification of Δ^*

In an important sense, none of the above approaches represents a satisfactory statistical framework for the design and analysis of active control trials. These approaches depend on specification of the minimal difference in efficacy Δ^* that one will be able to detect with high probability. If Δ^* is selected based on practical considerations such as patients available, the trial may not demonstrate equivalence. In general, the difference Δ should represent the largest difference that a patient is willing to give up in efficacy for the secondary benefits of the experimental treatment *E*. The difference Δ must be no greater than the efficacy of *C* relative to *P* and will in general be a fraction of that quantity Δ_c. Estimation of Δ_c requires review of clinical trials that established the effectiveness of *C* relative to *P*. Δ_c should not be taken as the maximum likelihood estimate of treatment effect from such trials because there is substantial probability that the true treatment effect in those trials was less than the ML*E*.

None of the approaches described previously deal with how Δ^* is determined. Fleming (1990) and Gould (1991, 1993) have noted that the design and interpretation of active control trials must utilize information about previous trials of the active control. Fleming proposed that the new treatment be considered effective if an upper confidence limit for the amount by which the new treatment may be inferior to the active control does not exceed a reliable estimate of the improvement of the active control over placebo or no treatment. Gould provided a method for creating a synthetic placebo control group in the active controlled trial based on previous trials comparing the active control to placebo. The next section presents a general Bayesian approach to the utilization of information from previous trials in the design and analysis of an active controlled trial (Simon, 1999).

3. BAYESIAN DESIGN AND ANALYSIS OF ACTIVE CONTROL TRIALS

3.1. Analysis

We use the following model for the active control trial:

$$Y=\alpha+\beta X+\gamma Z+\varepsilon$$

where Y denotes the response of a patient, $X=0$ for placebo or the experimental treatment and 1 for the control treatment, $Z=0$ for placebo or the control treatment and 1 for the experimental treatment, and ε is normally distributed experimental error with mean zero and variance σ^2. Hence the expected response for C is $\alpha+\beta$, the expected response for E is $\alpha+\gamma$, and the expected response for P is α.

Assuming that σ^2 is known and that the parameters α, β, γ have independent normal prior densities $N(\mu_\alpha, \sigma_\alpha^2)$, $N(\mu_\beta, \sigma_\beta^2)$, $N(\mu_\gamma, \sigma_\gamma^2)$, the posterior distribution of the parameters (α, β, γ) can be shown to be multivariate normal (Simon, 1999). The covariance matrix is

$$\Sigma=\frac{K}{\sigma^2}\begin{pmatrix} (1+r_\beta)(1+r_\gamma) & -(1+r_\gamma) & -(1+r_\beta) \\ -(1+r_\gamma) & r_\gamma+(1+r_\alpha)(1+r_\gamma) & 1 \\ -(1+r_\beta) & 1 & r_\beta+(1+r_\alpha)(1+r_\beta) \end{pmatrix} \tag{2}$$

where $r_\alpha=\sigma^2/\sigma_\alpha^2$, $r_\beta = \sigma^2/\sigma_\beta^2$, and $r_\gamma = \sigma^2/\sigma_\gamma^2$ and

$$K=r_a(1+r_\beta)(1+r_\gamma)+r_\beta(1+r_\gamma)+(1+r_\beta)r_\gamma.$$

The mean vector $\boldsymbol{\eta}=(\eta_\alpha, \eta_\beta, \eta_\gamma)$ of the posterior distribution is

$$\begin{aligned} \eta_\alpha &= \frac{r_\alpha(1+r_\beta)(1+r_\gamma)\mu_\alpha+r_\beta(1+r_\gamma)(\bar{y}_C-\mu_\beta)+r_\gamma(1+r_\beta)(\bar{y}_E-\mu_\gamma)}{K} \\ \eta_\beta &= \frac{r_\beta\{r_\gamma+(1+r_\alpha)(1+r_\gamma)\}\mu_\beta+r_\alpha(1+r_\gamma)(\bar{y}_C-\mu_\alpha)+r_\gamma(\bar{y}_C-\bar{y}_E+\mu_\gamma)}{K} \\ \eta_\gamma &= \frac{r_\gamma\{r_\beta+(1+r_\alpha)(1+r_\beta)\}\mu_\gamma+r_\alpha(1+r_\beta)(\bar{y}_E-\mu_\alpha)+r_\beta(\bar{y}_E-\bar{y}_C+\mu_\beta)}{K} \end{aligned} \tag{3}$$

where $\bar{y}_C$ and $\bar{y}_E$ are the observed mean responses in the active control trial for the control group and experimental treatment group, respectively.

Expression (3) indicates that the posterior mean of α is a weighted average of three estimates of α. The first estimate is the prior mean μ_α. The second estimate is the observed $\bar{y}_C$ minus the prior mean for β. This makes intuitive sense since the expectation of $\bar{y}_C$ is $\alpha+\beta$. The third estimate in the weighted average is the observed $\bar{y}_E$ minus the prior mean for γ. The expectation of $\bar{y}_E$ is $\alpha+\gamma$. The sum of the weights is K. The other posterior means are similarly interpreted.

The marginal posterior distribution of γ is normal with mean η_γ and variance the (3, 3) element of Σ given in (2). The parameter γ represents the contrast of experimental treatment versus placebo. One can thus easily compute the posterior probability that $\gamma>0$ which would be a Bayesian analog of a p value of a test of the null hypothesis that the experimental regimen is no more effective than placebo (if negative values of the parameter represent effectiveness).

The posterior distribution of $\gamma-k\beta$ is univariate normal with mean $\eta_\gamma-k\eta_\beta$ and variance $\Sigma_{33}+k^2\Sigma_{22}-2k\Sigma_{23}$. Consequently, one can also easily compute the posterior probability that $\gamma-k\beta\leq 0$. For $k=.5$, if $\beta<0$ this represents the probability that the experimental regimen is at least half as effective as the active control. Since there may be positive probability that $\beta>0$, it is more appropriate to compute the joint probability that $\beta<0$ and $\gamma-k\beta\leq 0$ to represent the probability that the experimental regimen is at least a kth as effective as the active control.

Often there will be no previous randomized trials on which to base a prior distribution for the effectiveness of the experimental treatment and it will be appropriate to use a noninformative prior for γ. The parameter α represents the expected response of untreated or placebo treated patients. This may be highly variable among trials. In the special case where a noninformative prior distributions are adopted for α and γ, setting σ_α and σ_γ to infinity in (2), the covariance matrix of the posterior distribution of the parameters takes the form

$$\Sigma = \sigma_\beta^2 \begin{pmatrix} 1+r_\beta & -1 & -(1+r_\beta) \\ -1 & 1 & 1 \\ -(1+r_\beta) & 1 & 1+2r_\beta \end{pmatrix}. \tag{4}$$

In this case the posterior distribution of β is the same as the prior distribution, the posterior distribution of γ is $N(\mu_\beta+\bar{y}_E-\bar{y}_C, \sigma_\beta^2+2\sigma^2)$ and the posterior distribution of α is $N(\bar{y}_C-\mu_\beta, \sigma_\beta^2+\sigma^2)$. It can be seen that the clinical trial comparing C to E contains information about α if an informative prior distribution is used for β.

One may permit correlation among the prior distributions. Let S denote the covariance matrix for the multinormal prior distribution for $(\alpha\ \beta\ \gamma)$. Then $\Sigma^{-1} = M + S^{-1}$, where

$$M=\frac{1}{\sigma^2}\begin{pmatrix} 2 & 1 & 1 \\ 1 & 1 & 0 \\ 1 & 0 & 1 \end{pmatrix} \tag{5}$$

and the posterior mean vector is the solution of $\Sigma^{-1}\eta=(1/\sigma^2)(y\cdot\ \bar{y}_C\ \bar{y}_E)' + S^{-1}\mu'$, where $\mu = (\mu_\alpha \quad \mu_\beta \quad \mu_\gamma)$ and $y\cdot = \bar{y}_C + \bar{y}_E$.

The above results can be applied to binary outcome data by approximating the log odds of failure by a normal distribution. Let Y denote the natural logarithm of the ratio of number of failures in a treatment arm of the trial divided by the number of nonfailures, for example, for the active control group $\bar{y}_C=\log\left(\frac{f_C}{n_C-f_C}\right)$. The standard approximation for the variance of the logit is $\sigma^2=\frac{n_C}{f_C(n_C-f_C)}$.

The approach can also be extended in an approximate manner to the proportional hazards model. Let the hazard be written as

$$\lambda(t)=\lambda_0(t)\exp(\beta X+\gamma Z)$$

where $\lambda_0(t)$ denotes the baseline hazard function and the indicator variables X and Z are the same as described at the start of Section 3. The data will be taken as the maximum likelihood estimate of the log hazard ratio for E relative to C for the active control study and will be denoted by y. For large samples y is approximately normally distributed with mean $\gamma-\beta$ and variance $\sigma^2=1/d_C+1/d_E$, where the d's denote the number of events observed on C and E, respectively. Using normal priors for β and γ as above, the same reasoning results in the posterior distribution of the parameters (β, γ) being approximately normal with mean $\eta=(\eta_\beta, \eta_\gamma)$ and covariance matrix $\Sigma=(\lambda_{ij})^{-1}$ with

$$\lambda_{11}=\frac{1}{\sigma^2}+\frac{1}{\sigma_\beta^2}$$

$$\lambda_{22}=\frac{1}{\sigma^2}+\frac{1}{\sigma_\gamma^2}$$

$$\lambda_{12}=-\frac{1}{\sigma^2}$$

and mean vector determined by

$$\Lambda\eta=\begin{pmatrix} \frac{\mu_\beta}{\sigma_\beta^2}-\frac{y}{\sigma^2} \\ \frac{y}{\sigma^2}+\frac{\mu_\gamma}{\sigma_\gamma^2} \end{pmatrix}.$$

If a noninformative prior is used for γ, then $\lambda_{22}=-\lambda_{12}$, and we obtain that the posterior distribution of β is $N(\mu_\beta, \sigma_\beta^2)$, the same as the prior distribution. In this case the posterior distribution of γ is $N(\mu_\beta+y, \sigma_\beta^2+\sigma^2)$. The posterior covariance of β and γ is $-\sigma_\beta^2$. Hence, the posterior probability that the experimental treatment is effective relative to placebo is $\Phi\left(-\frac{\mu_\beta+y}{\sqrt{\sigma_\beta^2+\sigma^2}}\right)$.

3.2. Design

A minimal objective of the active controlled trial is to determine whether or not the E is effective relative to P. Hence, we might require that if $\gamma=\beta$, then it should be very probable that the trial will result in data $\bar{y}-(\bar{y}_E, \bar{y}_C)$ such that $\Pr(\gamma<0|\bar{y}) > 0.95$, where $\gamma<0$ represents effectiveness of the experimental treatment. Thus, we want

$$\Pr\left(\frac{\eta_\gamma}{\sqrt{\Sigma_{33}}}\leq 1.645\right)>\xi \tag{6}$$

where η_γ, Σ_{33} are the posterior mean and variance of γ, the probability is calculated assuming $\gamma=\beta$ and that β is distributed according to its prior distribution, and ξ is some appropriately large value such as .90. In the special case where noninformative prior distributions are adopted for α and γ, this results in

$$\frac{-1.645\sqrt{1+2\sigma^2/\sigma_\beta^2}-\mu_\beta/\sigma_\beta}{\sqrt{2\sigma^2/\sigma_\beta^2}}=z_\xi \tag{7}$$

where z_ξ is the 100ξth percentile of the standard normal distribution. The sample size of the trial may be determined by finding the value of σ^2 that satisfies (7). σ^2 represents the variance of the means $\bar{y}_E$ and $\bar{y}_C$ and hence is inversely proportional to the sample size per treatment arm in the active controlled trial.

It is of interest that μ_β/σ_β is the "z value" for the evaluation of the active control versus placebo. The required sample size for the active control trial is very sensitive to that z value. For example, suppose that $\mu_\beta/\sigma_\beta=3$. This represents substantial evidence that the active control is indeed effective relative to placebo. In this case, for ξ=0.8 one requires that the ratio $r=2\sigma^2/\sigma_\beta^2=0.8$ in order for (7) to be satisfied. Since σ_β^2 is known and since $2\sigma^2$ represents the variance of the difference in mean responses between the treatment arms in the active controlled trial, the sample size per arm can be determined. Alternatively, if there is less substantial evidence for the effectiveness of the active control, for example $\mu_\beta/\sigma_\beta = 2$, then one requires that the ratio $r = 2\sigma^2/\sigma_\beta^2 = 0.10$ in order to satisfy (7). This represents eight times the sample size required for the case when $r = 3$. When the evidence for the effectiveness of the active control is marginal, then the active control design is neither feasible nor appropriate.

For the binary response approximation described previously, we have approximately $\sigma^2 = 1/npq$, where n is the sample size per treatment group in the active control trial. If there is one previous randomized trial of active control versus placebo on which to base the prior distribution of β, then we have approximately that $\sigma_\beta^2 = 2/n_0pq$ where n_0 denotes the average sample size per treatment group in that trial. Consequently, $2\sigma^2/\sigma_0^2 = n_0/n$. If $\mu_\beta/\sigma_\beta = 3$, then $n_0/n = 0.8$; that is, $n = 1.25n_0$, and the sample size required for the active control trial is 25% larger than that required for the trial, demonstrating the effectiveness of the active control. On the other hand, if $\mu_\beta/\sigma_\beta = 2$, then $n_0/n = 0.10$; that is, $n = 10n_0$.

Planning the trial to demonstrate that the new regimen is effective compared to placebo seems a minimal requirement. As indicated above, even establishing that objective may not be feasible unless the data demonstrating the effectiveness of the active control is definitive. One can be more ambitious and plan the trial to ensure with high probability that the results will support the conclusion that the new treatment is at least 100k% as effective as the active control when in fact the new treatment is equivalent to the active control. That is, we would require that $\Pr(\gamma < k\beta|\bar{y}) > 0.95$. In order to achieve this one obtains instead of (7) the requirement

$$\frac{-1.645\sqrt{(1-\mathrm{k})^2 + 2\sigma^2/\sigma_\beta^2} - (1-\mathrm{k})\mu_\beta/\sigma_\beta}{\sqrt{2\sigma^2/\sigma_\beta^2}} = z_\xi. \tag{8}$$

Equations (7) and (8) are quadratic equations in $\sqrt{r}$ and have the solution

$$\begin{aligned} \sqrt{\mathrm{r}} &= \frac{-\mathrm{B}+\sqrt{\mathrm{B}^2-4\mathrm{AC}}}{2\mathrm{A}} \\ \mathrm{A} &= 1.645^2 - \mathrm{z}_\xi^2 \\ \mathrm{B} &= -2\mathrm{z}(1-\mathrm{k})\mathrm{z}_\xi \\ \mathrm{C} &= (1-\mathrm{k})^2(1.645^2 - \mathrm{z}^2). \end{aligned} \tag{9}$$

3.3. Example

The Tamoxifen Prevention Trial evaluated the effectiveness of Tamoxifen for preventing breast cancer in high-risk women (Fisher et al., 1998). Tamoxifen was found to be effective, but also led to side effects, including increasing the risk of endometrial cancer. Consequently, there is interest in the identification of other antiestrogen drugs that are as effective as Tamoxifen for preventing breast cancer but with fewer side effects. The Tamoxifen trial randomized 13,388 women and found 175 invasive breast cancers in those assigned to the placebo group compared to only 89 in the Tamoxifen group. This is a total of 264 events. The investigators reported a risk ratio of 0.51 with an associated 95% confidence interval of 0.39–0.66.

Suppose one were planning an active control trial to evaluate a newer antiestrogen, such as Raloxifene, compared to Tamoxifen. One may use expression (9) to determine the size of the trial needed. Taking the logarithm of the risk ratio as approximately normally distributed, the point estimate and confidence interval reported yield a value of $z=\mu_\beta/\sigma_\beta$ of about 5. Using this value in (9) with $k=0$ and $z_\xi=1.28$ gives a value $r=2.38$. Since the precision of estimation of relative risk is approximately determined by the total number of events observed, this result indicates that the active control trial need only observe 1/(2.38) or 42% as many events as the initial trial in order to establish that the new treatment is effective compared to placebo. In order to establish that the new treatment is 80% as effective as Tamoxifen, when it is equivalent to Tamoxifen, one uses (9) with $k=0.8$ and obtains $r=0.095$. Consequently, the active control trial would have to contain 1/0.095 or 10.5 times as many events as the original trial. In order to establish that the new treatment is more effective than placebo and 50% as effective as Tamoxifen ($k=0.5$) requires $r=0.59$ or 1.695 times as many events as the original trial, or 431 events. The current trial comparing Raloxifene to Tamoxifen for the prevention of primary breast cancer is planned to observe 327 invasive breast cancers at the time of the definitive analysis. The Bayesian analysis described here suggests that this is sufficient to determine whether Raloxifene is effective relative to placebo but not sufficient to determine whether Raloxifene is at least 50% as effective as Tamoxifen.

4. CONCLUSION

In this chapter we have attempted to describe the serious limitations of active control trials and to indicate that the standard methods for planning and analysis of such trials are problematical and potentially misleading.

We have also described a new approach to planning and analysis of active control trials. The new approach is based on the premise that an active control trial is not interpretable unless one provides the quantitative evidence that the control treatment is effective. Active control trials are not practical unless there is very strong evidence for the effectiveness of the control treatment. Superiority trials are strongly preferable to active control trials whenever they are ethically possible.

REFERENCES

Blackwelder, W. (1982). Proving the null hypothesis in clinical trials. Controlled Clinical Trials 3:345–353.

Casagrande, J. T. and Pike, M. C. (1978). An improved formula for calculating sample sizes for comparing two binomial distributions. Biometrics 34:483–486.

Durrleman, S., Simon, R. (1990). Planning and monitoring of equivalence studies. Biometrics 46:329–336.

Fisher, B., Costantino, J. P., Wickerham, L., et al. (1998). Tamoxifen for Prevention of Breast Cancer: Report of the National Surgical Adjuvant Breast and Bowel Project P-1 Study. Journal of the National Cancer Institute 90: 1371–1388.

Fleming, T. (1990). Evaluation of active control trials in AIDS. Journal of Acquired Immune Deficiency Syndromes 3:S82–S87.

Freiman, J. A., Chalmers, T. C., Smith, H., Kuebler, R. R. The importance of beta the type II error and sample size in the design and interpretation of the randomized control trial: survey of 71 "negative" trials. New England Journal of Medicine 299:690–694.

Gould, A. (1991). Another view of active-controlled trials. Controlled Clinical Trials 12:474–485.

Gould, L. (1993). Sample sizes for event rate equivalence trials using prior information. Statistics in Medicine 12:2001–2023.

Makuch, R., Simon, R. (1978). Sample size requirements for evaluating a conservative therapy. Cancer Treatment Reports 62:1037–1040.

Rubenstein, L. V., Gail, M. H., Santner, T. J. (1981). Planning the duration of a comparative clinical trial with loss to follow-up and a period of continued observation. Journal of Chronic Diseases 34:469–479.

Simon, R. (1986). Confidence intervals for reporting results from clinical trials. Annals of Internal Medicine 105:429–435.

Simon, R. (1993). Why confidence intervals are useful tools in clinical therapeutics. Journal of Biopharmaceutical Statistics 3(2):243–248.

Simon, R. (1999). Bayesian design and analysis of active control clinical trials. Biometrics 55:484–487.

4

Adaptive Two-Stage Clinical Trials*

Michael A. Proschan
National Heart, Lung, and Blood Institute, National Institutes of Health, Bethesda, Maryland, U.S.A.

1. INTRODUCTION

A very important part of the planning of any clinical trial is the estimation of sample size and power. It is difficult because these depend not only on the size of the treatment effect one wishes to detect, but also on the values of certain nuisance parameters. For example, in a trial comparing two treatments with respect to a continuous measure like blood pressure change from baseline to end of study using a t test, power depends on both the difference in mean blood pressures between the treatment and control arms (the treatment effect) and the standard deviation (the nuisance parameter). In a trial with a dichotomous outcome such as 30 day mortality, one must specify the difference in event probabilities in the two arms (the treatment effect) and the overall event probability across the two treatments (the nuisance parameter).

Although the treatment effect and nuisance parameter are both critical components of power calculations, they are quite different in that the nuisance parameter must be accurately *estimated*, whereas the treatment effect is usually *assumed*. One usually specifies the minimum clinically

*This chapter was written by Michael Proschan in his private capacity. The views expressed in the chapter do not necessarily represent the views of NIH, DHHS, or the United States.

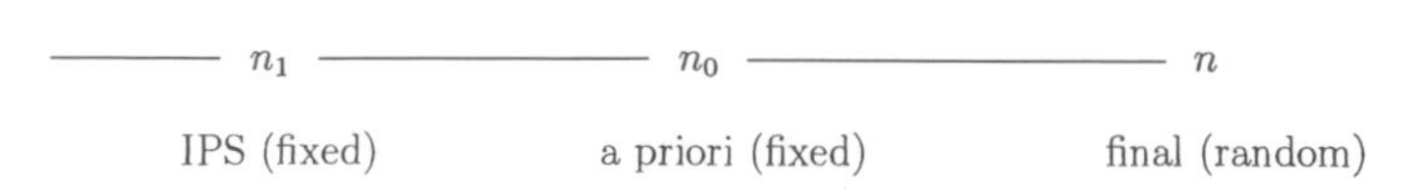

Figure 1 Per-arm sample sizes for two-stage trials.

relevant treatment difference (MCRD). If the actual treatment effect is smaller, then it is not clinically relevant, so the fact that we have low power to detect it is not troubling. It is much more troubling if the treatment effect is as expected, but power is jeopardized because the overall event probability is smaller than expected. One could do a pilot study to estimate the nuisance parameters, and then conduct a clinical trial in a separate, presumably much larger group of patients. A more efficient way is to use an *internal pilot study* (IPS) in which the patients used to estimate the nuisance parameters are also included in the final results of the larger trial.

In early trials of a given disease, an MCRD may not be known, so it must be *estimated* instead of *assumed*. The IPS in such cases is used to estimate both the nuisance parameters and the treatment effect. This is fundamentally different from the more common situation in which only nuisance parameters must be estimated. We will see that nuisance parameter estimates are essentially independent of the treatment effect estimate, so the fact that there was a two-stage design can be ignored when the results are analyzed. Such is not the case when both nuisance parameters and treatment effect are estimated in the IPS. Serious inflation of the type I error rate can occur if the analysis ignores the two-stage nature of the design.

2. REESTIMATION BASED ON A NUISANCE PARAMETER

For both the continuous and dichotomous outcome case, the format will be the same. One starts with an a priori estimate n_0 of the per-arm sample size. An IPS is performed with n_1 patients/arm, $n_1 \le n_0$, and then the final per-arm sample size n is determined. The IPS constitutes the first stage data, while the next $n_2 = n - n_1$ observations/arm make up the second stage data. Figure 1 illustrates the setup.

2.1. Continuous Outcome Case

Consider the continuous outcome setting with common variance σ^2. If we knew the variance, we could compute the sample size required per-arm to detect the MCRD, δ. For $100(1-\beta)\%$ power for a two-tailed test at level α, the required sample size per-arm is approximately

$$\psi(\sigma^2) = \frac{2\sigma^2(z_{\alpha/2} + z_\beta)^2}{\delta^2} \tag{1}$$

where z_α denotes the $100(1-\alpha)$th percentile of a standard normal distribution. In practice, a prior estimate ${\sigma_0}^2$ will have to be used, giving an estimated per-arm sample size of $n_0 = \psi({\sigma_0}^2)$.

We take a preliminary sample of n_1 observations in each arm and compute the pooled variance s_1^2. Based on this estimate, we revise the per-arm sample size from our initial estimate of n_0 to n. We may take $n = \psi(s_1^2)$, or $n = \psi(\sigma_*^2)$, where σ_*^2 is an estimate of the variance combining σ_0^2 and s_1^2. Note that n is a random variable, as is the second stage per-arm sample size, $n_2 = n - n_1$.

The treatment effect estimator using all of the data from the first and second stages is $\hat{\delta} = (n_1\hat{\delta}_1 + n_2\hat{\delta}_2)/n$, where $\hat{\delta}_i$ is the difference in treatment and control sample means for data of stage i, $i = 1,2$. Now ${s_1}^2$ is statistically independent of $\hat{\delta}_1$, so conditioned on $s_1^2, Z = (\hat{\delta} - \delta)/\sqrt{2\sigma^2/n}$ has a standard normal distribution. Because the conditional distribution of Z given s_1^2 is the same for all s_1^2, Z and s_1^2 are independent in this adaptive sample size setting, with Z having a standard normal distribution and s_1^2/σ^2 having the distribution of a chi-squared random variable divided by its degrees of freedom, $n_1 - 1$. It follows that under the null hypothesis, $T = Z/\sqrt{s_1^2/\sigma^2} = \hat{\delta}/\sqrt{2s_1^2/n}$ has a t distribution with $2(n_1 - 1)$ degrees of freedom. In other words, if we use the pooled variance from the IPS only, an exact p value may be obtained by referring T to a t distribution with $2(n_1 - 1)$ degrees of freedom. This result is due to Stein (1945).

Stein's procedure is not commonly used in clinical trials for at least two reasons. One is its perceived inefficiency in estimating the variance using only $2n_1$ of $2n$ observations. Another is that σ^2 may increase over time because of changes in the patient population, for example. Using only the first $2n_1$ patients could underestimate the true variability and increase the chance of a type I error. It is therefore more natural to use s^2, the pooled variance estimate based on all $2n$ observations. Unfortunately, the distribution of s^2 is not the same as if n had been fixed in advance. In fact, s^2 systematically underestimates σ^2. Wittes et al. (1999) have shown that $E(s^2) = \sigma^2 + (n_1 - 1)\operatorname{cov}\{s_1^2, 1/(n-1)\}$; the covariance term is negative because s_1^2 is an increasing function of ${s_1}^2$ and $1/(n-1)$ is a decreasing function of s_1^2. Still, the bias is so small that the type I error rate of this approximate t test is very close to α if the size of the internal pilot study is 20 or more (Wittes and Brittain, 1990; Birkett and Day, 1994; Wittes et al., 1999).

Those who worry about even small amounts of α inflation but want to use a better estimate of variance than Stein's can do so with a *restricted test*, whereby the final per-arm sample size is restricted to be at least as large as the originally planned n_0. Proschan and Wittes (2000) point out that instead of using the pooled variance from the IPS, one could augment each arm of the IPS with the first $n_0 - n_1$ observations from the corresponding arm in the second stage. The resulting test statistic has a null t distribution with $2(n_0 - 1)$ degrees of freedom instead of $2(n_1 - 1)$ degrees of freedom for Stein's procedure. This clear improvement is still unsatisfying because use of the first $n_0 - n_1$ observations per arm from the second stage is arbitrary; any set of $n_0 - n_1$ second stage observations could be used. Why not average over all possible augmentations of the IPS with $2(n_0 - n_1)$ observations from stage 2? Proschan and Wittes (2000) propose something very close to this. Their variance estimate reduces to $\hat{\sigma}^2 = \lambda s_1^2 + (1 - \lambda)\tilde{\sigma}^2$, where $\tilde{\sigma}^2 = \{(n-1)s^2 - (n_1 - 1)s_1^2\}/(n - n_1)$ and $\lambda = (n_1 - 1)/(n_0 - 1)$. They prove that referring $\hat{\delta}/\sqrt{2\hat{\sigma}^2/n}$ to a t distribution with $2(n_0 - 1)$ degrees of freedom has a type I error rate no greater than α.

2.2. Example: DASH

We illustrate these methods with the Dietary Approaches to Stop Hypertension Study (DASH). Three dietary patterns were compared with respect to change in diastolic blood pressure (DBP) from baseline to the end of 8 weeks of intervention in participants with blood pressures ranging from high normal to stage 1 hypertension ($80 \leq \text{DBP} \leq 95$). The control diet was similar to what many Americans eat; one of the active diets was rich in fruits and vegetables, while the other was rich in fruits and vegetables and low-fat dairy products. Adjustments were made for the two comparisons with control. Thus, to be significant, the approximate z statistic comparing an active diet to the control had to exceed 2.24, the critical value for a 2-tailed test at level .025. The standard deviation of DBP change was estimated to be about 5 mmHg, while the minimum treatment effect thought to have strong public health importance was $\delta = 2$ mmHg. For 85% power for a control comparison, approximately $n_0 = 2(2.24 + 1.04)^2(5)^2/2^2 = 135$ evaluable participants per arm were needed. Further details of the design of DASH may be found in Sacks et al. (1995).

At some point in the trial the issue was raised that the standard deviation may have been overestimated because it did not take into account the fact that a "funnel" was used prior to enrollment to eliminate participants whose blood pressures were too large or too small. Simulation results suggested that taking this funnel into account might decrease the standard deviation from 5 to 4.5. This would allow almost a 20% reduction in sample size to achieve the same power.

As it turned out, the standard deviation at an interim look was quite close to 5, so no changes were made in the sample size. For the sake of illustration, suppose hypothetically that after 68 observations in an active diet and 68 in the control diet, the variance pooled across these two diets were $s_1^2 = 4.5^2 = 20.25$, as hoped. The sample size could have been reduced to $n = 2(2.24 + 1.04)^2(4.5)^2/2^2 = 109$ evaluable participants per arm. At the end of the study, the ordinary t statistic could be used with $2(109 - 1) = 216$ degrees of freedom for the comparisons with control. If one wanted to be conservative and avoid even the slightest α inflation, one could use Stein's procedure. For example, if after 109 observations per arm the difference between the control and combination diet means were $\hat{\delta} = 2.1$, the t statistic would be $2.1/\sqrt{2(4.5)^2/109} = 3.45$, even if the pooled variance of all of the observations were $s^2 = 4.8^2 = 23.04$, for example. The Proschan–Wittes method cannot be used in this example because the goal was to see if the sample size could be reduced, and hence it was not a restricted design.

2.3. The Dichotomous Outcome Case

Suppose that the primary outcome of a clinical trial is the presence or absence of a short-term event such as 30-day mortality. Let p_C and p_T be the probabilities of experiencing such an event for patients in the control and treatment arms, respectively. Then $\delta = p_C - p_T$ is the treatment difference, and $\bar{p} = (p_C + p_T)/2$ is the average event probability over the two arms. Sample size per arm to achieve power $100(1 - \beta)$ for a two-tailed test at level α is given approximately by

$$n = \frac{[z_{\alpha/2}\sqrt{2\bar{p}(1-\bar{p})} + z_\beta\sqrt{p_C(1-p_C) + p_T(1-p_T)}]^2}{(p_C - p_T)^2}. \tag{2}$$

Here the nuisance parameter is $\bar{p}$, estimated by $\hat{p}_1$, the overall event proportion among the $2n_1$ observations in the IPS. Note that $\hat{p}_1$ is uncorrelated with $\hat{\delta}_1$, the difference in event proportions between the control and treatment arms in the IPS. If $2n_1$ is moderately large, then $\hat{p}_1$ and $\hat{\delta}_1$ are approximately bivariate normally distributed. If they were exactly bivariate normal, their lack of correlation would imply statistical independence. Thus, as in the continuous outcome case, the nuisance parameter estimate is approximately independent of the treatment effect estimator. Again it seems reasonable to treat the per-arm sample size n as if it had been fixed in advance and use an ordinary test of proportions on the $2n$ observations at the end of the study. Several authors have shown that the effect on the type I error rate of treating the final sample size as fixed is minimal. See, for example, Gould (1992) or Herson and Wittes (1993).

As with the continuous outcome case, there is a way to obtain an exact α level procedure for those who do not want even a slight inflation of the type I error rate. Instead of implementing the usual z test of proportions, one can condition on the total numbers of events at the first and second stages using, for example, the Mantel-Haenzel test. The p value is also conditional on these numbers of events, so the fact that the second stage sample size was driven by the first stage results becomes irrelevant.

2.4. DASH Example Embellished

Consider the DASH clinical trial described previously. Suppose that instead of treating the change in DBP as a continuous outcome, the DASH investigators had compared the proportions of patients in each arm whose DBP decreased by 3 mmHg or more. Call these patients "responders." Further assume that the investigators were interested in detecting a doubling of the proportion of responders in an active diet relative to control. Suppose, hypothetically, that from the first 100 participants evaluated in the control and 100 in an active arm, 60 responded. Then $\bar{p} = 60/200 = .30$. Treat this as a population parameter and set $(p_C + p_T)/2 = .30, p_T = 2p_C$. This yields $p_C = .20, p_T = .40$. Substituting into (2) and using 85% power and the adjusted two-tailed alpha level of .025 ($z_{\alpha/2} = 2.24$) yields 112 participants per arm. Thus, only 12 more participants would be needed in each arm.

Suppose that the results were as shown in Table 1. Overall, $\hat{p}_C = 30/112 = .268$ and $\hat{p}_T = 41/112 = .366$. The ordinary test of proportions on the entire data yields a p value of .11. This analysis treats the sample size

Table 1 Hypothetical Results for the First 100 Participants/Arm (1st 2×2 Table), the Next 12 Participants/Arm (2nd 2×2 Table), and the Total of 112/Arm (Last 2×2 Table) in the Embellishment of the DASH Example Considering Responders (R) and Nonresponders (NR)

	R	NR	R	NR	R	NR
C	25	75	5	7	30	82
T	35	65	6	6	41	71

of 128 per arm as if it had been fixed in advance. As stated above, this is highly accurate, producing only very slight α inflation. We could avoid any inflation by conditioning on the total numbers of events at stages 1 and 2. For example, the two-tailed p value using the exact distribution of the Mantel-Haenzel statistic is .15.

3. SAMPLE SIZE REESTIMATION BASED ON TREATMENT EFFECT

As mentioned earlier, it is highly desirable to base sample size on the minimal clinically relevant treatment difference, but this is not always possible. For example, in heart disease trials using an angiographic endpoint such as the average change in minimum lumen diameter over many different segments of a coronary artery, it is not clear what size treatment difference would result in clinical benefit. In these cases one may wish to use the IPS to estimate both the nuisance parameter and the treatment effect. This is different from the nuisance parameter situation in that it is inherently a one-tailed testing situation; one would not be interested in determining the number of additional observations to prove the treatment harmful. Thus, one-tailed testing is assumed in this section. In practice one might use one-tailed $\alpha = .025$ instead of .05.

Unlike the earlier scenarios in which only the nuisance parameters had to be estimated, the treatment effect at the end of the study is highly correlated with the parameters estimated at the first stage. Thus, the random per-arm sample size n contains very relevant information about the size of the treatment effect; acting as though it were fixed in advance can lead to serious inflation of the type I error rate. Proschan and Hunsberger (1995) show that depending on how one chooses the second stage sample size, the actual type I error rate can be as high as $\alpha + \exp(-z_\alpha^2/2)/4$. Thus, for a .025 (.05) level one-tailed test, the actual type I error rate can be as great as .06 (.11).

One can avoid inflation of the type I error rate by using a larger critical value at the end of the study. For example, suppose one takes $n_2(z_1)$ additional observations per-arm based on the IPS z score z_1, but then uses critical value $c = c(z_1, n_2)$. The actual type I error rate is

$$\int_{-\infty}^{\infty} CP_0(n_2, c|z_1)\phi(z_1)dz_1 \qquad (3)$$

where ϕ is the standard normal density function and $CP_0\,(n_2, c|z_1)$ denotes the conditional probability, computed under the null hypothesis, that the z

score using all $2(n_1 + n_2)$ observations will exceed c, given z_1. Now suppose that prior to the study we had selected a rule $A(z_1)$ dictating how much conditional type I error rate to use, given z_1, such that

$$\int A(z_1)\phi(z_1)\,dz_1 = \alpha. \tag{4}$$

$A(z_1)$ is called a *conditional error (CE) function*. Further suppose that regardless of the additional number of observations per arm, n_2, we could find a critical value $c = c(z_1, n_2)$ to make $CP_0(n_2, c|z_1) = A(z_1)$. Then by (3) and (4), the procedure would have level α.

Proschan and Hunsberger (1995) have shown that it is always possible to find such a c:

$$c = \frac{\sqrt{n_1}z_1 + \sqrt{n_2}z_A}{\sqrt{n_1 + n_2}} \tag{5}$$

where z_A is short-hand notation for $\Phi^{-1}\{1 - A(z_1)\}$. One may then select n_2 such that $CP_\delta(n_2, c)$, computed under the alternative hypothesis of treatment effect δ, reaches a desired level $1 - \beta$:

$$n_2 = \frac{2(z_A + z_\beta)^2}{\delta^2}. \tag{6}$$

The formula for n_2 is easy to interpret when one recognizes that the conditional error function approach is mathematically equivalent to the following procedure: Having observed z_1, take n_2 additional observations per arm and perform a z test on only the second stage data, rejecting the null hypothesis if that z score exceeds the critical value corresponding to significance level $A(z_1)$. The sample size formula (6) yielding conditional power $1 - \beta$ is the sample size corresponding to unconditional power $1 - \beta$ in a z test applied only to the second stage data.

Similarly, for any given value n_2, the conditional power assuming that the true treatment effect is δ is the same as the unconditional power in a trial at level $A(z_1)$ with n_2 observations per arm:

$$CP = 1 - \Phi\left(z_A - \sqrt{n_2/2}\;\delta/\sigma\right). \tag{7}$$

As any conditional error function $A(z_1)$ may be used, the procedure is very general. In fact, as Proschan (2000) points out, CE functions and two-stage tests are really synonymous; associated with any two-stage test statistic T is a CE function $A(z_1) = \Pr(T \text{ is significant} \mid Z_1 = z_1)$. Thus, it might be easier to consider good two-stage tests and see what CE functions they induce rather than directly trying to find good CE functions. Once we determine the induced CE function, we can use (7) to choose a second-stage sample size yielding the desired conditional power.

How do we choose a reasonable two-stage test? If the second stage sample size were fixed in advance, things would be very easy; we would be testing whether the mean of (Z_1, Z_2) was $(0, 0)$ against a specific alternative proportional to $(\sqrt{n_1}, \sqrt{n_2})$. The problem is that we do not know n_2 a priori, so we do not know the alternative direction. We only know that, because $n_2 \geq 0$, the alternative lies somewhere in the positive quadrant $Q^+ = \{(z_1, z_2): z_1 \geq 0, z_2 \geq 0\}$. Tests powerful against the positive quadrant alternative are therefore appealing.

One such test is due to O'Brien (1984). The null hypothesis is rejected if $(z_1 + z_2)/\sqrt{2} > z_\alpha$. This is the optimal test statistic for the fixed sample size setting with $n_2 = n_1$, but it can be used even if one changes n_2 after seeing z_1.

To find the induced CE function, note that the amount of conditional type I error rate one uses after seeing $Z_1 = z_1$ is

$$A(z_1) = \Pr(Z_1 + Z_2 > \sqrt{2}\, z_\alpha | Z_1 = z_1) = 1 - \Phi(\sqrt{2}\, z_\alpha - z_1). \qquad (8)$$

This is a member of what Proschan and Hunsberger (1995) called the linear class of CE functions, even though it is $z_A = \sqrt{2} z_\alpha - z_1$ that is linear in z_1. The induced CE function is used, in part, to reexpress the rejection region via (5) in terms of $(\sqrt{n_1} z_1 + \sqrt{n_2} z_2)/\sqrt{n}$, the usual z score on all $2(n_1 + n_2)$ observations. Investigators would naturally want to compare the two-stage test to the more familar one-stage test with the same number of observations; they would feel legitimately uneasy if a two-stage procedure rejected the null hypothesis while the one-stage procedure did not.

The above procedure is a no-cost extension of the fixed sample size test; if one decides to use the originally planned second stage sample size, the test is equivalent to rejecting the null hypothesis when the usual fixed-sample z statistic exceeds z_α. The advantage is that at the first stage one could choose to change the second stage sample size.

One would probably not continue to the second stage if $z_1 < 0$. Furthermore, it makes no sense to reject at the end of the second stage if $z_2 < 0$; if the evidence was not convincing at stage 1, how could it be more convincing having observed a negative trend since stage 1? Thus, it is a good idea to modify the above procedure. One stops at stage 1 without rejection of H_0 if $z_1 < 0$, and with rejection if $z_1 > k$, where $k = 2.79$ for $\alpha = .025$ and $k = 2.36$ for $\alpha = .05$. If $0 \le z_1 \le k$, one proceeds to stage 2 and rejects if $z_1 + z_2 > k$. The "linear" CE function is shown as the solid line in Figure 2 for $\alpha = .025$.

Another test that could be used is the likelihood ratio test for the positive quadrant alternative. One rejects the null hypothesis if $z_1 \ge k$ or $z_2 \ge k$ or $\sqrt{z_1^2 + z_2^2} > k$ and $(z_1, z_2) \in Q^+$. Eliminating $z_1 < 0$ and modifying k to maintain an α-level procedure yields the rejection region $z_1 \ge k$ or $0 \le z_1 \le k$ and $z_2 > \sqrt{k^2 - z_1^2}$. What is the induced CE function? For $z_1 < 0$ there is no chance of rejecting the null hypothesis, while for $z_1 > k$ there is probability 1 of rejecting the null hypothesis. For z_1 in the continuation region $[0, k]$, the null probability of rejecting H_0 is $\Pr(Z_2 > \sqrt{k^2 - z_1^2}) = 1 - \Phi(\sqrt{k^2 - z_1^2})$. Thus, the induced conditional error function is

$$A_{\text{cir}}(z_1) = \begin{cases} 0 & \text{if } z_1 \le 0 \\ 1 - \Phi\left(\sqrt{k^2 - z_1^2}\right) & \text{if } 0 < z_1 \le k \\ 1 & \text{if } z_1 > k. \end{cases} \tag{9}$$

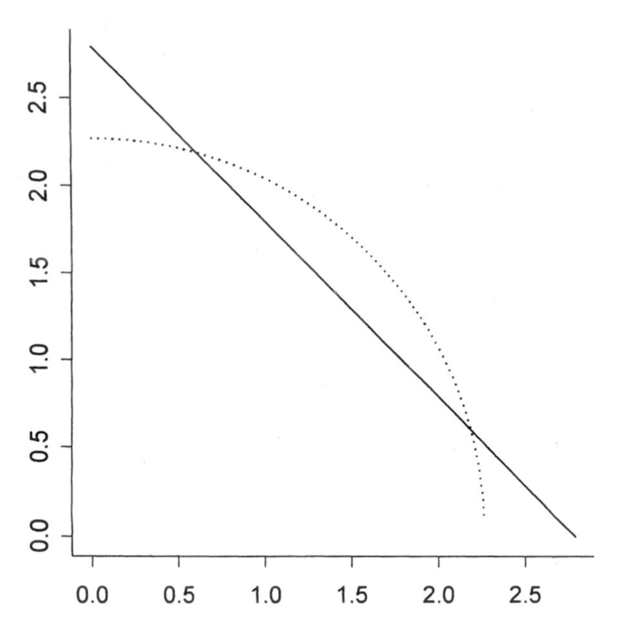

Figure 2 Linear and circular conditional error functions for $\alpha = .025$.

Table 2 Values of k for Different Values of the Overall Significance Level α and the First Stage Futility Level α_0 for the Circular CE Function Approach

	α_0								
α	.10	.15	.20	.25	.30	.35	.40	.45	.50
.025	2.13	2.17	2.19	2.21	2.22	2.23	2.25	2.26	2.27
.050	1.77	1.82	1.85	1.88	1.89	1.91	1.93	1.94	1.95

For a one-tailed alpha of .025(.05) $k = 2.27$ (1.95). Proschan and Hunsberger (1995) called $A_{\text{cir}}(z_1)$ a "circular" CE function because over the continuation region $[0, k]$ z_A is the equation of a circle centered at the origin with radius k. The dotted curve in Figure 2 shows the circular CE function. Again it is convenient to express the rejection region in terms of the usual z score for $2(n_1 + n_2)$ observations using (5).

The circular CE function procedure stops for futility if $z_1 < 0$, but it can be modified to stop for futility for other values of z_1. It is easier to interpret if we rephrase this as follows. We stop for futility when the first-stage p value, p_1, exceeds some number α_0; $\alpha_0 = .5$ corresponds to the $z_1 < 0$ case already considered. For smaller values of α_0, the value of k required for an α-level procedure decreases. Table 2 gives the value of k for different values of α and α_0.

If one proceeds to the second stage, the critical value for z is given by (5). The circular CE function has the property that the critical value at the second stage is no greater than k, the critical value at stage 1. Furthermore, among all two-stage tests with the same continuation region as the circular CE function, the circular CE function is the only one that can guarantee this for all possible values of n_2 (see Proschan, 2003).

3.1. Example

Suppose that a clinical trial in patients with coronary heart disease compares a cholesterol reducing drug to placebo with respect to angiographic changes from baseline to end of study. Specifically, coronary arteries are first divided into segments; for each segment the difference in minimum lumen diameter from baseline to end of study is computed, and the average difference over all segments of a patient is the outcome measure. It is not known what constitutes a clinically relevant change, but another similar study showed an effect size of about one third of a standard deviation. The sample size required for 90% power to detect a similar effect size is about 190 patients per arm, or 380 total. After 95 are evaluated in each arm, we compute the estimated effect size, namely the difference in sample means divided by the square root of the pooled estimate of variance. Which method we use must be specified in advance.

If we use the circular conditional error function approach, we stop the trial and declare a significant treatment effect at the first stage if $z_1 > 2.27$. We stop for lack of treatment effect if $z_1 < 0$. If $0 \le z_1 \le 2.27$, we proceed to the second stage. Suppose that the first-stage z score were 1.5. This corresponds to an estimated effect size of about .218 standard deviations instead of the originally anticipated one third of a standard deviation. The value of the conditional error function is $A(1.5) = 1 - \Phi(\sqrt{2.27^2 - 1.5^2})$, so $z_A = \sqrt{2.27^2 - 1.5^2} = 1.704$. To have 80% conditional power under the empirically estimated treatment effect, we use Eq. (6): $n_2 = 2(1.704 + .84)^2/.218^2 = 273$. Thus, we would need 273 more patients per-arm, making the total sample size $2(95 + 273) = 736$. Given that the originally projected sample size was 380, such a large increase may be prohibitive. Instead one might prefer to see the conditional power for different total sample sizes using equation (7). If we stick with the originally planned sample size of 190 per arm, so $n_2 = 190 - 95 = 95$, conditional power under the empirical estimate will be $1 - \Phi\{1.704 - \sqrt{95/2}(.218)\} = .42$. Increasing the sample size to 250 per arm (a second stage sample size of 155 per arm) increases the conditional power to about .59. These calculations are all under the empirical estimate of treatment effect. After the first stage, we might want to compute power under an alternative that is not as optimistic as what was originally hypothesized, but not as pessimistic as what has been observed so far. For example, we might prefer to use an effect size of one fourth of a standard deviation. At any rate, suppose we decided to take 200 more per arm. If the z score for the second half of the data were 1.9, then $z_1^2 + z_2^2 = 1.5^2 + 1.9^2 = 5.86$ exceeds $2.27^2 = 5.15$, so the null hypothesis would be rejected. Results would probably be reported in the following equivalent way. The full-data z score is $(95 + 200)^{-1/2}\{\sqrt{95}(1.5) + \sqrt{200}(1.9)\} = 2.42$. The critical value (5) is $(95 + 200)^{-1/2}\{\sqrt{95}(1.5) + \sqrt{200}(1.704)\} = 2.25$; therefore the null hypothesis is rejected.

Bauer and Köhne (1994) considered a much more general setting in which the first-stage data was used not only to modify sample size, but to make more drastic alterations such as changing the test statistic. Their method is based on Fisher's product of independent p values. Recall that p values are uniformly distributed under the null hypothesis for any test statistic with a continuous distribution function. If p_1 and p_2 are independent p values, then $-2\ \ln(p_1 p_2)$ has a chi-squared distribution with 4 degrees of freedom under the null hypothesis. The null hypothesis is rejected if $T = p_1 p_2 < c_\alpha = \exp\{-\chi^2_{4,\alpha}/2\}$, where $\chi^2_{4,\alpha}$ is the upper α point of a chi-squared distribution with 4 degrees of freedom; $c_\alpha = .004$ or .009 for $\alpha = .025$ or $\alpha = .05$, respectively.

Fisher's test can be applied to first- and second-stage p values even if the second-stage sample size n_2 depends on p_1. The reason is that p_1 is uniformly distributed, and for given p_1, n_2 becomes fixed and p_2 is uniformly distributed. Because p_2 has the same (uniform) conditional distribution for any given value of p_1, p_1 and p_2 are independent uniforms, and Fisher's product of p values test is valid. Bauer and Köhne imply that their procedure can be used even if one changes the test statistic after seeing the first stage data, but some care is needed (Liu, Proschan, and Pledger, 2002).

Note that if $p_1 < c_\alpha$, there is no point in continuing the study since $p_1 p_2$ is assured of being less than c_α. Bauer and Köhne also consider a variant in which one stops at the first stage without rejecting the null hypothesis if $p_1 > \alpha_0$. By allowing the possibility of stopping early for futility, one can decrease the level of evidence required to declare statistical significance at stage 1. Table 3 shows α_1, the p value required to declare significance at stage 1 as a function of α and α_0. For example, for $\alpha = .025$ and $\alpha_0 = .5$, $\alpha_1 = .010$. Thus the continuation region is $.010 \leq p_1 \leq .5$, which corresponds to $0 \leq z_1 \leq 2.32$.

Note the similarity between the Bauer-Köhne continuation region and that of the circular CE function with $\alpha_0 = .5$. Wassmer (1998) showed that the power functions were also quite close. This is because of the similarity of the induced CE functions. An advantage of the Bauer-Köhne procedure is that it is exact. One need not make the assumption that the sample size is large enough to estimate the variance accurately.

Table 3 Values of α_1, the Required p-Value to Declare Significance at Stage 1 for the Bauer-Köhne Procedure That Stops for Futility at Stage 1 if $p_1 > \alpha_0$. (If $\alpha_1 \leq p_1 \leq \alpha_0$, One Proceeds to Stage 2 and Rejects the Null Hypothesis if $p_1 p_2 < c_\alpha$.)

		α_0								
α	c_α	.10	.15	.20	.25	.30	.35	.40	.45	.50
.025	.004	.019	.017	.015	.014	.013	.012	.012	.011	.010
.050	.009	.043	.038	.035	.032	.030	.028	.026	.025	.023

4. CONCLUSIONS

Clinical trials must be large enough to have reasonable power to detect treatment differences. Unfortunately, the information needed to determine the sample size is not always available or accurate; other studies upon which estimates are based may not be sufficiently similar to the one being planned. It therefore becomes appealing to use part of the current trial data to estimate the parameters needed to determine sample size. Often this involves estimation of only nuisance parameters, because one can usually specify a minimum clinically relevant treatment difference. When only nuisance parameters are estimated during the IPS, one can essentially ignore the two-stage nature of the design when it is time to analyze the results. This is true for both continuous and dichotomous outcomes.

In some cases the IPS is used to estimate treatment effects as well. Much more caution is required. The two-stage nature of the design must be taken into account when results are analyzed. Adaptive sample size estimation based on treatment effect is usually one-tailed; one would not want to increase the sample size to show harm. Under an alternative hypothesis, the mean of (Z_1, Z_2) lies somewhere in the positive quadrant, so tests of the positive quadrant alternative are attractive. Two such tests are O'Brien's and the likelihood ratio test (LRT). The properties of these and other tests depend on their induced conditional error functions. The O'Brien and LRT tests induce the linear and circular CE functions, respectively. An advantage of the linear CE function is that if one maintains the originally planned sample size, the test reduces to the usual fixed sample size test. An advantage of the circular CE function is that the critical value at the end of the study can be no greater than that of the first stage. Conditional power and sample size to achieve a given conditional power may be obtained using the formulas for fixed sample size trials conducted at level $A(z_1)$ instead of α.

REFERENCES

Bauer, P., Köhne, K. (1994). Evaluation of experiments with adaptive interim analyses. Biometrics 50:1029–1041.

Birkett, M. A., Day, S. J. (1994). Internal pilot studies for estimating sample size. Statistics in Medicine 13:2455–2463.

Gould, A. (1992). Interim analyses for monitoring clinical trials that do not materially affect the type I error rate. Statistics in Medicine 11:55–66.

Herson, J., Wittes, J. (1993). The use of interim analysis for sample size adjustment. Drug Information Journal 27:753–760.

Liu, Q. Proschan, M. A., Pledger, G. W. (2002). A unified theory of two-stage adaptive designs. Journal of the American Statistical Association 97:1034–1041.

O'Brien, P. C. (1984). Procedures for comparing samples with multiple endpoints. Biometrics 40:1079–1087.

Proschan, M. A. (2003). The geometry of two-stage tests. Statistica Sinica 13:163–177.

Proschan, M. A., Wittes, J. (1999). An improved double sampling procedure based on the variance. Biometrics 56:1183–1187.

Sacks, F. M., Obarzanek, E., Windhauser, M. M., Svetkey, L. P., Vollmer, W. M., McCullough, M., Karanja, N., Lin, P., Steele, P., Proschan, M. A., Evans, M. A., Appel, L. J., Bray, G. A., Vogt, T. M., Moore, T. J., for the DASH Investigators. (1995). Rationale and design of the Dietary Approaches to Stop Hypertension (DASH) trial. Annals of Epidemiology 5:108–118.

Stein, C. (1945). A two-sample test for a linear hypothesis whose power is independent of the variance. Annals of Mathematical Statistics 16:243–258.

Wassmer, G. (1998). A comparison of two methods for adaptive interim analyses in clinical trials. Biometrics 54:696–705.

Wittes, J., Brittain, E. (1990). The role of internal pilot studies in increasing the efficiency of clinical trials. Statistics in Medicine 9:65–72.

Wittes, J., Schabenberger, O., Zucker, D., Brittain, E., Proschan, M. (1999). Internal pilot studies I: Type I error rate of the naive t-test. Statistics in Medicine 18:3481–3491.

5

Design and Analysis of Cluster Randomization Trials

David M. Zucker
Hebrew University, Jerusalem, Israel

1. INTRODUCTION

In the great majority of clinical trials, randomization is performed at the level of the individual subject. In certain trials, however, the appropriate unit of randomization is some aggregate of individuals. This form of randomization is known as cluster randomization or group randomization. Cluster randomization is employed by necessity in trials in which the intervention is by nature designed to be applied at the cluster level. Examples of this type of trial include trials of community-based interventions, such as the Community Health Trial for Smoking Cessation (COMMIT) (Gail et al., 1992; COMMIT Research Group, 1995), and trials of school-based interventions, such as the Child and Adolescent Trial for Cardiovascular Health (CATCH) (Zucker et al., 1995; Luepker et al., 1996). Cluster randomization is also sometimes employed for convenience of trial administration in trials in which the intervention is applied at the level of the individual. An example of this situation is the trial design in which clinics are assigned to the various experimental arms, with all patients in a given clinic receiving the treatment to which the clinic was assigned (Simon, 1981).

The cluster randomization design poses special issues in the areas of design, logistics, sample size calculation, and statistical analysis. This point was raised in the epidemiological literature by Cornfield (1978), and has received increasing attention since then. The purpose of this chapter is to review these special issues. Comprehensive discussion of cluster randomization trials is provided in the recent monographs of Murray (1998) and Donner and Klar (2000). In this chapter, emphasis is placed on the following aspects: (1) the rationale for taking the cluster as the unit of analysis: (2) statistical handling of individuals who drop out of the trial: (3) analytical methods that are both statistically efficient and statistically rigorous, in the sense of scrupulously protecting the type 1 error level: (4) sample size calculation for cluster randomized trials, taking into account intracluster correlation.

2. GENERAL DESIGN CONSIDERATIONS

2.1. Unit of Randomization and Analysis

Randomization of experimental units is designed to provide three key benefits: (1) avoidance of investigator bias in the allocation process, (2) experimental arms that are appropriately balanced with respect to both known and unknown factors that may affect response, and (3) a basis for analyzing the study results without statistical modeling assumptions. The analytical benefit arises because the randomization itself provides the statistical structure whereby the study results may be judged in principle through the use of a randomization test, though in common practice through the use of a normal-theory test that approximates the randomization test (Fisher, 1935; Kempthorne, 1952).

To preserve the analytical benefit, the statistical analysis must follow the form of randomization. In a cluster randomization trial, it is particularly important to "analyze as you randomize." Under cluster randomization, the mean response in each experimental arm is subject to two sources of variation: variation from cluster to cluster and variation across individuals within a cluster. Donner et al. (1981) have described the increased variance of the sample mean in each experimental arm that results from between-cluster variation in terms of a variance inflation factor (IF) involving the intraclass correlation coefficient (ICC): if the clusters are all of the same size n, then $\text{IF} = 1 + (n - 1)\,\text{ICC}$. An analysis in which the unit of analysis is the individual rather than the cluster fails to account properly for the between-cluster variation and therefore is liable to produce misleading results. In effect, the treatment effects become confounded with the natural cluster-to-cluster variability, and serious inflation in the Type I error level may result (Zucker, 1990; Glass and Stanley, 1970). To avoid this error, the unit of analysis must be the cluster.

To provide statistically rigorous results, a cluster randomization trial must include an adequate number of clusters. Many cluster randomization studies are conducted with a very small number of clusters per arm, such as two or four. Such studies cannot yield statistically definitive conclusions about treatment benefit because it is impossible for a randomization-based analysis of such a trial to yield a statistically significant result. Application of a normal-theory procedure such as ANOVA to such data rests on bald assumptions with no clear justication: for a trial of this small size, the usual central limit theorem argument supporting a normal-theory analysis as an approximation to a randomization-based analysis does not apply. A trial of such small size often will be a very useful means of assessing the feasibility of implementing the intervention and obtaining preliminary indications of the likelihood that the intervention will succeed, but such a trial cannot provide a definitive basis for evaluating the benefit of the intervention. By contrast, studies such as the CATCH trial (Zucker et al., 1995, Luepker et al., 1996), involving 96 schools, the COMMIT trial (Gail et al., 1992; COMMIT Research Group, 1995), involving 11 matched pairs of communities, and the Jerusalem Study of Hygiene Education in Kindergartens (Rosen, 2003), involving 40 kindergartens, include an adequate number of units to permit a meaningful statistical analysis. In COMMIT, in view of the relatively small number of units, the intervention effect was assessed using a randomization-based permutation test rather than a normal-theory test.

Some authors, for example Hopkins (1982), suggest that one may perform a statistical test for between-cluster variation, and that if the test result is not statistically significant one may take the unit of analysis to be the individual. This procedure is problematic for at least two reasons. Firstly, the test for between-cluster variation tends to have very low power when the number of clusters is small. As a result, even under the classical nested ANOVA assumptions, the procedure has inflated Type I error (Bozivich et al., 1956; Hines, 1996). Secondly, the procedure relies on the classical nested ANOVA assumptions that between-cluster and within-cluster effects are all normally distributed and the within-cluster dependence can be completely described by an additive cluster effect. In general, especially for trials with a small number of clusters, there is no definite basis for these assumptions. Thus, it is preferable to keep the cluster as the unit of analysis in all cases.

2.2. Sampling Methodology and Handling of Participant Migration

A further statistical issue in the analysis of long-term school-based or community-based trials is of how to identify individuals from the school or community for measurement and statistical analysis. This issue involves into two aspects: (1) determining how to sample individuals for measurement and (2) defining the primary study population for statistical analysis purposes.

There are two main approaches to sampling individuals for measurement. In the cohort approach, a sample of the individuals initially entered into the study (possibly all such individuals) is selected to be measured throughout the duration of the study. In the cross-sectional approach, separate samples of individuals are taken at each measurement time point. Hybrid schemes combining these two sampling approaches also may be considered.

The main advantage of the cohort approach is that within-individual correlation can be exploited to enhance precision. A major advantage of the cross-sectional approach is that the measurement load is more evenly distributed across individuals. This feature of the cross-sectional design can be an important one from a logistic standpoint when the design calls for multiple repeated measurements, and is particularly beneficial in situations where there is serious concern that the act of measurement itself can influence participants' subsequent behavior. When every individual in a pre-defined study population is to be measured, the cohort and cross-sectional approaches obviously coincide.

The main issue in defining the primary study population for the purpose of analysis is how to handle outmigrating and inmigrating individuals. This issue is closely related to the issue of how to handle patients in a classical clinical trial with individual-level randomization who switch from the assigned intervention to another therapy during the course of the trial, i.e., dropouts and dropins. In the clinical trials field, there is a generally well-accepted "intention to treat" principle that states that patients should be handled in the analysis according to their original assignment, regardless of the therapy subsequently received (Friedman et al., 1996; Pocock, 1983). In school-based or community-based intervention research, the following represent three possible options for defining the primary study population:

1. Include individuals who were in the school or community and measured at the beginning of the trial regardless of what

happened afterwards, with suitable tracking of outmigrating individuals.
2. Include individuals who were in the school or community at both the beginning of the trial and at the measurement point in question.
3. Include individuals who happen to be present in the school or community at the specific measurement time in question.

The first approach is analogous to the intention to treat approach in clinical trials. The other two approaches represent two different forms of "on-treatment" analysis. The advantages and disadvantages of the intent to treat approach as compared with the on-treatment approaches are similar to those in the classical individual-level randomization clinical trial. The main point calling for special mention is that bias can arise not only as the result of an entire cluster being eliminated from analysis, but also as the result of certain individuals within the various clusters being eliminated from or added to the analysis. Such a bias threat exists because the behavior leading to inclusion or exclusion from analysis, e.g., migration, may be influenced by the intervention. The bias threat posed by migration is analogous to the well-recognized bias threat posed by missing data in sample surveys (see Cochran, 1977).

An extended discussion of the migration issue is given in the CATCH statistical design paper (Zucker et al., 1995). The most appropriate strategy is to perform analyses using a variety of approaches to handling migrators, with the outlook that the truth probably lies somewhere in the middle of the range spanned by the various approaches. In concluding whether or not the study provides definite statistical evidence of efficacy, primary emphasis should be given to the intent to treat approach.

2.3. Some Further Considerations

In a trial with individual-level randomization, there is generally no need for special close cooperation with organizations outside the trial group itself. It suffices to secure the cooperation of each individual participant. By contrast, in the typical cluster randomization trial the trial group must gain the cooperation of various administrative offices. For example, in a school-based intervention trial, it is necessary to gain the approval and cooperation of school district administrators, school principals, and teachers. Also, in implementing and assessing the intervention, in the typical clinical trial the participant visits the study clinic, but in many cluster randomization trials, study staff must go out into the field.

Frequently, the cluster randomization design is used to assess behavioral intervention programs, because such programs often are developed for implementation at a school or community level. Susser (1995) has observed that an number of major behavior-oriented cluster randomization trials have failed to exhibit an intervention effect; this observation raises concern about this type of trial. Susser discusses possible explanations for the negative results seen in these trials. One possibility suggested is that the treatment effect may be diluted by a general population trend toward adopting the behavior change in question or by exposure of the control group to a extant program of similar nature. Another possibility suggested is that the type of behavioral change sought may be unlikely to occur in a substantial proportion of individuals over the relatively short time frame of a clinical trial. In considering a trial of a school-based or community-based behavioral change program, it is wise to take due account of the possibility of dilution effects and to consider carefully how large an intervention effect realistically can be expected over the time frame of the trial.

3. STATISTICAL ANALYSIS STRATEGIES

In this section and the next we discuss statistical methods and sample size considerations for the analysis of a single outcome variable measured at the end of the study on a specified cohort of individuals in each cluster (aside from missing data), with the possibility of using baseline measurements on these individuals as covariates. The structure of the resulting data set is formally the same as that arising from repeated measures studies, in that each involves sampling of a number of units and observation on a number of subunits within each unit. For a cluster randomization study, the unit is the cluster and the subunit is the individual; in a repeated measures study the unit is the individual and the subunit is the measurement time point. Because of this common structure, the analytical methods used for the two types of study are similar.

3.1. Unadjusted Analyses

Let Y_{ijk} denote the response for individual ijk, with i indexing the experimental arms, j indexing the clusters within an arm, and k indexing the individuals within a cluster. We consider first the case in which the number of clusters within each group is moderate to large (say about 30 clusters per arm). For a continuous response, it is appropriate to analyze the data using the conventional mixed ANOVA model

$$Y_{ijk} = \mu + a_i + b_{j(i)} + \varepsilon_{k(ij)} \tag{1}$$

where μ represents the overall response level, a_i is a fixed parameter representing the effect of treatment i, $b_{j(i)}$ is a random cluster effect term assumed distributed $N(0, \sigma_b^2)$, and $\varepsilon_{k(ij)}$ is an individual error term assumed distributed $N(0, \sigma_\varepsilon^2)$, with all random variables assumed independent.

The variance of an individual response Y_{ijk} is $\sigma^2 = \sigma_b^2 + \sigma_\varepsilon^2$. The intraclass correlation coefficient (ICC) is given by $\rho = \sigma_b^2/\sigma^2$.

Let n_{ij} denote the number of individuals in cluster ij. When the n_{ij} are all equal, then the model (1) may be analyzed by the classical mixed ANOVA procedure described in basic experimental design texts such as that of Winer (1971). This procedure is equivalent to applying the classical two-sample t test or one-way fixed ANOVA model to the cluster means $\overline{Y}_{ij\cdot}$. When the n_{ij} are not equal, the theoretically most efficient approach is to apply maximum likelihood or restricted maximum likelihood analysis, as described by Laird and Ware (1982) and Jennrich and Schluchter (1986). These methods, which require iterative fitting for the parameter estimation, are available in major statistical computation packages such as SAS (PROC MIXED) and BMDP (5V). Alternatively, one may use a moment-based method, for which closed-form expressions are available. We describe a typical moment-based method, for simplicity for the case of two experimental arms. Denote the overall treatment means by $\overline{Y}_{i\cdot\cdot}$. Define a cluster mean square MSC and a error mean square MSE by the following formulas (*cf.* Henderson, 1953):

$$\text{MSC} = \frac{1}{J-1}\sum_{ij} n_{ij}\,(\overline{Y}_{ij\cdot} - \overline{Y}_{i\cdot\cdot})^2$$

$$\text{MSE} = \frac{1}{N-J}\sum_{ijk}(Y_{ijk} - \overline{Y}_{ij\cdot})^2,$$

where J denotes the total number of clusters and N the total number of observations in the analysis. These expressions reduce to the classical mean square expressions when the n_{ij} are equal. The intraclass correlation ρ is estimated by

$$\hat{\rho} = \frac{\text{MSC} - \text{MSE}}{\text{MSC} + (n^* - 1)\text{MSE}}$$

with

$$n^* = \bar{n} - \frac{1}{\bar{n}J(J-1)} \sum_{ij} (n_{ij} - \bar{n})^2$$

where $\bar{n} = N/J$. We set $\hat{\rho} = 0$ if MSC < MSE. The variance σ^2 of a given response is estimated by $\hat{\sigma}^2 = \text{MSE} / (1 - \hat{\rho})$. The expected response $\mu_i = \mu + a_i$ in arm i is estimated by

$$\hat{\mu}_i = \sum_j \frac{w_{ij} \bar{Y}_{ij\cdot}}{W_i}$$

where $w_{ij} = n_{ij}/[1 + (n_{ij} - 1)\hat{\rho}]$ and $W_i = \Sigma_j w_{ij}$. The two arms are then compared using the t statistic

$$t = \frac{\hat{\mu}_1 - \hat{\mu}_2}{\sqrt{\hat{\sigma}^2 (W_1^{-1} + W_2^{-1})}} \tag{2}$$

which is regarded as t distributed with $J - 2$ degrees of freedom.

The idea behind the estimate $\hat{\mu}_i$ is as follows. The variance of $\bar{Y}_{ij\cdot}$ is $\sigma^2[1 + (n_{ij} - 1)\rho]/n_{ij}$. In the estimate $\hat{\mu}_i$, the cluster mean $\bar{Y}_{ij\cdot}$ is weighted according to the reciprocal of its variance, which represents the amount of information contained in cluster ij.

For a binary (0–1) response representing the occurrence of some event, the ANOVA model (1) is not applicable, but methods similar in form may be used. Here $\mu_i = E[Y_{ijk}]$ is the event probability for an individual in arm i and the intraclass correlation coefficient $\rho = \text{Cov}(Y_{ijk}, Y_{ijk'})/\text{Var}(Y_{ijk})$, $k \neq k'$, becomes the Cohen (1960) kappa coefficient, which may be expressed as $\rho = [\Pr(Y_{ijk} = 1, Y_{ijk'} = 1) - \mu_i^2]/[\mu_i(1 - \mu_i)]$. When the n_{ij} are equal, one may again apply the usual two-sample t test or the one-way fixed ANOVA F-test to the cluster means $\bar{Y}_{ij\cdot}$. When the n_{ij} differ, one may employ a model for binary data with random effects as described below in the discussion of adjusted analyses. Alternatively, one may employ the moment-based method described above for the continuous response case. For the case of binary data, the expression for MSE simplifies to the following (Fleiss, 1981, sec. 13.2):

$$\text{MSE} = \frac{1}{N - J} \sum_{ij} n_{ij} \bar{Y}_{ij\cdot}(1 - \bar{Y}_{ij\cdot}).$$

The foregoing methods are easily extended to the case of stratified analysis; Donner and Donald (1987) discuss such extension of the moment-based method for the case of a binary response.

When the number of units per arm is small, a permutation-based analysis is preferable. Recently, efficient statistical software for permutation tests has become available (Hirji et al., 1987; Reboussin and DeMets, 1996); Cytel's Stat-Xact is a prominent software package for such tests. When the n_{ij} are equal, a permutation test may be applied to the cluster means $\overline{Y}_{ij\cdot}$. When the n_{ij} differ, a more powerful test is obtained by factoring in the weights w_{ij}. For the permutation approach to go through, the calculation of the weights w_{ij} must be modified by replacing the estimate ρ by an estimate that does not distinguish between the experimental arms: specifically, in the expression for MSC, one must replace the cluster mean $\overline{Y}_{i\cdot\cdot}$ by the overall mean $\overline{Y}_{\cdots}$. Braun and Feng (2001) discuss weighted permutation tests. As these authors show, the optimal procedure is to apply a permutation test to the scores $U_{ij} = w_{ij}(\overline{Y}_{ij\cdot} - \hat{\mu})$, with $\hat{\mu} = \sum_{ij} w_{ij}\overline{Y}_{ij\cdot}/\sum_{ij} w_{ij}$.

3.2. Adjusted Analyses

We now consider methods that allow covariate adjustment. In cluster randomization trials one may have both cluster-level covariates (e.g., location of school, urban or rural) and individual-level covariates (e.g., ethnicity of the student). A proper analysis scheme must account for both types of covariates and for cluster-to-cluster variability. Below we present the two most popular analytical approaches, namely the mixed model approach and the GEE approach. In addition, we present a two-stage analysis strategy that allows for inference that is robust to mis-specification of the model. We then provide a brief discussion. The presentation here is adapted from Zucker et al. (1995). We let $\mathbf{X}_{ijk}$ denote the vector of covariates, including both cluster-level and individual-level covariates, for individual ijk.

Mixed Model Approach

For a continuous response, the standard mixed linear model is given by the following simple generalization of the model (1):

$$Y_{ijk} = \mu + a_i + b_{j(i)} + \beta^T \mathbf{X}_{ijk} + \varepsilon_{k(ij)} \tag{3}$$

where the $b_{j(i)}$ and $\varepsilon_{k(ij)}$ satisfy the same assumptions as in the model (1). Inference for this model is discussed by Laird and Ware (1982) and Jennrich and Schluchter (1986). The computations may be accomplished in SAS PROC MIXED or BMDP5V.

For a binary response, the corresponding model is

$$\text{Prob}(Y_{ijk} = 1) = G(\mu + a_i + b_{j(i)} + \beta^T \mathbf{X}_{ijk}) \tag{4}$$

where G is a continuous, strictly increasing distribution function and the $b_{j(i)}$ are i.i.d. with some specified distribution. The most common version of this model takes G to be the logistic distribution $G(u) = e^u/(e^u + 1)$ and the $b_{j(i)}$ to be normal. One then obtains logistic regression with a normal random effect (Longford, 1994). This model may be fit using the the recent SAS procedure PROC NLMIXED.

In principle, it is possible to allow cluster-to-cluster variation in the regression coefficients corresponding to the individual-level covariates. This extension is discussed in the references cited. The extension, however, is usually of less interest in cluster randomization studies than in repeated measures studies, where, for example, one commonly postulates a unit-specific intercept and slope. In cluster randomization studies with a number of repeated measurements over time, however, this extension is of importance (Murray et al., 1998).

GEE Approach

An alternative approach is the generalized estimating equations (GEE) approach advanced by Liang and Zeger (1986) (see also Prentice, 1988). In this approach a model is postulated for the marginal expectation $E[Y_{ijk} \mid \mathbf{X}_{ijk}]$, and estimating equations are developed for the model parameters that take into account the presumed form of the dependence of the observations within a cluster. Variance estimates for the parameter estimates are obtained that are robust to mis-specification of the dependence structure. Software developed by M. Karim, a student of Zeger and Liang, has been available for some time; recently, the method has been incorporated into SAS PROC GENMOD.

The models for $E[Y_{ijk}|\mathbf{X}_{ijk}]$ are fairly standard. For continuous data the typical model is

$$E[Y_{ijk}|\mathbf{X}_{ijk}] = \mu + \beta^T \mathbf{X}_{ijk}; \tag{5}$$

for binary data the typical model is

$$E[Y_{ijk}|\mathbf{X}_{ijk}] = G(\mu + \beta^T \mathbf{X}_{ijk}) \tag{6}$$

for a suitable distribution function G such as the logistic.

Zeger et al. (1988) discuss the relationship between the mixed model approach and the GEE approach. The mixed model approach is more relevant when interest focuses on the effect of intervention at the cluster level, whereas the GEE approach is more relevant when interest focuses on the intervention effect on a general population level averaging across clusters. In cluster randomization studies, both levels of analysis could be of interest. The two levels of analysis coincide for the linear statistical models typically used for a continuous response, but are distinct for the nonlinear models typically used for a binary response.

Two-Stage Analysis Strategy

Following Gail et al. (1988), either of the foregoing analytical approaches may be modified to yield an analysis that is robust to violations of the underlying model assumptions. The procedure operates in two stages. In the first stage, a model of the form discussed above is fit, but *omitting* the treatment effect term a_i. In the second stage, residuals Z_{ijk} are defined by

$$Z_{ijk} = Y_{ijk} - \hat{E}[Y_{ijk}|\mathbf{X}_{ijk}]$$

where the second term represents the expectation of Y_{ijk} evaluated at the model parameter estimates. These residuals are then subjected to an analysis of the form described in the subsection on unadjusted analyses.

For the continuous-data case, under either the mixed model (3) or the GEE model (5), we have simply $\hat{E}[Y_{ijk}|\mathbf{X}_{ijk}] = \hat{\mu} + \hat{\beta}^T\mathbf{X}_{ijk}$. For the binary-data case, under the GEE approach the estimated expectation is obtained simply by substituting the estimated μ and β into (6). Under the mixed model approach, the situation is more complex. The expectation $E[Y_{ijk}|\mathbf{X}_{ijk}]$ is given by

$$E[Y_{ijk}|\mathbf{X}_{ijk}] = \int G(\mu + b + \beta^T\mathbf{X}_{ijk})f(b)\ db$$

where $f(b)$ denotes the density function of $b_{j(i)}$. Generally it is not possible to evaluate the integral in closed form, and resort must be made to numerical methods related to those used in the fitting algorithm itself. Numerical integration may be employed relatively straightforwardly, because the integral in the present context is one dimensional. Alternatively, an approximation may be used. A very simple approximation is given by

$$E^{(1)} = G(\mu + \beta^T\mathbf{X}_{ijk})$$

a more refined approximation is given by

$$E^{(2)} = E^{(1)} + \sigma_b^2[G''(\mu + \beta^T\mathbf{X}_{ijk})]^2.$$

Discussion

For defining the analysis scheme for a cluster randomization trial, we have discussed the mixed model and GEE approaches, with the possibility of testing for treatment effect directly within the framework of the selected analytical approach or by means of the two-stage analysis procedure. If the response variable is a continuous one analyzed using a linear model, and the number of randomized units is large, the various analytical options are broadly equivalent. With a binary response, and in other cases involving a nonlinear model, the two-stage procedure is preferable for testing treatment effect because it provides a valid test for treatment effect without relying on the correctness of the model assumptions. When the number of randomized units is small, the analytic strategy of choice in all cases is to implement the two-stage procedure (applied either to the mixed model or the GEE model) in conjunction with an exact permutation test. This strategy provides a test with a guaranteed type 1 error rate under the null hypothesis that the intervention has no influence whatsoever on the response.

4. SAMPLE SIZE CALCULATION

Sample size calculation for cluster randomization trials is discussed in Donner et al. (1981). The main point of note is the need to take into account the variance inflation factor (IF) arising from the within-cluster dependence. In sample size formulas for continuous or binary data based on the usual asymptotic normal approximation, the sample size must be multiplied by the IF. Consider, for example, a two-arm trial with equal allocation of clusters to arms and with (approximately) the same number n of observations per cluster, with two-sided testing with Type I error level α and power $1-\beta$. The formula for the total number of clusters J for a continuous endpoint is

$$J = 4n^{-1}[1 + (n-1)\rho]\frac{(z_{\alpha/2} + z_{\beta})^2\sigma^2}{\delta^2} \tag{7}$$

where σ^2 is the variance of an individual response, δ is the difference to be detected, z_λ is the $(1 - \lambda)$ normal quantile, and ρ is the intraclass correlation coefficient. The corresponding formula for a binary endpoint is

$$J = 2n^{-1}[1 + (n-1)\rho](z_{\alpha/2} + z_{\beta})^2\frac{p_1(1-p_1) + p_2(1-p_2)}{(p_1 - p_2)^2} \tag{8}$$

where p_i is the event probability for a given individual in arm i and ρ is the kappa coefficient as defined in Section 3.1. In either case, the total number of individuals is Jn. In power calculations based on the noncentral t distribution, the noncentrality parameter must be divided by the IF.

Typically the ICC is relatively small. But if the ICC is moderate to large, substantial effort may be saved with modest loss of efficiency by subsampling individuals within the clusters. Let m denote the total cluster size. Then, for given ρ, the relative efficiency (RE) of measuring only n individuals in each cluster as compared with measuring all individuals in each cluster is given as

$$RE = \frac{\rho + \dfrac{(1-\rho)}{m}}{\rho + \dfrac{(1-\rho)}{n}}.$$

That is, the number of clusters J needed if n individuals in each cluster are measured is $1/RE$ times the number of clusters needed if all m individuals in each cluster are measured. In cases with large enough ρ the cost of adding further clusters may be offset by the reduced measurement cost engendered by sampling.

To calculate the sample size, one needs to specify not only the usual parameters such as σ^2 and δ or p_1 and p_2 but also the ICC. In some situations, a prior data set is available that includes data on the outcome of interest under a cluster structure identical or similar to the cluster structure that will exist in the planned study. In this case, a prior estimate of the ICC is readily obtained. Otherwise, one must make some educated guess about the ICC. It is often useful to examine ICCs obtained in other settings and to make a guess of the ICC in the planned study based on the range of ICCs in the other settings and a judgment of which of the other settings is likely to have a level of within-cluster dependence similar to that in the setting at hand. Donner and Klar (1994) have presented ICC's for a range of public health settings.

5. EXAMPLE: THE CATCH TRIAL

As as example of a cluster randomized trial, we describe the Child and Adolescent Trial for Cardiovascular Health (CATCH). Details concerning the design of this trial are reported in Zucker et al. (1995), and the main trial results are reported in Luepker et al. (1996). The CATCH study investigated a school-based educational and environmental intervention aimed at promoting heart-healthy habits in elementary school children.

Because the intervention was implemented the school level, a cluster randomization design was mandatory.

The trial involved randomization of 96 schools, of which 40 were assigned to the control group C, 28 were assigned to receive the school-based intervention S, and 28 were assigned to receive the school-based intervention plus a supplementary family-based intervention ($S+F$). The main trial comparison was that between the combination of S and $S+F$ groups and the control group.

The intervention was aimed at changing a number of behaviors, principally fat and salt consumption and physical exercise. The primary trial endpoint was taken to be serum total cholesterol, because it was felt that dietary and exercise habit measures would be susceptible to reporting bias, whereas cholesterol would be free of such bias but responsive enough to reflect true diet and exercise changes. Various diet, exercise, and other endpoints were included as secondary endpoints.

The primary study cohort was defined to be those students who underwent a baseline cholesterol measurement. Provisions were made to track outmigrating students and to attempt to measure cholesterol in these students at the end of the study.

The sample size was determined by the following slightly extended version of the formula (7):

$$J = [CS\gamma(1-\gamma)]^{-1}[1+(S-1)\rho_1+(C-1)S\rho_2]\frac{(z_{\alpha/2}+z_\beta)^2\sigma^2}{\delta^2} \qquad (9)$$

where C denotes the number of classrooms in a school, S denotes the number of students per classroom with available data, ρ_1 denotes the within-classroom correlation, ρ_2 denotes the within-school correlation for students in different classrooms in the same school, and γ denotes the proportion of clusters assigned to the intervention arm.

The CATCH calculations assumed 3–4 classrooms per school (3.5 on average) and 17 students with available data per class. On the basis of past studies the standard deviation σ was estimated to be 28 mg/dl. The correlations ρ_1 and ρ_2 were estimated on the basis of a variance components analysis of a small data set on cholesterol levels among schoolchildren in a prior observational study conducted by one of the study centers in CATCH. The estimates were $\rho_1 = 0.023$ and $\rho_2 = 0.003$. The projected treatment difference on cholesterol (S and $S+F$ versus C) was determined to be 5.1 mg/dl. A conservative adjustment factor was incorporated to account for possible missing data bias; see Zucker et al. (1995) for details. The effect of the adjustment was to reduce the difference δ to be detected from 5.1 mg/dl to an effective difference, after the adjustment, of 2.9 mg/dl. The intervention ($S+F$ and S) to control C allocation ratio was 7:5 (to enhance the power of the $S+F$ versus S comparison), so that $\gamma = 0.583$. Substituting these parameters into the formula (9) yields a sample size requirement of 102 schools total for 90% power at the two-sided 0.05 level. Based on administrative considerations, the final sample size was taken to be 96 schools total.

The sample size calculation incorporated both school and classroom effects because at the design stage it was felt important to do so. As regards the analysis, with school-level assignment the randomization theory of statistical testing requires school to be the primary unit of analysis. However, the theory does not require incorporation of classroom as a factor for the analysis to be valid in terms of type I error. In fact, the final CATCH analysis did not include classroom as a factor.

The serum cholesterol results were analyzed using a mixed linear model of the form (3), with experimental arm, CATCH center, baseline cholesterol level, and a number of relevant covariates as fixed effect terms and school as a random effect. The post-study mean cholesterol levels were 168.3 mg/dl for treatment (S and $S+F$) and 169.5 mg/dl for control; the treatment-control difference was not statistically significant. On the other hand, nominally statistically significant though modest differences were found on dietary and physical activity measures. As possible explanations for the negative finding on cholesterol, the investigators point up the smaller than projected dietary changes and the effects of puberty.

In regard to cooperation with study procedures, the percentage of students in the study schools who had a baseline cholesterol measurement and were entered into the primary CATCH cohort was 60% as opposed to the projected 80%. Among the students in the primary cohort, 72% continued in CATCH schools up to the end of the study. Of these, 90% underwent the final cholesterol measurement. Of the students who migrated out of CATCH schools, 50% underwent the final cholesterol measurement. Thus, overall, 79% of the students in the primary CATCH cohort had a final cholesterol measurement, representing a data completeness level not too far from the projected 85%.

6. SUMMARY

A cluster randomization design is necessary when assessing a cluster-level intervention and sometimes convenient in other clinical trial settings. When cluster randomization is employed, the primary unit of analysis must be the cluster to preserve validity of the type I error. Though it is uncommon for entire clusters to drop out from the trial, dropout at the individual level is quite common, and a intention-to-treat approach to analysis is called for to avoid dropout bias. The analysis plan and sample size determination must be appropriately tailored to account for the role of the cluster as the primary analysis unit. Suitable approaches are available for ensuring a valid analysis while allowing adjustment for both cluster-level and individual-level covariates.

REFERENCES

Braun, T., Feng, Z. (2001). Optimal permutation tests for the analysis of group randomized trials. Journal of the American Statistical Association 96:1424–1432.

Bozivich, H., Bancroft, T. A., Hartley, H. O. (1956). Power of analysis of variance test procedures for certain incompletely specified models. Annals of Mathematical Statistics 27:1017–1043.

Cochran, W. G. (1977). Sampling Techniques. 3rd ed. New York: John Wiley.

Cohen, J. (1960). A coefficient of agreement for nominal data. Educational and Psychological Measurement 20:37–46.

COMMIT Research Group. Community Intervention Trial for Smoking Cessation (COMMIT): I. Cohort results from a four-year community intervention. American Journal of Public Health 85:183–192.

Cornfield, J. (1978). Randomization by cluster: A formal analysis. American Journal of Epidemiology 108:100–102.

Donner, A., Birkett, N., Buck, C. (1981). Randomization by cluster: Sample size requirements and analysis. Americal Journal of Epidemiology 114:906–914.

Donner, A., Donald, A. (1987). Analysis of data arising from a stratified design with cluster as the unit of randomization. Statistics in Medicine 6:43–52.

Donner, A., Klar, N. (1994). Methods for comparing event rates in intervention studies when the unit of allocation is a cluster. American Journal of Epidemiology 140:279–289.

Donner, A., Klar, N. S. (2000). Design and Analysis of Cluster Randomization Trials in Health Research. London: Arnold.

Fisher, R. A. (1935). The Design of Experiments. Edinburgh: Oliver and Boyd. 8th ed. New York: Hafner, 1966.

Fleiss, J. L. (1981). Statistical Analysis of Rates and Proportions. 2nd ed. New York: John Wiley.

Friedman, L. M., Furberg, C. D., DeMets, D. L. (1996). Fundamentals of Clinical Trials. 3rd ed. St. Louis MO: Mosby—Year Book.

Gail, M.H., Byar, D.P., Pechacck, T.F., Corle, D.K. (1992). Aspects of the statistical design for the Community Health Trial for Smoking Cessation (COMMIT). Controlled Clinical Trials 13:6–21.

Gail, M. H., Tan, W. Y., Piantadosi, S. (1988). Tests for no treatment effect in randomized clinical trials. Biometrika 75:57–64.

Glass, G. V., Stanley, J. C. (1970). Statistical Methods in Education and Psychology. Englewood Cliffs, NJ: Prentice-Hall.

Henderson, C. R. (1953). Estimation of variance and covariance components. Biometrics 9:226–252.

Hines, W. G. S. (1996). Pragmatics of pooling in ANOVA tables. American Statistician 50:127–139.

Hirji, K. F., Mehta, C. R., Patel, N. R. (1987). Computing distributions for exact logistic regression. Journal of the American Statistical Association 82: 1110–1117.

Hopkins, K. D. (1982). The unit of analysis: Group means versus individual observations. American Educational Research Journal 19:5–19.

Jennrich, R. I., Schluchter, M. D. (1986). Unbalanced repeated-measures models with structured covariance matrices. Biometrics 42:805–820.

Kempthorne, O. (1952). The Design and Analysis of Experiments. New York: John Wiley.

Laird, N. M., Ware, J. H. (1982). Random-effects models for longitudinal data. Biometrics 38:963–974.

Liang, K. Y., Zeger, S. L. (1986). Longitudinal data analysis using generalized linear models. Biometrika 73:13–22.

Longford, N. (1994). Logistic regression with random coefficients. Computational Statistics and Data Analysis 17:1–15.

Luepker, R. V., Perry, C. L., McKinlay, S. M., Nader, P. R., Parcel, G. S., Stone, E. J., Webber, L. S., Elder, J. P., Feldman, H. A., Johnson, C. C., Kelder, S. H., Wu, M. (1996). Outcomes of a field trial to improve children's dietary patterns and physical activity: The Child and Adolescent Trial for Cardiovascular Health (CATCH). Journal of the American Medical Association 275:768–776.

Murray, D. M. (1998). Design and Analysis of Group-Randomized Trials. Oxford: Oxford University Press.

Murray, D. M., Hannan, P. J., Wolfinger, R. D., Baker, W. L., Dwyer, J. H. (1998). Analysis of data for group-randomized trial with repeat measures on the same group. Statistics in Medicine 17:1581–1600.

Pocock, S. J. (1983). Clinical Trials: A Practical Approach. New York: John Wiley and Sons.

Prentice, R. (1988). Correlated binary regression with covariates specific to each binary observation. Biometrics 44:1033–1048.

Reboussin, D. M., DeMets, D. L. (1996). Exact permutation inference for two sample repeated measures data. Communications in Statistics, Theory and Methods 25:2223–2238.

Rosen, L. J. (2003). The effect of a health promotion program on hygiene behavior and illness-related absenteeism. Ph.D. dissertation. School of Public Health, Hebrew University of Jerusalem. In preparation.

Simon, R. (1981). Composite randomization designs for clinical trials. Biometrics 37:723–731.

Susser, M. (1995). Editorial: The tribulations of trials—intervention in communities. American Journal of Public Health 85:156–158.

Winer, B. J. (1971). Statistical Principles in Experimental Design. 2nd ed. New York: McGraw-Hill.

Zeger, S. L., Liang, K. Y., Albert, P. A. (1988). Models for longitudinal data: a generalized estimating equations approach. Biometrics 44:1049–1060.

Zucker, D. M. (1990). An analysis of variance pitfall: The fixed effects analysis in a nested design. Educational and Psychological Measurement 50:731–738.

Zucker, D. M., Lakatos, E., Webber, L. S., Murray, D. M., McKinlay, S. M., Feldman, H. A., Kelder, S. H., Nader, P. R. (1995). Statistical design of the Child and Adolescent Trial for Cardiovascular Health (CATCH). Controlled Clinical Trials 16:96–118.

6

Design and Analysis of Clinical Trials with Multiple Endpoints*

Nancy L. Geller
National Heart, Lung, and Blood Institute, National Institutes of Health, Bethesda, Maryland, U.S.A.

1. INTRODUCTION AND NOTATION

In many clinical trials, there are several endpoints of comparable importance, rather than one primary endpoint. In cholesterol-lowering trials, for example, we may be interested in LDL and HDL or LDL and the ratio of total cholesterol to HDL and tryglycerides. In patients with coronary heart disease, we may be interested in both resting and exercise ejection fractions. In blood pressure lowering trials, we might be interested in diastolic and systolic blood pressure or mean arterial pressure and pulse pressure. In stroke treatment there are a number of scales used to measure recovery and no one scale is believed to assess all dimensions. We later will consider an example using four of these scales, the Barthel Index, NIH Stroke scale, Glasgow Outcome score, and the modified Rankin score. In lung diseases, we may be interested in several lung function tests such as FEV_1, FVC, PI. In behavioral studies, we may be interested in several scales for quality of life. Recent advances in DNA technology have led investigators to undertake

---

* This chapter was written by Nancy L. Geller in her private capacity. The views expressed in the chapter do not necessarily represent the views of NIH, DHHS, or the United States.

exploratory studies, seeking genes which are over- or underexpressed in (say) a diseased population compared to a control. The number of genes which are examined is often in the thousands.

The examples illustrate that restricting ourselves to one primary endpoint when designing or analyzing a clinical study may be inappropriate. Further, the multiple endpoints one might consider are correlated with one another. Here we consider methodology for situations where there are multiple primary endpoints in a clinical study. We concentrate on clinical trials, although the methods are applicable to other studies as well.

Let $\mathbf{X}_{ij}$ $i = 1, 2, j = 1, 2, \ldots, n_i$, be independent vectors of length K representing the jth observation of the ith sample. We assume that $\mathbf{X}_{ij}$ has a multivariate normal distribution with mean μ_i and known variance-covariance matrix Σ_0.

We are interested in testing a null hypothesis that two K-dimensional mean vectors of k endpoints are equal against an alternative hypothesis that the difference in mean vectors is a vector of positive constants:

$$H_{0\{1,2,\ldots,K\}}: \boldsymbol{\mu}_2 = \boldsymbol{\mu}_1$$
$$H_{A\{1,2,\ldots,K\}}: \boldsymbol{\mu}_2 - \boldsymbol{\mu}_1 = \boldsymbol{\delta}\lambda$$

where $\boldsymbol{\mu}_i$, $i = 1, 2$, is a $K \times 1$ column vector of the true means and $\boldsymbol{\delta}$ is a column vector of specified positive treatment differences (of length K) and λ is a positive scalar. We may think of the second sample as representing a new treatment, the first sample as representing a control treatment, and the alternative as specifying that the new treatment is better than control on all endpoints. We develop one-sided tests, although extensions to two-sided alternatives (that one treatment is superior to the other, without specifying which) are straightforward.

We subscript the null and alternative hypotheses by $\{1, 2, \ldots, K\}$ to indicate hypotheses involving all K endpoints. Later we will consider testing null hypotheses on various subsets of endpoints. We will also mention extensions to more than two samples.

2. SOME HYPOTHESIS TESTS FOR MULTIPLE ENDPOINTS

In this section, we describe a number of the statistics which have been proposed for testing null hypotheses involving multiple primary endpoints.

2.1. Bonferroni Methods

Perhaps the simplest methods perform univariate tests on each of the K endpoints and adjust the p value in one of a number of ways. The original method used the Bonferroni inequality, performing univariate (one-sided) tests on each endpoint at level α/K. This maintains an overall type I error α, but is conservative, with the degree of conservatism increasing with K and as the correlation increases (Pocock, Geller, and Tsiatis, 1987).

A number of modifications have been proposed (Holm, 1979; Hochberg, 1988; Simes, 1986) to decrease the conservatism of the Bonferroni procedure. Holm's sequentially rejective procedure performs the univariate tests on each endpoint and orders the univariate p values from smallest to largest, denoted by $P(1) \leq P(2) \leq \cdots \leq P(\mathrm{K})$. If $P(1) > \alpha/K$, Holm's procedure stops and we do not reject any of the null hypotheses. If $P(1) \leq \alpha/K$, Holm's procedure rejects the corresponding null hypothesis; then if $P(2) > \alpha/(K\text{-}1)$, Holm's procedure stops and rejects only the first null hypothesis, but not the others; if $P(2) \leq \alpha/(K\text{-}1)$, Holm's procedure rejects also the corresponding null hypothesis, etc. Holm's procedure is clearly less conservative (and hence more powerful) than the original Bonferroni procedure, yet still protects the type I error.

Simes (1986) proposed rejecting $H_{0\{1,\ 2,\ \ldots,\ K\}}$ if $P(i) < i\alpha/K$ for at least one i. Since the rejection region contains the Bonferroni rejection region, Simes's procedure is always more powerful than Bonferroni's. However, Simes only proved his procedure maintained α when the test statistics were independent. Sarkar and Chang (1997) proved that Simes's procedure maintained α when the distribution of the vector of test statistics was positively dependent under the null hypothesis. The assumption of positive dependence needed for the Simes's procedure cannot be verified until the data are seen.

Procedures of the Bonferroni type are appealing because they are simple and distribution-free. The Bonferroni and Holm procedures require at least one endpoint to be highly significant to reject $H_{0\{1,\ 2,\ \ldots,\ K\}}$. In the case of five endpoints, each with p value .02, the Bonferroni and Holm procedures would not reject $H_{0\{1,\ 2,\ldots,\ K\}}$, yet if all of the endpoints go in the same direction, the null hypothesis is not likely to be true. The Bonferroni and Holm procedures do not use the information about the relationship between endpoints and so lose power. Resampling methods improve on this.

2.2. Resampling Methods (Westfall and Young, 1993; Troendle, 1995, 1996)

Consider the univariate comparisons on the K individual endpoints and order the test statistics T_i. Let $t(1) \leq t(2) \leq \cdots \leq t(K)$ be the ordered values of the T_i and $H_{0(1)}, H_{0(2)}, \ldots, H_{0(K)}$ be the corresponding ordered null hypotheses. Determine constants $q_1, q_2 \ldots, q_K$ and sequentially accept hypotheses $H_{0(1)}, H_{0(2)}, \ldots$ until the first time $t(i) > q_i$, at which point reject $H_{0(I)}, \ldots, H_{0(K)}$. The constants q_i are determined so that the probability of rejecting any true hypothesis under any parameter configuration is at most α. In effect this procedure can be viewed as an exact version of Holm's procedure. An algorithm (which uses permutational resampling) determines the constants and it is shown (under certain conditions) that the familywise error is strongly controlled asymptotically.

An overall adjusted p value for a subset of hypotheses on single endpoints is available from this procedure. The adjusted p value is the smallest overall significance level α for which the given subset of hypotheses would be rejected by the multiple test procedure using the observed test statistics.

2.3. Linear Combinations of Endpoints

Several statistics which are linear combinations of the endpoints have been suggested. Assume first that the underlying data have a normal distribution with known covariance matrix Σ and that there are $n_i = N$ patients assigned to each treatment. We consider three linear combination tests for testing $H_{0\{1, 2, \ldots, K\}}$ versus $H_{A\{1, 2, \ldots, K\}}$. Each test statistic has a standard normal distribution and $H_{0\{1, 2, \ldots, K\}}$ would be rejected for large values of the test statistic.

Let Y be the column vector of differences in means for the K endpoints (second sample minus first sample), $\Sigma = (\sigma_{im})$ the covariance matrix of Y, and $\sigma_{mm} = \sigma_m^2$, the variance of the mth mean difference. The ordinary least squares (OLS) statistic (O'Brien, 1984) is a function of the average of Y_m/σ_m, which is then properly normalized:

$$Z_{\mathrm{OLS}} = \frac{(N/2)^{1/2} J^T Y}{(J^{\mathrm{T}} \Sigma J)^{1/2}}$$

where $J = (\sigma_1^{-1}, \sigma_2^{-1}, \ldots, \sigma_K^{-1})^T$.

The generalized least squares (GLS) statistic (O'Brien, 1984) is a weighted average of the Y_m/σ_m:

$$Z_{\text{GLS}} = \frac{(N/2)^{1/2}\delta^{\text{T}}\Sigma^{-1}\text{Y}}{(\delta^{\text{T}}\Sigma^{-1}\delta)^{1/2}}$$

where δ = alternative vector (fixed). Here Y is weighted by $\delta^{\text{T}}\,\Sigma^{-1}$. A third linear combination, the centered linear combination (CLC) statistic, was suggested by Tang, et al. (1993):

$$Z_{\text{CLC}} = \frac{(N/2)^{1/2}J_1^T D^{1/2}Y}{(J_1^{\text{T}}D^{1/2}\Sigma D^{1/2}J_1)^{1/2}}$$

where $J_1 = (1, 1, \ldots, 1)^{\text{T}}$ and $D = \text{diag}[(\Sigma^{-1})_{11}, \ldots, (\Sigma^{-1})_{KK}]$, the matrix with the same diagonal elements as Σ^{-1} and off-diagonal elements 0. Z_{CLC} was suggested because among all linear combinations, this choice of coefficients maximizes the minimum power over the positive orthant.

All of the linear combination statistics are appealing because they are simple. Tang et al. (1989a) showed that O'Brien's GLS statistic has a power advantage over the univariate statistics that comprise it in the following sense. Suppose δ, α, and $1 - \beta$ are fixed. Suppose we calculate the required sample sizes based on each of the K endpoints. If we also calculate the required sample size based on the GLS test, the required sample size for the GLS test is at most the minimum of the sample sizes required if any one endpoint were used to set sample size for the trial. The other linear combinations are not known to have the same power advantage. Of course the disadvantage is that if a trial were designed using O'Brien's GLS test, there would be limited power to detect differences in individual endpoints.

A disadvantage of the GLS test is that it does not always have positive coefficients. This implies that the GLS test is inadmissible and that peculiar results might emerge from the combination of a large negative test statistic with a negative coefficient (Pocock, Geller, and Tsiatis 1986; Follmann, 1995; Perlman and Wu, 1999). Both the OLS and the CLC will always have positive coefficients and therefore are to be preferred.

2.4. Wald-Type Test for Multiple Binary Outcomes

Lefkopoulou and Ryan (1992) considered an experiment involving two treatment groups where K binary variables were recorded for each subject. Let X_{ijm} represent the mth response, m = $1, 2, \ldots, K$ in the ith group for the jth subject, $j = 1, 2, \ldots, n_i$. For two groups, $i = 1$ (conventional treatment group) and 2 (experimental group). Assume that the observation vectors for each subject are independent, with mean vector $E(X_{ijm}) = \mu_{im}$ and $\text{var}(X_{ijm}) = \mu_{im}(1 - \mu_{im})$. The outcomes within a subject may be correlated.

For multiple binary outcomes, assume a linear logistic model for the probabilities of a favorable outcome, that is, μ_{im} satisfies

$$\text{logit}\ \mu_{im} = \alpha_m + \beta(i - 1)$$

where α_m allows for a different control level for each of the endpoints and β is the intervention effect coefficient for each of the endpoints. Thus β represents a single log odds for the endpoints.

Generalized estimating equations were used to obtain a Wald-type test to test the null hypotheses that the set of endpoints were equal in the two treatment groups against the alternative hypothesis

$$H_A\colon \beta > 0.$$

The test statistic is asymptotically χ^2 with 1 d.f. The methodology also allows the estimation of β which is interpreted as the odds ratio of improvement on all of the endpoints with experimental treatment relative to conventional treatment. 95% (or other) confidence limits for the odds ratio can be obtained.

When the correlations between the pairs of endpoints are equal ($\alpha_m = \alpha$ for $m = 1, 2, \ldots, K$) the Lefkopoulou/Ryan statistic coincides with O'Brien's OLS (and GLS in this case).

The Lefkopoulou/Ryan statistic was developed in the context of studies on laboratory offspring and was more general than developed here, e.g., it applies to more than two treatments and a different number of endpoints for each subject. Tilley et al. (1996) discussed use of the Lefkopoulou/Ryan statistic in the context of the stroke clinical trial described below.

2.5. Likelihood Ratio Tests

Likelihood Ratio and Approximate Likelihood Ratio Test

The distribution of the likelihood ratio test of $H_{0\{1, 2, \ldots, K\}}$ versus

$$H_{A\{1, 2, \ldots, K\}}\colon \mu_1 - \mu_2 \geq 0$$

with strict inequality holding for at least one endpoint was obtained by Kudo (1963) when the covariance matrix was known. Perlman (1969) obtained corresponding results with unknown covariance matrix. Because evaluating these distributions for purposes of application were difficult, Tang et al. (1989b) proposed the approximate likelihood ratio (ALR) test. When Σ is a known diagonal matrix, the ALR statistic coincides with the LR statistic and can be evaluated as

$$\frac{N}{2}\Sigma(Y_i^+)^2$$

where Y_i^+ is the maximum of Y_i and 0 and the summation is over the K endpoints. For a general covariance matrix, the mean vector Y must be transformed before the statistic is calculated. Let A be a square matrix such that $A'A = \Sigma^{-1}$. Note that A is not unique and $Z = (N/2)^{1/2} AY$ is a vector of independent normal variables with unit variance. The ALR test, $g(Z)$ is

$$g(Z) = \Sigma(Z_i^+)^2$$

where Z_i is the ith component of Z, Z_i^+ is the maximum of Z_i and 0, and the summation extends over the K endpoints. A is chosen so that $g(Z)$ suitably approximates the likelihood ratio statistic of $H_{0\{1,2,\ldots,K\}}$ versus $H_{A\{1,2,\ldots,K\}}$. The method to choose A is given in the appendix of Tang et al., 1993. Tang et al. (1989b) showed that the null hypothesis distribution of $g(Z)$ is a weighted sum of χ^2 random variables. They compared the power performance of the ALR test, O'Brien's GLS test and Hotelling's T^2. The performance in terms of power hinges on the closeness of the true direction of the alternative to the model direction. They note that the ALR test ignores differences going in the wrong direction and so urge caution when using one-sided multivariate testing.

The X_+^2 Test

Follmann (1996) proposed rejecting $H_{0\{1,2,\ldots,K\}}$ in favor of $H_{A\{1,2,\ldots,K\}}$ using Hotelling's T^2 at the 2α level as long as the sum of the difference in mean vectors is positive. This simple test has type I error equal to α, even when the variance-covariance matrix is unknown. The test has reasonable power when the mean vector is positive and not in a prespecified direction.

2.6. Nonparametric Tests

A number of authors have suggested other global tests, some of which are very briefly described here.

Rank Tests

An alternative approach which does not require the normality assumption is the rank sum statistic proposed by O'Brien (1984). O'Brien suggested ranking the X_{ijm} over all i and j for each m, summing the ranks for each subject, then ranking the subject sums and applying a Mann-Whitney-Wilcoxon test. While this procedure is very simple, it must be noted that it does not consider the correlation between either the endpoints or their ranks. Another rank test has recently been investigated by Huang and Hall (2002), where the covariance of the ranks is included.

One-Sided Bootstrap Tests

Bloch, Lai, and Tubert-Bitter (2001) consider alternatives of the form

$$H_A\colon \mu_{1m} > \mu_{2m} \qquad \text{for some } m$$

and

$$\mu_{1m} > \mu_{2m} - \varepsilon_m \qquad \text{for all } m$$

i.e., treatment 1 is superior to treatment 2 on at least one of the endpoints and all of the other endpoints for treatment 1 are noninferior to those of treatment 2.

They consider the intersection of the rejection region for the likelihood ratio test of H_0 (Hotelling's T^2) with the rejection region for the non-inferiority region (a set of univariate tests). They show that this results in a level α test and generate its bootstrap distribution. Because they are using the bootstrap, the normality assumption required by many of the other tests is not needed. Although numerically intense, this formulation is shown to have high power and type I error close to alpha under various distributions, such as a mixture of normals and a normal-exponential mixture.

3. A STEP-DOWN CLOSED PROCEDURE FOR DETERMINING WHICH ENDPOINTS DIFFER FOLLOWING A GLOBAL TEST

When dealing with multiple endpoints, aside from establishing an overall treatment effect, investigators are always interested in which individual endpoints differ. The theory of multiple comparison procedures adapts nicely to this setting.

Let $Z_{\{1,2,\ldots,K\}}$ denote any global test statistic based on all K endpoints. Let $Z_{\mathbf{F}}$ denote the same test statistic based on the subset **F** of the K endpoints. If the type I error for the global test $Z_{\{1,2,\ldots,K\}}$ is α and simultaneously there is control at level α for each test $Z_{\mathbf{F}}$ for all subsets **F**, we say that the type 1 error is *strongly* controlled (protected) at level α. If there is control at level α only for $Z_{\{1,2,\ldots,K\}}$ we say that the type I error is protected *weakly* (at level α).

3.1. Lehmacher et al.'s Procedure

Lehmacher, Wassmer, and Reitmeir (1991) proposed a step-down closed procedure to determine which of the k endpoints differ in the two treatment groups. Suppose $Z_{\{1,2,\ldots,K\}}$ is conducted at level α at the end of a trial and $H_{0\{1,2,\ldots,K\}}$ is rejected. A step-down closed procedure very similar to that used for multiple comparisons can be applied to find if individual endpoints differ. Consider $Z_{(2,3,\ldots,K\}}$, $Z_{\{1,3,4,\ldots,K\}}, \ldots, Z_{\{1,2,\ldots,K-1\}}$. Whenever one of these rejects at level α, form the global test statistics on each subset of $K-2$ endpoints and test at level α. Whenever the null hypothesis on $K-2$ endpoints is rejected, step down again. Whenever we do not reject, declare that set of endpoints not significantly different and do not continue stepping down. Once a set of endpoints does not differ by one path, endpoints in that set are not considered if they arise via another path.

This step-down closed procedure yields strong control of α and provides a method to find individual endpoints which differ. The procedure may be applied using any of the test statistics described above. Of course, it is possible that a global test statistic rejects $H_{0\{1,2,\ldots,K\}}$ but no individual endpoints differ. This may be an issue of power, but also may be an issue of the correlation between the pairs of endpoints.

3.2. A Procedure with Weak Control of the Overall Type I Error

When $H_{0\{1,2,\ldots,K\}}$ is rejected, we may be interested in testing equality of individual endpoints irrespective of the outcome of the step-down procedure. Such a procedure yields only weak control of the overall type I error; that is, the probability of rejecting the true global null hypothesis that the mean vectors are equal is α, but the type I error for a true subset of the global null hypothesis is not maintained at α.

4. GROUP SEQUENTIAL METHODS IN TRIALS WITH MULTIPLE ENDPOINTS

Several of the aforementioned test statistics have been considered in a group sequential setting. Suppose we undertake analysis of $H_{0\{1,\,2,\ldots,\,K\}}$ at time t based on a global statistic $Z^{(t)}$.

4.1. Asymptotically Normally Distributed Test Statistics with Known Covariance Matrix

With known Σ, Tang et al. (1989a) and Tang et al. (1993) observed that the "ordinary" two-sample group sequential theory could be applied to the linear combination statistics. In 1997 Jennison and Turnbull provided an elegant general theory for application of group sequential procedures for (asymptotically) normally distributed test statistics. The linear combination statistics fall under the Jennison and Turnbull theory (c.f. Jennison and Turnbull, 2000, chaps. 11, 15) as does the (square root of the) Wald-type test of Lefkopoulou and Ryan (1993) as developed here. When the covariance matrix is unknown, it may be estimated from the data, but the implication is that resulting tests are no longer exact.

4.2. Nonnormally Distributed Test Statistics

For test statistics which are not asymptotically normally distributed, a group sequential theory may need to be developed. Jennison and Turnbull (1999) suggest that the sequences of p-values based on normally distributed test statistics provide an adequate approximation in many cases. The ALR statistic of Tang et al. (1989b) and Tang et al. (1993) is an example of a multiple endpoint test statistic with known nonnormal distribution, where, indeed, the sequences of nominal p values for group sequential testing are very close to those of normally distributed test statistics.

4.3. Step-Down Procedures for Group Sequential Trials with Multiple Primary Endpoints

Tang and Geller (1999) extended the Lehmacher et al. (1991) procedure of Section 3 to group sequential trials. Suppose $Z^{(t)}{}_{1,\,2,\ldots,\,K}$ denotes a multiple endpoint test statistic at time t and we have a group sequential boundary $c^{(t)}{}_{1,\,2,\ldots,\,K}$ for $Z^{(t)}{}_{1,\,2,\ldots,\,K}$ at time t.

Proposition 1. The following procedure preserves strong control of the type I error:

Step 1. Conduct interim analyses to test the null hypothesis $H_{0\{1, 2, \ldots, K\}}$ based on a group sequential boundary $\{c^{(t)}{}_{1, 2, \ldots, K}, \mathrm{t} = 1, 2, \ldots, g\}$.

Step 2. When $H_{0\{1, 2, \ldots, K\}}$ is rejected, say at time t^*, stop the trial and apply the step-down closed testing procedure to test all the other null hypotheses $H_{0\mathbf{F}}$, using $Z_{\mathbf{F}}^{(\mathrm{t}^*)}$ and boundaries $c_{\mathbf{F}}^{(\mathrm{t}^*)}$, where **F** is a subset of the indices 1, 2, ..., k.
The procedure in Proposition 1 does not allow for continuation of the trial once a stopping boundary is crossed. However, this is possible using an alternative closed step down procedure given in Proposition 2.

Proposition 2. The following procedure preserves strong control of the type I error:

Step 1. Conduct interim analyses to test the null hypothesis $H_{0\{1, 2, \ldots, K\}}$ based on a group sequential boundary $\{c^{(\mathrm{t})}_{1, 2, \ldots, K}, t = 1, 2, \ldots, g\}$.

Step 2. When $H_{0\{1, 2, \ldots, K\}}$ is rejected, say at time t*, apply the step-down closed testing procedure to test all the other null hypotheses H_{0F} using $Z_{\mathbf{F}}^{(\mathrm{t}^*)}$ and boundaries $c_{\mathbf{F}}^{(\mathrm{t}^*)}$, where **F** is a subset of the indices 1, 2, ..., K.

Step 3. If any hypothesis is not rejected, continue collecting data in the trial to the next interim analysis, at which time the closed testing procedure is repeated, with the previously rejected hypotheses automatically rejected without retesting.

Step 4. Reiterate step 3 until all hypotheses are rejected or the last stage is reached.

In Table 1, we give an illustration of Proposition 2 for four endpoints. All testing is conducted at a fixed significance level α. In this example, the global null hypothesis was rejected at the first analysis time t_1, but no three-endpoint hypotheses were rejected at time t_1. Therefore more data were collected on all endpoints and at time t_2, a second analysis was conducted on the four three-endpoint hypotheses. It is convenient to superscript the hypotheses to indicate the time at which the hypotheses are tested. Of the three endpoint hypotheses at time t_2,

Table 1 Illustration of a Group Sequential Step-Down Procedure Using Proposition 2

Null hypothesis	Test statistic	t_1	t_2	t_3
$H_{0,\ \{1,2,3,4\}}$	Z_{1234}	x	—	—
$H_{0,\ \{1,2,3\}}$	Z_{123}	o	o	o
$H_{0,\ \{2,3,4\}}$	Z_{234}	o	o	o
$H_{0,\ \{1,3,4\}}$	Z_{134}	o	x	—
$H_{0,\ \{1,2,4\}}$	Z_{124}	o	o	o
$H_{0,\ \{1,2\}}$	Z_{12}	—	—	—
$H_{0,\ \{1,3\}}$	Z_{13}	—	x	—
$H_{0,\ \{1,4\}}$	Z_{14}	—	o	o
$H_{0,\ \{2,3\}}$	Z_{23}	—	—	—
$H_{0,\ \{2,4\}}$	Z_{24}	—	—	—
$H_{0,\ \{3,4\}}$	Z_{34}	—	o	o
$H_{0,\ \{1\}}$	Z_1	—	o	x
$H_{0,\ \{2\}}$	Z_2	—	—	—
$H_{0,\ \{3\}}$	Z_3	—	o	o
$H_{0,\ \{4\}}$	Z_4	—	—	—

x = test and reject; o = test and do not reject; — = test not done.

only $H^{(t2)}_{0\{1,\ 3,\ 4\}}$ was rejected, so at time t_2 the step-down procedure was conducted on the three pairs of endpoints {1, 3}, {1, 4} and {3, 4}. Since $H^{(t2)}_{0\{1,\ 3\}}$ was rejected, we conducted the hypothesis tests of $H^{(t2)}_{0\{1\}}$ and $H^{(t2)}_{0\{3\}}$. These were not rejected. We continued collecting data on all endpoints so that at time t_3, we could retest the null hypotheses on endpoints {1, 2, 3}, {2, 3, 4}, and {1, 2, 4}. At time t_3, we also retested $H^{(t3)}_{0\{1,\ 4\}}$ and $H^{(t3)}_{0\{3,\ 4\}}$. $H^{(t3)}_{0\{1,\ 4\}}$ and $H^{(3)}_{0\{3,\ 4\}}$ were not rejected and so we did not step down. Because $H^{(t2)}_{0\{1,\ 3\}}$ was rejected and $H^{(t2)}_{0\{1\}}$ and $H^{(t2)}_{0\{3\}}$ were not rejected, at time t_3 we also tested $H^{(t3)}_{0\{1\}}$ and $H^{(t3)}_{0\{3\}}$. Of these, the first was rejected. The conclusion was that there was a difference in endpoint 1, but not in the other three endpoints.

The complexity of the example of Table 1 illustrates that in practice, the use of Propositions 1 and 2 require certain care. Further, the stopping rule, that is, whether Proposition 1 or 2 will be used, should be decided when the study is planned. This is especially important in using Proposition 2, where one must consider if ethics allow continuing collecting data when a global null hypothesis is rejected. Of course, if single endpoint hypotheses are rejected at an interim analysis, there is no need to continue to collect that endpoint if the trial continues. In contrast to

Proposition 1, Proposition 2 allows continuation of data collection until a difference in at least one individual endpoint is found (or full sample size is reached).

5. AN EXAMPLE: THE NINDS STROKE TRIAL

The NINDS tissue Plasminogen Activator (*t*-PA) trial (sponsored by the National Institute of Neurologic Disorders and Stroke, or NINDS) randomized patients within 6 hours of onset of (nonhemorrhagic) stroke to intravenous *t*-PA or placebo. Recombinant *t*-PA is a thrombolytic agent or "clot buster, " which was believed to be effective in ischemic stroke, although intracerebral hemorrhage had been reported in early trials. Details are found in *The New England Journal of Medicine* (1995) 333, 1581–1587.

Accrual took place between January 1991 and October 1994. The trial was designed with 320 patients in order to have 95% power to detect a 20% improvement in the Bartel Index (Bartel) at 90 days (16% versus 36%) when hypothesis testing was conducted at the $\alpha = .05$ level. Three hundred and thirty-three patients were randomized, and, aside from the Bartel, three other stroke scales at 90 days were of interest, the modified Rankin scale (mod RS), the National Institutes of Health Stroke Scale (NIHSS) and the Glasgow scale (Glasgow). We refer to endpoints 1, 2, 3, 4 to refer to the Bartel, mod RS, NIHSS and the Glasgow scales, respectively.

While the trial was ongoing, the data and safety monitoring board met and decided that for the new treatment to be acceptable, the trial should show a "clear and substantial evidence of an overall improvement." Therefore the endpoints were dichotomized to define "improvement" and the test statistic used for the trial was the Wald test of Lefkopoulou and Ryan based on the four dichotomized endpoints. Two-sided testing was conducted. The results were published in December 1995, indicating the superiority of *t*-PA over placebo with a p value of .008 based on the Lefkopoulou/Ryan statistic. The univariate test results reported by the investigators on the individual endpoints are shown in Table 2. The odds ratio for favorable outcome in *t*-PA group relative to placebo was 1.7 with 95% C.I. 1.2 to 2.6.

We performed a reanalysis of the NINDS *t*-PA trial using the original study data (and two-sided testing to be consistent), assuming that it had been designed as a group sequential trial with analyses planned

Table 2 Results of the t-PA Trial as Reported[a]

	Percent with favorable outcome		
	t-PA	Placebo	Univariate *p* value
Bartel	50	38	.026
Modified RS	39	26	.019
Glasgow	44	32	.025
NIHSS	31	20	.033

[a] Stratification on center and time since onset of stroke.

after the first 100 and 200 patients and at the end of the trial (333 patients) using an O'Brien and Fleming boundary and the Lefkopoulou/Ryan statistic. This implies that the analysis times would be .3, .6, 1.0. The analyses reported here are not adjusted for time of entry and center, whereas those in the *New England Journal of Medicine* paper were.

The Reboussin et al. (1998) program was used to generate two-sided symmetric O'Brien and Fleming boundaries. For three interim analyses, overall $\alpha = .05$ and analysis times .3, .6, and 1.0, Table 3 gives the critical values.

Positive values of the test statistic favor tPA over placebo. For the first interim analysis, at time $t_1 = .3$, $Z^{(t1)}_{1,2,3,4} = 0.77$ (nominal p value .44). Since $Z^{(t1)}_{1,2,3,4}$ did not exceed the first critical value, 3.93, $H_0^{(t1)}$ would not be rejected and the trial would continue. At the second interim analysis at time $t_2 = .6$, $Z^{(t2)}_{1,2,3,4} = 1.44$ (nominal $p = .15$). Since $Z^{(t2)}_{1,2,3,4}$ did not exceed 2.67, $H_0^{(t2)}$ would not be rejected and the trial would continue. At the third and final analysis ($t_3 = 1$), $Z^{(t3)}_{1,2,3,4} = 2.62$ (nominal $p = .0087$). Since $Z^{(t3)}_{1,2,3,4}$ exceeds the third critical value, 1.98, $H_0^{(t3)}$ would be rejected.

Proposition 1 was then used to determine which of the four endpoints differed. The results are shown in Table 4. At the third and final analysis, all hypotheses were rejected by the closed step-down

Table 3 Two-Sided Critical Values, Increment in α, and Cumulative α for Interim Analyses at Times .3, .6, and 1

Time	Critical values	α(i)−α(i−1)	Cumulative α
.3	± 3.9286	.00009	.0009
.6	± 2.6700	.00753	.00762
1	± 1.9810	.04238	.5000

Table 4 Results of the Step-Down Procedure (Reanalysis of the *t*-PA Trial)

Comparison	Z-value (nominal *p* value)	Decision
1. Compare global test statistic based on four endpoints to 1.981.	2.62 (.087)	Reject
2. Step down to all comparisons of three endpoints. Compare each Z to 1.981.		
NIHSS, Bartel, modified RS	2.63 (.009)	Reject
NIHSS, Bartel, Glasgow	2.63 (.009)	Reject
NIHSS, Modified RS, Glasgow	2.59 (.010)	Reject
Bartel, Modified RS, Glasgow	2.50 (.012)	Reject
3. Step down to all comparisons of two endpoints. Compare each Z to 1.981.		
NIHSS, Bartel	2.58 (.010)	Reject
NIHSS, Modified RS	2.61 (.009)	Reject
NIHSS, Glasgow	2.52 (.012)	Reject
Bartel, Modified RS	2.50 (.012)	Reject
Bartel, Glasgow	2.45 (.014)	Reject
Modified RS, Glasgow	2.46 (.014)	Reject
4. Step down to all comparisons of individual endpoints. Compare Z to 1.981.		
Bartel	2.28 (.023)	Reject
Modified RS	2.46 (.014)	Reject
Glasgow	2.35 (.019)	Reject
NIHSS	2.29 (.022)	Reject

procedure. Thus the conclusion was that t-PA was superior to placebo with respect to each of the four stroke scales (with strong control of α). The t-PA investigators reported the global test and the single endpoint nominal p values without performing the intermediate tests. This resulted in weak control of α.

6. EXTENSIONS TO MORE THAN TWO SAMPLES

Follmann et al. (1994) and more recently Hellmich (2001) considered monitoring single endpoint trials which had two or more treatment arms. The spending function approach was generalized and one is allowed to drop treatments which are inferior. Hellmich proved the strong family-wise error control of the sequentially rejective approach proposed by Follmann et al. for the Pocock and O'Brien and Fleming spending function. We observe here that these results would hold whether the trial had a single or multiple endpoints.

Suppose we have A treatment arms which will be compared on multiple endpoints. We test

$$H_{0\{1,2,\ldots,K\}}\colon \mu_1 = \mu_2 = \cdots = \mu_A$$

against an alternative hypothesis, e.g.,

$$H_{A\{1,2,\ldots,K\}}\colon \mu_s - \mu_t = \delta(>0) \qquad \text{for at least one s and all } t \neq s.$$

One can envision different schemes for monitoring such a trial combining the methodology of Hellmich and that here. For this alternative hypothesis and multivariate normally distributed data, one could use a group sequential version of the F test proposed by O'Brien (1984). For other alternative hypotheses, one might use the chi-squared or F tests proposed by Jennison and Turnbull (1991) or Lauter (1996).

For any alternative, one could monitor arms as suggested by Hellmich (2001) until the trial is stopped and follow this by a step-down procedure to determine which endpoints differ. Alternately, one could monitor arms-then-endpoints during the course of the trial. The advantages and disadvantages of various schema have not been investigated. When one is allowed to drop either arms or endpoints during the course of a trial, care needs to be taken that the results are interpretable by clinicians as well as statisticians.

There are other limitations to implementing such methodology at present. There are a limited number of test statistics for combining endpoints of different types (continuous, discrete, censored) and properties of different test statistics in complex settings are not well studied. The adequacy of using the group sequential boundaries of the "normal theory" as approximations when parameters are estimated may be unknown. Further research into the multiple arm and multiple endpoints problem is needed.

7. DISCUSSION

Methodology has been given in this chapter for determining which endpoints differ in a clinical trial with multiple endpoints when group sequential monitoring will occur. We combine step-down procedures with group sequential methods to determine which individual endpoints differ. The theory has many missing pieces, leaving room for further research.

Several points need to be considered in undertaking a clinical trial with multiple endpoints. One-sided hypothesis testing has inherent limitations (whether on one or more endpoints). Endpoints with small univariate test statistics can dilute the significance of the global test statistics. Indeed, the number of endpoints and their correlation structure will determine whether the trial will stop or continue. Examples can be given to show we can cross a boundary with K endpoints, but not with any subset of them, as well as the reverse. Thus, one needs to consider carefully the selection of the multiple endpoints in a particular situation. In particular in designing a trial using multiple endpoints, the plans for analysis, including the test statistic, should be chosen in advance.

ACKNOWLEDGMENTS

We are grateful to the *t*-PA investigators for the use of their data as an example and to Ms. Mei Lu for undertaking the calculations on that data set which are reported here and to Drs. Dean Follmann and Dei-In Tang for comments on this chapter.

REFERENCES

Bloch, D. A., Lai, T. L., Tubert-Bitter, P. (2001). One sided tests in clinical trials with multiple endpoints. Biometrics 57:1039–1047.

Follmann, D. (1995). Multivariate tests for multiple endpoints in clinical trials. Statistics in Medicine 14:1163–1176.

Follmann, D. (1996). A simple multivariate test for one-sided alternatives. Journal of the American Statistical Association 91:854–861.

Follmann, D. A., Proschan, M. A., Geller, N. L. (1994). Monitoring pairwise comparisons in multi-armed clinical trials. Biometrics 50:325–336.

Hellmich, M. (2001). Monitoring clinical trials with multiple endpoints. Biometrics 57:892–897.

Hochberg, Y. (1988). A sharper Bonferroni procedure for multiple tests of significance. Biometrika 75:800–802.

Holm, S. (1979). A simple sequentially rejective multiple test procedure. Scandanavian Journal of Statistics 6:65–70.

Huang, P., Hall, W. J. (2002). Multivariate rank tests for comparing several responses between two samples. Presented at the Eastern North American Region of the Biometrics Society meeting, March 2002.

Jennison, C., Turnbull, B. W. (1991). Exact calculations for sequential t, χ^2 and F tests. Biometrika 78:133–141.

Jennison, C., Turnbull, B. W. (1997). Group-sequential analysis incorporating covariate information. Journal of the American Statistical Association 92:1330–1341.

Jennison, C., Turnbull, B. W. (1999). Group sequential methods with applications to clinical trials. Boca Raton, FL: Chapman & Hall/CRC.

Kudo, A. (1963). A multivariate analogue of the one-sided test. Biometrika 50:403–418.

Lauter, J. (1996). Exact t and F tests for analyzing studies with multiple endpoints. Biometrics 52:964–970.

Lefkopoulou, M., Ryan, L. (1993). Global tests for multiple binary outcomes. Biometrics 49:975–988.

Lehmacher, W., Wassmer, G., Reitmeir, P. (1991). Procedures for two-sample comparisons with multiple endpoint controlling the experimentwise error rate. Biometrics 47:511–521.

O'Brien, P. C. (1984). Procedures for comparing samples with multiple endpoints. Biometrics 40:1079–1087.

Perlman, M. D. (1969). One-sided testing problems in multivariate analysis. Annals of Mathematical Statistics 40:549–567.

Perlman, M. D., Wu, L. (1999). The emperor's new tests, with Comments. Statistical Sciences 14:355–381.

Pocock, S. J., Geller, N. L., Tsiatis, A. A. (1987). The analysis of multiple endpoints in clinical trials. Biometrics 43:487–498.

Reboussin, D. M., DeMets, D. L., Kim, K., Lan, K. L. G. (1998). Programs for computing group sequential boundaries using the Lan-DeMets method Version 2. http://www.biostat.wisc.edu/landemets/.

Sarkar, S. K., Chang, C. -K. (1997). The Simes method for multiple hypothesis testing with positively dependent test statistics. Journal of the American Statistical Association 92:1601–1608.

Simes, R. J. (1986). An improved Bonferroni procedure for multiple tests of significance. Biometrika 73:751–754.

Tang, D. -I., Geller, N. L. (1999). Closed testing procedures for group sequential clinical trials with multiple endpoints. Biometrics 55:1188–1192.

Tang, D. -I., Geller, N. L., Pocock, S. J. (1993). On the design and analysis of randomized clinical trials with multiple endpoints. Biometrics 49:23–30.

Tang, D. -I., Gnecco, C., Geller, N. L. (1989a). Design of group sequential clinical trials with multiple endpoints. Journal of the American Statistical Association 84:776–779.

Tang, D. -I., Gnecco, C., Geller, N. L. (1989b). An approximate likelihood ratio test for a normal mean vector with nonnegative components with application to clinical trials. Biometrika 76:577–583.

The National Institute of Neurological Disorders and Stroke rt-PA Stroke Study Group (1995). Tissue plasminogen activator for acute ischemic stroke. New England Journal of Medicine 333:1581–1587.

Tilley, B. C., Marler, J., Geller, N., Lu, M., Legler, J., Ryan, L., Grotta, J. (1996). Use of a global test for multiple outcomes in stroke trials with application to the National Institute of Neurological Disorders and Stroke t-PA stroke trial. Stroke 27:2136–2141.

Troendle, J. F. (1995). A stepwise resampling method of multiple hypothesis testing. Journal of the American Statistical Association 85:370–378.

Troendle, J. F. (1996). A permutational step-up method of testing multiple outcomes. Biometrics 52:846–859.

Westfall, P. H., Young, S. S. (1993). Resampling-Based Multiple Testing: Examples and Methods for P-Value Adjustment, vol. I. New York: John Wiley.

7
Subgroups and Interactions*

Dean Follmann
National Institute of Allergy and Infectious Diseases, National Institutes of Health, Bethesda, Maryland, U.S.A.

1. INTRODUCTION

Clinical trials are generally not designed to identify if the benefit of treatment differs as a function of patient characteristics. The anticipation is that each randomized group will respond relatively homogeneously and a single pronouncement regarding benefit will suffice for the entire cohort. While one might well expect that different patients will respond somewhat differently, we will not be led astray with a single pronouncement unless some subset of patients is actually harmed by treatment. Thus it seems that for the primary goal of a standard clinical trial, subgroup analyses should be undertaken to confirm that a single pronouncement is justified.

In practice, however, clinical trials involve a substantial investment in resources and there is proper interest in examining the data in some detail. Such exploratory analyses can be useful in suggesting new questions which might be answered in future trials. Estimating how the effect of treatment varies with baseline characteristics may be of interest for a variety of reasons, even if treatment harms no one. For example, some pa-

* This chapter was written by Dean Follmann in his private capacity. The views expressed in the chapter do not necessarily represent the views of NIH, DHHS, or the United States.

tients may appear to receive marginal benefit. Such an observation might lead one to consider a trial for this subgroup where an alternative treatment is evaluated. Also, while clinical trials are designed to answer a clinical question, they can provide insights to nonclinical questions. For example, a treatment may benefit all patients, but there may be a strong differential in this benefit as a function of a baseline covariate. Identifying such a differential may provide insight into the biology of the disease or the mechanism of action of the treatment.

In this chapter we provide a survey of statistical techniques for subgroup analyses and interaction. Our view is that one perspective is appropriate for the paper reporting the main results of the clinical main while another perspective is reasonable for secondary papers. Several excellent papers on the use and abuse of subgroup analyses have been written (see e.g., Yusuf et al. 1991, Oxman and Guyatt 1992, Bulpitt 1988, Simon 1982). They chiefly provide a strong justification for the "main results" view and emphasize the danger in making strong conclusions based on exploratory subgroup analyses. Another useful dichotomy of subgroup analyses has been proposed by Peto (1995) who distinguishes between qualitative interactions, where the treatment is actually harmful to some subgroup of patients and beneficial to other, and quantitative interactions, where the magnitude of treatment benefit varies, but the sign does not. Peto argues that the former are clinically important and rare, while the latter are clinically unimportant and common.

This chapter is organized as follows. We begin by developing standard approaches to subgroups and interaction in a simple setting. We then develop in some detail nonstandard approaches to tests of interaction. We end by discussing some practical issues that were encountered in the AVID clinical trial.

2. STANDARD APPROACHES

Throughout we assume a randomized two-armed clinical trial. To keep matters simple, we will assume that the primary endpoint is continuous, such as diastolic blood pressure (DBP). Our basic arguments apply to other endpoints with obvious modifications. Let Y_i be the endpoint measured on the ith subject where $i = 1, \ldots,$ n. We will use $Z = 1(0)$ to identify the treatment (control) group, and use $\mathbf{X}$ to denote a vector of covariates, e.g. prognostic variables or subgroup identifiers. We assume an equal number of patients in each treatment group.

A standard approach for assessing if treatment has an overall effect is to write

$$Y_i = \beta_0 + \beta_1 Z_i + \varepsilon_i \tag{1}$$

where ε_i is an error term with mean 0 and variance σ^2. For simplicity, we will assume that σ^2 is known. The effect of treatment is $E[Y_i|Z_i = 1] - E[Y_i|Z_i = 0] = \beta_1$, and a test of treatment effect is achieved by testing whether $\beta_1 = 0$.

Subgroup analyses are conducted by applying this model to subsets of the randomized cohort. For example, one might apply (1) to men and women separately. Writing this in a concise form we have

$$Y_i = \beta_0 + \beta_1 Z_i + \beta_2 X_i + \beta_3 X_i Z_i + \varepsilon_i \tag{2}$$

where $X_i = 1$ identifies men. Here the treatment effect among men is given by $\beta_1 + \beta_3$ while the treatment effect among women is β_1. In general, the X_i in (2) can be continuous, or vector valued, even though the term "subgroup" may not be meaningful in these cases. In this more general setting, (2) describes how the effect of treatment varies with X_i.

Figure 1a–c gives graphical examples of three possibilities for (2). In all figures, the symbols denote the mean response at $X = 0$ or 1, while the lines denote the mean response for a continuous $X \in [0, 1]$. Large values of the response indicate a more favorable outcome. In Figure 1a, the benefit of treatment at $X = 0$ is the same as the benefit at $X = 1$. In Figure 1b, there is an interaction, but it is a "quantitative" interaction where there is somewhat greater benefit of treatment at $X = 1$ compared to $X = 0$, but treatment is beneficial at both levels of X. Finally, Figure 1c presents a "qualitative" interaction, where treatment is beneficial at $X = 0$ but harmful for $X = 1$.

At times, one might wish to report the treatment effects separately for different subgroups. This may be because one has an a priori reason to suspect a strong differential, or it may be because the effect in some subgroups is of interest in its own right, e.g., men and women. In this case, it may be appropriate to examine the effects in the subgroups, though more to support the overall conclusion. Occasionally, a study may be adequately powered for a subgroup. For example, the PATHS clinical trial (Cushman et al., 1994) examined the effect of reduced alcohol consumption on the change in DBP, among drinkers with mild to moderate hypertension. In the design of the study a separate power calculation was done for the moderate hypertensive subgroup. In such a case, the results in the adequately powered subgroup are intended to be presented separately. In

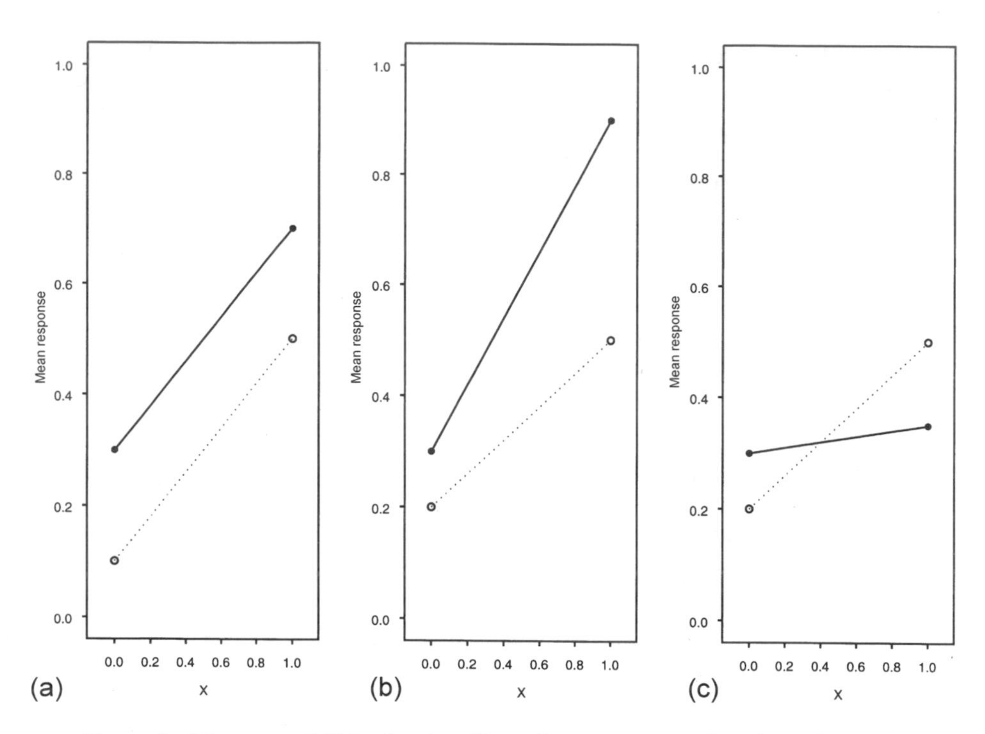

Figure 1 Three possibilities for the effect of treatment as a function of X. Solid circles and lines denote the treatment group; open circles and dashed lines denote the control group. Larger values of the response are more desirable.

general, subgroups need to be interpreted within the context of the trial, other studies, and the biological phenomena being investigated (Yusuf et al., 1991).

Treating a single trial as if it were two separate trials, one for each subgroup, when in fact it was designed as a single study can be very misleading. This point is forcefully made by reexpressing an observation made by Peto (1995). Imagine a clinical trial which has a continuous endpoint and uses the standardized mean difference to test treatment efficacy. Suppose that the mean difference is 2 and the standard error of this difference is known to be 1 so that the overall test of significance, is 2. The p value is just less than .05, so treatment appears efficacious. We're also very interested in two equally sized subgroups, e.g., men and women, and decide to report these separately. We perform the calculations and discover that in men, the test statistic (mean difference divided by standard error) is

$3/\sqrt{2}$ and thus men have a p value of about .03. The overall result and the result in men imply that the test of treatment effect in women is $1/\sqrt{2}$ with associated p value of about .48. It may seem that the answer is clear that men benefit while women do not. However, the chance of seeing a discrepancy in the treatment effects between men and women at least as large as the observed value (i.e., $|3 - 1|/\sqrt{2}$) is about 1 in 3, provided the true effect of treatment is the same in men and women. Even with an overall significant result, simply looking at subgroup p values is likely to suggest heterogeneity in response which may well be due to chance. As argued by Peto (1995), Yusuf et al. (1991), and others, we would generally expect the overall result to provide a better estimate of the effect within subgroups.

Another problem results from trying to identify subgroups for which the treatment effect is significant, when the overall treatment is nonsignificant but with a trend towards significance. It is natural enough to think that surely treatment must have worked somewhere and to feel obliged to identify where. Such tendencies should be avoided. For such trials, the overall type I error has already been used up so that it is unclear what the type I error for subgroups even means here. Nonetheless, such subgroup analyses are sometimes done. Suppose we have two equal sized subgroups, use the standardized mean difference to test efficacy, have equal treatment effects in each subgroup, and, for simplicity, a one-sided hypothesis. Figure 2 graphs the conditional probability of having a p value in one of the two subgroups less than .05 given the overall p value. (Since the overall p value is nonsignificant, it is impossible to have both subgroup p values less than .05, thus this is the probability of one subgroup p value less than .05 and the other subgroup p value greater than .05.) Thus Figure 2 graphs the probability of incorrect discordant conclusions about the treatment effect in the two subgroups. With an overall p value of just greater than .05, the chance of having one subgroup p value less than .05 and the other greater than .05 is nearly .5. Even with an overall p value of .25, the chance of finding one significant and one nonsignificant subgroup is about .10. If several mutually exclusive subgroupings are analyzed the chance of "identifying" a significant subgroup can be quite large. As pointed out by Bulpitt (1988), subgroup analyses showing harm or benefit when a trial does not reveal an overall effect may be particularly misleading.

A statistical method to guard against overinterpreting the results of a trial within subgroups is provided by a test of interaction. In the context of model (2) this amounts to testing whether $\beta_3 = 0$. (In words, we see whether the treatment effect among women equals the treatment effect among men.) Subgroup analyses provide the estimate of treatment effect within a subgroup, albeit with a lot of noise due to the small sample sizes.

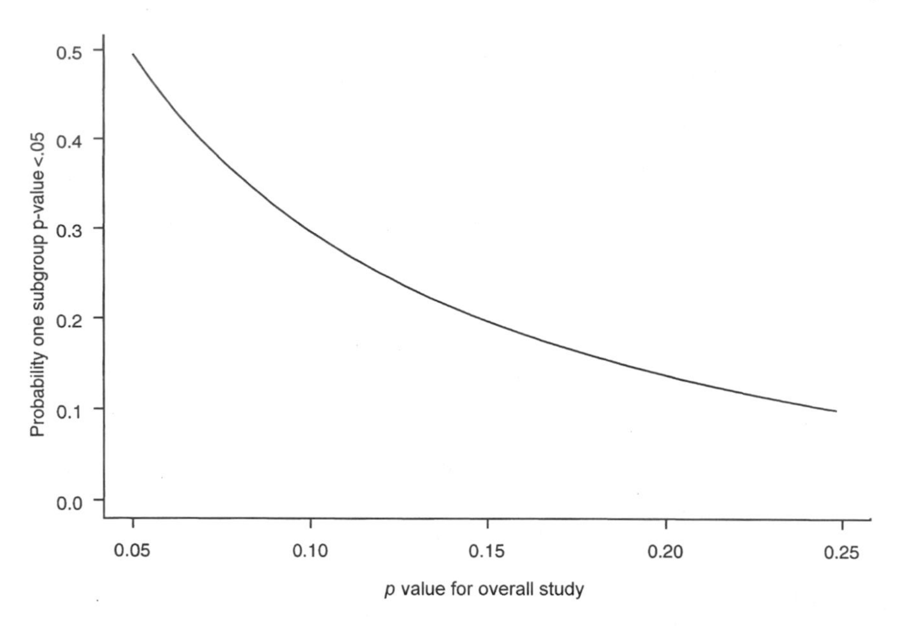

Figure 2 The chance of finding a subgroup with a p value less than .05 conditioned on the p value of the overall trial. Calculation based on two equally sized subgroups with continuous Gaussian response.

A test of interaction is used to determine whether the effect of treatment differs between subgroups. The p value for a test of interaction in the illustration due to Peto is about $1/3$, buttressing the idea than men and women do not differ. Given that a trial is designed for the entire group, it seems more prudent to investigate a differential treatment effect by a test of interaction, than by looking at subgroups in isolation. When reporting the main results of a study, tests of interaction can be used to support the relative homogeneity of treatment effect.

2.1. Power of Tests of Interaction

It is often mentioned that the power for a test of interaction is substantially less than for the test of the overall main effect. The test statistic for the null hypothesis $\beta_1 = 0$ in (1) is

$$\frac{\overline{Y}_1 - \overline{Y}_0}{\sqrt{\sigma^2 4/n}} \tag{3}$$

where $\overline{Y}_j$ is the sample mean in group j. Assuming equal numbers of men and women, with exactly half of each in the treatment group, the test statistic for $\beta_3 = 0$ in (2)

$$\frac{\overline{Y}_{11} - \overline{Y}_{10} - (\overline{Y}_{01} - \overline{Y}_{00})}{\sqrt{\sigma^2 16/n}} \tag{4}$$

where $\overline{Y}_{j\ell}$ is the sample mean for the people in treatment group j with covariate $X = \ell$.

The variance of the numerator of the test statistic for interaction (4) is 4 times greater than that for the test of overall effect (3). If a trial has power equal to .90 to detect an overall effect of treatment equal to δ, the trial will have power equal to about .37 to detect an interaction of size δ. If men and women are not equally numbered, the denominator in (4) is larger and the power is less. Power is .9 to detect interactions of size 2δ. Of course, there is no inherent reason why δ should be a plausible or meaningful difference for the interaction: δ is chosen to be clinically meaningful for the test of overall effect.

In principle one might have marked heterogeneity among patients, and such a differential in treatment effect might be anticipated. However if such marked heterogeneity were recognized during the planning of the trial, one might well choose not to include those patients with the relatively small anticipated treatment effect. The generally poor power of tests of interaction should encourage skepticism when interpreting interactions that are statistically significant. In the design of a standard clinical trial, one's prior opinion is that the result of the study should be applicable to the entire randomized cohort and one should need reasonably strong evidence to be dissuaded from this opinion. For the main results paper, examining interactions and subgroups should be done, but more for assurance that nothing unexpected has occurred.

2.2. Multiplicity

In practice, many characteristics of patients are measured at baseline. If several of these covariates are examined using tests of interaction, as is commonly done, the chance of seeing at least one significant at $p = .05$ is increased, even if the true treatment effect is constant over all baseline covariates. The exact probability of at least one p value less than .05 depends on the number of tests conducted and the correlation between the test statistics. Suppose K tests are conducted which are all independent of each other. The probability of at least one p value less than .05 is $1 - .95^K$. If the tests are so dependent that they are all identical, the probability of at least one p value less than .05 is .05. In practice, the test statistics will have a correlation between 0 and 1 and the true probability of at least one significant p value will lie between 1 - $.95^K$ and .05.

To more accurately gauge the extent of the multiplicity problem, we conducted a small simulation. We imagined a large clinical trial where K tests of interaction were conducted. Since this imaginary trial was large and the treatment effect constant over all subgroups and covariates, the K tests of interaction were approximately univariate normal with mean 0 and variance 1. While in practice the correlation between the various tests would be different, for simplicity we assumed that all tests of interaction had a common correlation ρ. For various values of K and ρ, we generated 100,000 imaginary clinical trials, and recorded the percentage of times that at least one of the test exceeded 1.96 in absolute value. Figure 3 (left panel) presents the results. For 32 independent tests, there is about an 80% false positive rate. This decreases with decreasing number of tests and also decreases as the correlation increases.

A simple correction for this problem of multiplicity is the Bonferroni correction. Recall that

$$P(R_1 \cup \cdots \cup R_K) \leq P(R_1) + \cdots + P(R_K)$$

where R_k denotes rejection of the null hypothesis using covariate k. To ensure that the probability of at least one type I error, i.e., $P(R_1 \cup \cdots \cup R_K)$, is at most α we require $P(R_k) \leq \alpha/K$ for each k. Thus if K tests are conducted, one requires a p value smaller than $.05/K$ to declare significance. Figure 3 (right panel) illustrates the degree of conservatism for this procedure when all tests have equal correlation. We see that the correction is not very conservative provided the common correlation is less than about .4. The degree of conservatism increases with the number of covariates and the correlation. Pocock, Geller, and Tsiatis (1987) make a similar conclusion, but based on an exact calculation rather than simulation.

A simple improvement on the Bonferroni method is the sequentially rejective Bonferroni procedure of Holm (1979). Here one orders the K p values from smallest to largest, say $p_{(1)} \leq p_{(2)} \leq \cdots \leq p_{(K)}$. The smallest p value, $p_{(1)}$ is compared to $.05/K$. If $p_{(1)} \leq .05/K$, we reject the null hypothesis for the associated hypothesis and then compare the second smallest p value $p_{(2)}$ to $.05/(K-1)$. If $p_{(2)} \leq .05/(K-1)$, we then compare the third smallest p value to $.05/(K-2)$ and continue on in this fashion until we cannot reject. This sequentially rejective procedure provides the same protection of the probability of at least 1 type I error, but is more powerful than the Bonferroni method, because smaller critical values are used.

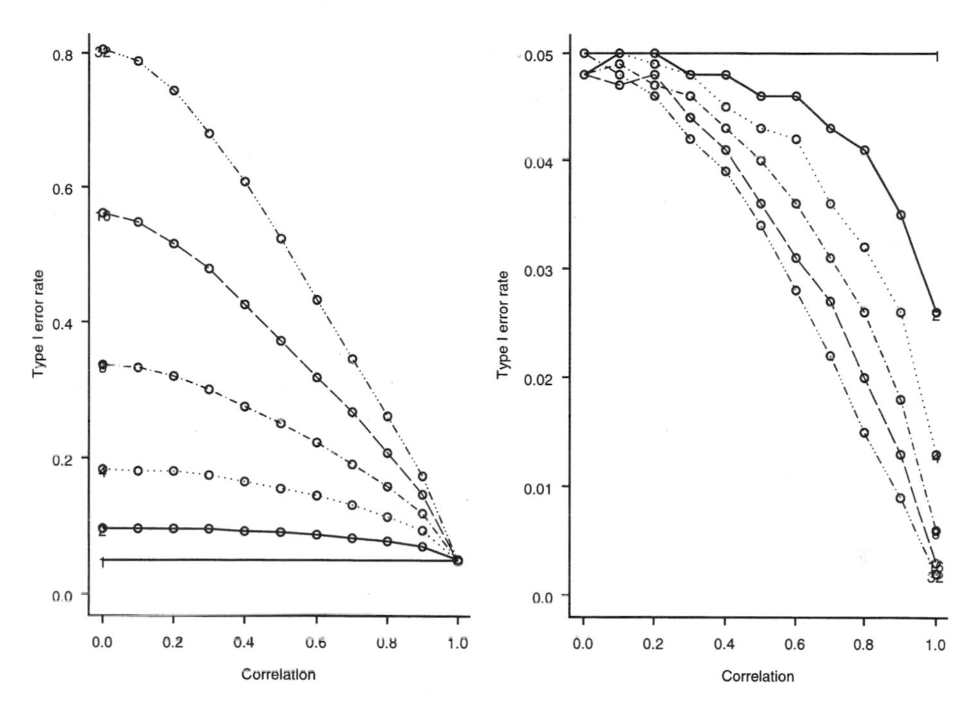

Figure 3 Simulated rejection rates for $K = 2, 4, 8, 16, 32$ tests of interaction as a function of the common correlation between tests. Curves based on interpolation between values at correlation = 0, .1, .2, . . . , .9, 1.0. For the left (right) panel, we reject if any test has a p value smaller than .05 (.05/K). Simulations done under the null hypothesis.

Subgroups and multiplicity were of major concern in the Bypass Angioplasty Revascularization Investigation (BARI) (BARI Investigators, 1996). This study randomized patients with multivessel coronary artery disease in need of revascularization to either coronary-artery bypass graft (CABG) or percutaneous transluminal coronary angioplasty (PTCA). The primary endpoint was total mortality. In the design of the study, five factors were prespecified: severity of angina three possibilities), number of diseased vessels (two or three), left ventricular (LV) function (normal/abnormal), the complexity of the lesions (class C lesion absent/present), and the combination of number of diseased vessels and LV function (four possibilities). These five factors these resulted in 3, 2, 2, 2, and 4 subgroups, respectively.

As is common, BARI was monitored by an independent Data Safety Monitoring Board (DSMB) while the study was ongoing. The DSMB monitored mortality differences between the two groups, overall and for the five factors. While tests of interaction could have been used here, it was decided to monitor within subgroups. In 1992, the DSMB requested that the treatment effect in diabetics and nondiabetics also be monitored as additional subgroups. Due to the concern about multiplicity, a p value of .005 was decided upon as a threshold for the test of treatment effect in the diabetic subgroup.

Before the study was completed, a striking result was observed in the diabetic subgroup: the 5 year survival for CABG as 80.6 percent compared to 65.5 percent for PTCA (nominal $p = .0024$). This was less than the threshold of .005 and these results were disseminated before the completion of followup for the main trial by a Clinical Alert. Because diabetics were chosen as a subgroup a priori and because of the concern about multiplicity, the primary results paper suggested that the result in the diabetic subgroup should be confirmed in other populations. Overall, the 5 year survival rates were 89.3 (CABG) and 86.3 (PTCA), $p = .19$.

After BARI was over, a permutation method was was used to provide an exact p value for the result observed in diabetics, controlling for the multiple subgroups. Based on the 5 initial variables plus the diabetic variable, there were a total of 15 overlapping subgroups. Within each subgroup, a standardized log-rank test statistic was used so that there were 15 test statistics, $T_1, \ldots, T_{15}$. A Bonferroni correction applied to these 15 tests would require a p value less than .05/15 or .0033 to declare significance. Since the nominal p value in diabetics was .0024, a Bonferroni adjusted p value is $15 \times .0024 = .036$. However, the Bonferroni correction is conservative and a simple permutation method was used to provide an exact adjustment for the multiplicity. Under this method, the treatment and control labels were permuted a large number of times and for a generic permutation, say the bth, the vector of test statistics $T_1^{(b)}, , \ldots, T_K^{(b)}$, was calculated as well as $M^b = \max(|T_1^{(b)}|, \ldots, |T_K^{(b)}|)$. By simulation, Brooks et al. (1997) estimated a permutation p value for the diabetic subgroup of .026, i.e. the maximum associated with the original vector of test statistics, $M = \max(|T_1|, \ldots, |T_K|)$, was at the 97.4th percentile of the M^bs. In this analysis, the Bonferroni correction is not very conservative. Strictly speaking, this permutation procedure tests the strong null that treatment has no effect whatsoever, i.e. no overall effect, and no effect in any subgroup. See, e.g., Edgington (1995).

Though we have focused on the impact of multiplicity on testing, multiplicity also has an impact on estimation. If several variables are examined for interactions or subgroups and the single variable with the most extreme value is selected, the estimate of the effect of treatment associated with this variable is likely to be biased. Suppose that K subgroups are examined, and the subgroup with the most extreme estimate of treatment effect singled out. This will provide a biased (away from 0) estimate of treatment effect in that subgroup. The amount of bias depends on the configuration of the true treatment effects in the K subgroups, e.g. $\delta_1, \ldots, \delta_K$. If $\delta_k = \delta$ for all k, the bias is most extreme. Harrell, Lee, and Mark (1996) discuss strategies which produce statistical models with accurate estimates of treatment effect while allowing for differential effects across subgroups or covariates.

3. OTHER APPROACHES TO INTERACTION

In terms of statistical methodology, the standard approaches to subgroups and interaction are quite straightforward as both can be effected by fitting model (2). In this section, we discuss some other methods that may be useful in certain settings.

3.1. Tests of Qualitative Interaction

As argued by Peto and others, quantitative interactions are likely to exist, but are unlikely to be clinically important. Here, treatment causes no harm at any value of X, but may be relatively better for certain values of X compared to other values of X (see Fig. 1b). Unless there were values of X for which treatment was basically the same as control, and treatment were associated with some nontrivial side effects, the clinical implication of a quantitative interaction would be that treatment should be given to anyone satisfying the inclusion criteria of the trial.

On the other hand, qualitative interaction where treatment causes harm for certain values of X is quite clinically important (see Fig. 1c). It seems important therefore to check for qualitative interaction when reporting the main results of the trial. There are two ways of doing this. First, one could check for harm in various subgroups. However, if apparent harm is observed in a specific subgroup (e.g., $p < .05$) it may be due to chance, for reasons of multiplicity as well as the arguments given by Peto (1995). Therefore it seems more logical to perform a formal test of interaction here.

A standard test of interaction [$H_0 : \beta_3 = 0$ in (2)] does not make a distinction between quantitative and qualitative interaction. Thus if β_3 is rejected we only know there is evidence of an interaction, not necessarily a qualitative interaction. If detecting qualitative interaction is of prime concern, it makes sense to apply a non-standard test, specifically derived to detect qualitative interactions. Gail and Simon (1985) proposed such a test which we outline below.

Suppose that there are $k = 1, \ldots, K$ mutually exclusive subgroups. Within each subgroup, let D_k be the estimate of treatment effect. The D_k's are assumed to be normally distributed with mean δ_k and known variance σ_k^2. Gail and Simon's procedure is appropriate even if the D_k's are approximately normal and accurate estimates of $\sigma_k{}^2$ are used. Let $\boldsymbol{\delta} = (\delta_1, \ldots, \delta_K)$. The null hypothesis of no qualitative interaction means that the elements of δ are either all positive (treatment always helpful) or all negative (treatment always harmful). Let $\mathbf{O}^+$ denote the positive orthant $\{\boldsymbol{\delta} \mid \delta_k \geq 0, k = 1, \ldots, K\}$ and $\mathbf{O}^- = -\mathbf{O}^+$ the negative orthant. A likelihood ratio test for

$$H_0: \boldsymbol{\delta} \in \mathbf{O}^+ \cup \mathbf{O}^-$$

versus the complement of H_0 is constructed by taking the ratio of maximized likelihoods under H_A and H_0 and rejecting for large values of this ratio. This reduces to rejecting H_0 if

$$\sum \left(\frac{D_k^2}{\sigma_k^2} \right) I(D_k > 0) > c \qquad \text{and} \qquad \sum \left(\frac{D_k^2}{\sigma_k^2} \right) I(D_k < 0) > c$$

where $I(A)$ is the indicator function for the event A and c is chosen so that the type I error rate is α. Gail and Simon provide critical values for this test for various values of K and α.

A generalization of this test is discussed by Russek-Cohen and Simon (1993), whereby the estimates of treatment effect in the K subsets are allowed to be correlated. Correlated estimates arise in a variety of practical settings. For example, suppose $X \in [0, 1]$ is a continuous covariate and that model (2) is fit. The hypothesis of no qualitative interaction means that the sign of the treatment effect $(\beta_1 + \beta_3 X)$ does not change over $X \in [0, 1]$, or more simply, that the signs of δ_1, δ_2 are the same, where $(\delta_1, \delta_2) = (\beta_1, \beta_1 + \beta_3)$. Thus the setup of Gail and Simon applies, but the estimates of δ_1, δ_2 are correlated.

The approach of Gail and Simon should work best if the treatment is superior to the control for some subgroups and vice versa for other subgroups, but we don't have an idea about the number of harmful subgroups. If control is harmful for only one of a few subgroups while treatment is superior for the remaining subgroups, a more powerful procedure can be developed. Piantadosi and Gail (1993) develop a range test for this setting where the null hypothesis of no qualitative interaction is rejected if both

$$\max \frac{D_k}{\sigma_k} > c' \qquad \text{and} \qquad \min \frac{D_k}{\sigma_k} < -c'.$$

They evaluate the power of this procedure and conclude that for $K = 2$ or 3, there is little difference between the range test and the LRT. For $K > 3$, however, the different tests have more of a differential in performance. If, e.g., $\boldsymbol{\delta} \propto (-1, 1, 1, 1, 1, 1)$, then the range test is preferred, while if $\boldsymbol{\delta} \propto (-1, -1, -1, 1, 1, 1)$ the approach of Gail and Simon is preferred.

3.2. Multivariate Approaches to Interaction

In many settings, it is reasonable to postulate that the effect of treatment may depend on the severity of the underlying disease (see, e.g., Peto 1995; Smith, Egger, and Phillips 1997; Gueyffier et al. 1997; or Friedman, Furberg, and DeMets 1996). Examining for interaction along disease severity may yield insights regarding the mechanism of action of the treatment. For example, sicker patients may benefit more than healthier patients, or sicker patients might benefit less than healthier patients.

A straightforward way to proceed is to identify baseline covariates which are related to severity and to separately test each one for an interaction with treatment. Frequently, however, severity of disease is not really captured by a single variable, but is better determined by a combination of factors. Suppose that a severity score $S_i = \boldsymbol{\beta}' \mathbf{X}_i$ were available on each patient, where $\mathbf{X}_i$ is a vector of baseline covariates and $\boldsymbol{\beta}$ is a vector of parameters. One could imagine that $\boldsymbol{\beta}$ was estimated with an ancillary data set using the model

$$Y_i = \boldsymbol{\beta}'\mathbf{X}_i + \varepsilon_i.$$

If β were known, it would be a simple matter to replace X_i with S_i in (2) and and perform a test of interaction in the usual way.

In practice there is probably no ancillary data set and, to pursue this tack, one needs to both estimate $\boldsymbol{\beta}$ and test for interaction simultaneously. Follmann and Proschan (1999) proposed such a procedure. One postulates

$$Y_i = \beta_0 + \beta_1 Z_i + \boldsymbol{\beta}_2'\mathbf{X}_i + \theta\boldsymbol{\beta}_2'\mathbf{X}_i Z_i + \varepsilon_i \tag{5}$$

where β_0, β_1, $\boldsymbol{\beta}_2$, θ are parameters to be estimated. Under this model, the parameter vector for $\mathbf{X}_i$ in the treatment group ($\theta\boldsymbol{\beta}_2$) is assumed proportional to the parameter vector for $\mathbf{X}_i$ in the control group ($\boldsymbol{\beta}_2$). To test for an interaction along the univariate quantity $\boldsymbol{\beta}_2'\mathbf{X}$, Follmann and Proschan derive the likelihood ratio test for H_0: $\theta = 1$ versus H_α: $\theta \neq 1$.

A simple way to calculate the test statistic is to fit the model

$$Y_i = \beta_{0j} + \boldsymbol{\beta}_{2j}'\mathbf{X}_i + \varepsilon_i \tag{6}$$

in group $j = 0, 1$. Let $\hat{\boldsymbol{\beta}}_{2j}$ be the estimated parameter vector in group $j = 0, 1$, and let $\hat{\Sigma}$ be the average of the control and treatment estimates of the covariance of $\hat{\boldsymbol{\beta}}_{2j}$. Decompose $\hat{\Sigma}$ as $\hat{\Sigma} = \hat{\Sigma}^{1/2}\,[\hat{\Sigma}^{1/2}]'$, and define $\boldsymbol{U}_j = \hat{\Sigma}^{-1/2}\,\hat{\boldsymbol{\beta}}_{2j}$. Minus twice the log of the ratio of likelihoods is

$$T = \frac{\|\mathbf{U}_1 - \mathbf{U}_0\|^2}{2} - \|\mathbf{U}_1 - \hat{\boldsymbol{\mu}}_1\|^2 - \|\mathbf{U}_0 - \hat{\boldsymbol{\mu}}_0\|^2$$

where

$$\hat{\boldsymbol{\mu}}_0 = \frac{a\mathbf{U}_1 + \mathbf{U}_0}{a^2 + 1}$$

$$a = \frac{(R - 1/R) + \sqrt{(R - 1/R)^2 + 4\cos^2(\theta)}}{2\cos(\theta)}$$

$$\hat{\boldsymbol{\mu}}_1 = a\hat{\boldsymbol{\mu}}_0$$

$$R = \frac{\|\mathbf{U}_1\|}{\|\mathbf{U}_0\|}$$

$$\cos(\theta) = \frac{\mathbf{U}_0.\mathbf{U}_1}{\|\mathbf{U}_0\|\,\|\mathbf{U}_1\|}$$

and $\|\boldsymbol{w}\| = \sqrt{w_1^2 + \cdots + w_k^2}$, where $w = (w_1, \ldots, w_k)$. Under the null hypothesis T has an asymptotic chi-square distribution with one degree of freedom and we reject H_0 for large values provided $\boldsymbol{\beta}_2 \neq \mathbf{0}$, If $\boldsymbol{\beta}_2$ is too close to $\mathbf{0}$, or the sample size too small, the chi-square approximation may not be accurate.

The procedure of Follmann and Proschan (1999) will work best if treatment interacts with S_i, or, put another way, if $\boldsymbol{\beta}_{20} \propto \boldsymbol{\beta}_{21}$. If the interactive effect is concentrated in a few elements of $\mathbf{X}_i$, e.g. the element-wise division of $\boldsymbol{\beta}_{20}/\boldsymbol{\beta}_{21} = (a, 1, 1, 1, 1)$, then examining each element of $\mathbf{X}_i$ in turn should be more powerful. Simulations studies confirmed this point.

A different multivariate approach to interaction is suggested by Shuster and van Eys (1983) whereby the vector of covariates $\mathbf{X}_i$ is examined for a region of indifference between treatments and regions of superiority for treatment or control. The case of a single prognostic variable is instructive. Here we fit

$$Y_i = \beta_0 + \beta_1 Z_i + \beta_2 X_i + \beta_3 Z_i X_i + \varepsilon_i. \tag{7}$$

At a specific $X_i = x$, the treatment effect is

$$\Delta(x) = \beta_1 + \beta_3 x.$$

The solution for $\Delta(x) = 0$, say $\hat{x_0}$ is given by $-\hat{\beta}_1/\hat{\beta}_3$. They propose using Fieller's theorem to construct confidence intervals for x_0, say (X_{0L}, X_{0U}). Within the confidence interval, neither treatment is preferred, while outside of the interval, either treatment or control is preferred. Of course, either of the regions outside (X_{0L}, X_{0U}) may be vacuous since X has a restricted range.

Shuster and van Eys discuss generalizing this method to the multivariate setting. Confidence regions for the solutions to $\Delta(x) = 0$ are described. However, there is a multiplicity problem to this approach, as pointed out by Gail and Simon (1985), and the procedure can be very anticonservative.

4. AVID TRIAL

In this section, we apply some of the principles and methods outlined in this chapter to the Antiarrhythmics versus Implantable Defibrillators (AVID) Trial (AVID Investigators, 1997). The AVID study was a randomized clinical trial that enrolled patients with either ventricular fibrillation (VF) or serious sustained ventricular tachycardia (VT). Patients were randomized to treatment by either an implantable cardioverter-defibrillator (ICD) or by an antiarrhythmic drug (AAD). The primary endpoint was all cause mortality. The study planned on enrolling 1200 patients, but was stopped early due to a substantial reduction in mortality associated with the ICD. At study's end, 1016 patients had been randomized.

An important aspect of the AVID study was whether the ICD would be homogeneous in terms of benefit. Thus subgroup analyses were planned at the outset for the following important categories: age, left ventricular ejection fraction (LVEF), arrhythmia due to coronary artery disease (CAD = 1 yes, CAD = 0 no), and type or arrhythmia (VF = 1 due to VF, VF = 0 due to VT). In the main results paper, hazard ratios were graphed for subgroups created on the basis of these four variables.

Three subgroups were created for age (< 60, ≥70, and 60–69), while LVEF was dichotomized (LVEF > .35, LVEF ≤ .35), as were CAD and VF.

Figure 4 displays the hazard ratios along with 95% confidence intervals for these subgroups. The hazard ratios are calculated from a Cox regression model with

$$\lambda(t) = \lambda_0(t)\exp(\beta Z_i)$$

where Z_i identifies treatment group. The above Cox model is applied repeatedly within each subgroup. There are some subgroups for which the confidence interval overlaps 1. If one incorrectly viewed AVID as being separate trials in each of these subgroups, one would conclude that it is not beneficial for LVEF > .35, for causes of arrhythmia other than CAD, and for patients with VT. Such an interpretation does not make sense as the

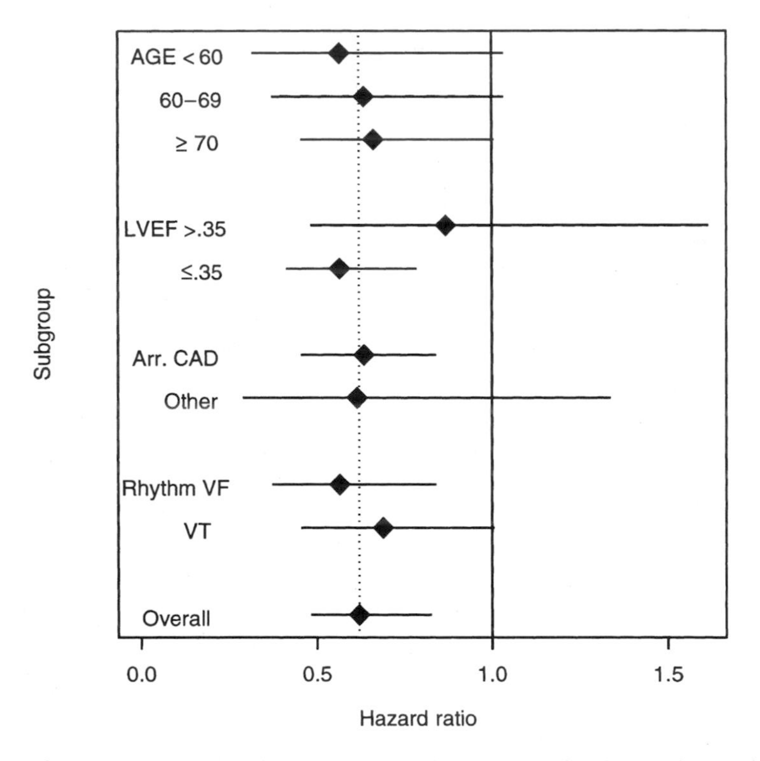

Figure 4 Hazard estimates with confidence bars for four subgroupings of the trial participants of the AVID study. Overall hazard given by dashed vertical line.

study was not designed as separate trials. Indeed, it is not particularly surprising that ICD shows no benefit in each age subgroup. If enough small subgroups are created, tests of treatment effect in each have low power.

A proper interpretation of Figure 4 evaluates the confidence intervals relative to the overall estimated hazard. None of the subgroup confidence intervals excludes .62 suggesting that the effect of treatment is relatively homogeneous. To buttress this impression, we conducted standard tests of interaction for each of the four subgroupings: age, LVEF, CAD, VF. Age and LVEF were treated as continuous covariates, while CAD and VF were binary covariates. For each test of interaction, we fit the Cox regression model:

$$\lambda(t) = \lambda_0(t)\ \exp(\beta_1 Z_i + \beta_2 X_i + \beta_3 X_i Z_i)$$

where X_i was one of the four covariates. Based on this model we tested whether β_3 was equal to 0. The p value for each of the four tests of interaction was at least .10. On the basis of the standard analysis, the effect appears homogeneous as a function of prespecified baseline covariates.

We next apply the other tests of interaction discussed in this chapter. For each of the four methods of subgrouping in Figure 4, the test of Gail and Simon can be applied. However, since the estimate of the log hazard ratio is always negative the condition

$$\sum\left(\frac{D_k^2}{\sigma_k^2}\right) I(D_k > 0) > c \qquad \text{and} \qquad \sum\left(\frac{D_k^2}{\sigma_k^2}\right) I(D_k < 0) > c$$

is satisfied for no c and the test will not reject for any α. The test of Piantadosi and Gail (1993) similarly cannot reject. Intuitively this makes sense. To conclude that a qualitative interaction exists we need to assure ourselves that the point estimates for some subgroups lie well within the region where treatment is harmful while the point estimates for other subgroups lie well within the region where treatment is beneficial. If all point estimates lie in the same region, there is little evidence of a qualitative interaction.

While examining these factors each in turn does not suggest an interaction, it could be that risk varies with the severity of disease. We thus also calculated the test of Follmann and Proschan (1999). The value of the test statistic is .209 which has a p-value of .65. All in all, the main result of AVID seems to be that there is really no evidence of harm of the ICD for anyone and the results of the study can be applied to the overall cohort.

After the main results of AVID were reported, dozens of other manuscripts were prepared. Some of these analyses focused on the effect of subgroups or specifically investigated the effect of treatment as a function of a baseline covariate. A good example of the latter is given by the paper by Domanski et al. (2000) which evaluated the effect of treatment as a function of left ventricular dysfunction. They demonstrated that while the effect of treatment did not interact with baseline ejection fraction, the effect did appear to be somewhat diminished for patients with well preserved LV function. They suggest that further studies of ICD versus antiarrhythmic drugs may be of interest.

5. DISCUSSION

In this chapter we have tried to provide a perspective on conducting tests of interaction and subgroup analyses in clinical trials. In reporting the main results of a clinical trial, it makes sense to be cautious in such analyses. Subgroup analyses should be performed to confirm the lack of clinically important heterogeneity. In secondary papers, exploratory analyses of the effect of treatment for different subgroups may yield useful scientific insights.

ACKNOWLEDGMENTS

I would like to thank Maria Mori Brooks, Al Hallstrom, and Nancy Geller for help in preparing this chapter.

REFERENCES

AVID Investigators (1997). A comparison of antiarrhythmic-drug therapy with implantable defibrillators in patients resuscitated from near-fatal ventricular arrhythmias. The New England Journal of Medicine 337:1576–1583.

BARI Investigators (1996). Comparison of coronary bypass surgery with angioplasty in patients with multivessel disease. The New England Journal of Medicine 335:217–225.

Brooks, M. M., Rosen, A. D., Holubkov, R., Kelsey, S. F., Detre, K. (1997). Treatment comparisons controlling for multiple testing. Controlled Clinical Trials 18:81S.

Bulpitt, C. J. (1988). Subgroup analysis. The Lancet 31–34.

Cushman, W. C., Cutler, J. A., Bingham, S., Harford, T., Hanna, E., Dubbert, P., Collins, J., Dufour, M., Follmann, D. A. (1994). Prevention and treatment of hypertension study (PATHS): Rationale and design. American Journal of Hypertension 7:814–823.

Domanski, M. J., Sakseena, S., Epstein, A. E., Hallstrom, A. P., Brodsky, M. A., Kim, S., Lancaster, S., Schron, E. (2000). Relative effectiveness of the implantable cardioverter-defibrillator and antiarrhythimc drugs in patients with varying degrees of left ventricular dysfunction who have survived malignant ventricular arrhythmias. Journal of the American College of Cardiology 34: 1090–1095.

Edgington, E. S. (1995). Randomization Tests. New York: Marcel Dekker.

Follmann, D. A., Proschan, M. A. (1999). A multivariate test of interaction for use in clinical trials. Biometrics 55:1151–1155.

Friedman, L., Furberg, C., DeMets, D. (1996). Fundamentals of Clinical Trials. St. Louis: Mosby.

Gail, M., Simon, R. (1985). Testing for qualitative interations between treatment effects and patient subsets. Biometrics 41:361–372.

Gueyffier, F., Boutitie, F., Boissel, J.-P., Pocock, S., Coope, J., Cutler, J., Ekbom, T., Fagard, R., Friedman, L., Perry, M., Prineas, R., Schron, E. (1997). Effects of antihypertensive drug treatment on cardiovascular outcomes in women and men. Annals of Internal Medicine 126:761–767.

Harrell, F. E., Lee, K. L., Mark, D. B. (1996). Tutorial in biostatistics: Issues in developing models, evaluating assumptions and adequacy, and measuring and reducing errors. Statistics in Medicine 15:361–387.

Holm, S. (1979). A simple sequentially rejective multiple test procedure. Scandanavian Journal of Statistics 6:65–70.

Oxman, A. D., Guyatt, G. H. (1992). A consumer's guide to subgroup analyses. Annals of Internal Medicine 116:78–84.

Peto, R. (1995). Statistical aspects of cancer trials. In: Price, P., Sikoa, K., eds. Treatment of Cancer. 3rd ed. London: Chapman and Hall, pp. 1039–1043.

Piantadosi, S., Gail, M. H. (1993). A comparison of the power of two tests of qualitative interaction. Statistics in Medicine 12:1239–1248.

Pocock, S. J., Geller, N. L., Tsiatis, A. A. (1987). The analysis of multiple endpoints in clinical trials. Biometrics 43:487–498.

Russek-Cohen, E., Simon, R. M. (1993). Qualitative interactions in multifactor studies. Biometrics 49:467–477.

Shuster, J., van Eys, J. (1983). Interaction between prognostic factors and treatment. Controlled Clinical Trials 4:209–214.

Simon, R. (1982). Patient subsets and variation in therapeutic efficacy. British Journal of Clinical Pharmacology 14:473–482.

Smith, G. D., Egger, M., Phillips, A. N. (1997). Meta-analysis: Beyond the grand mean? British Medical Journal 315:1610–1614.

Yusuf, S., Wittes, J., Probstfield, J., Tyroler, H. A. (1991). Analysis and interpretation of treatment effects in subgroups of patients in randomized clinical trials. Journal of the American Medical Association 266:93–98.

8

A Class of Permutation Tests for Some Two-Sample Survival Data Problems

Joanna H. Shih and Michael P. Fay
National Cancer Institute, National Institutes of Health, Bethesda, Maryland, U.S.A.

1. INTRODUCTION

In clinical trials with right-censored failure time responses, inference goals often focus on comparing the survival distributions of different treatment groups, and the ordinary logrank test (Mantel, 1966) is most commonly used for testing the treatment difference. The appeal of the test comes from its simplicity and being nonparametric in the sense that it does not require specifying the parametric form of the underlying survival distributions. The logrank test is a score test and has full Pitman efficiency under the proportional hazards alternative (Kalbfleisch and Prentice, 1980, p. 106). However, it may lose efficiency under different alternative models. The goal of this chapter is to consider modifications to this standard situation, and to address them with a unifying approach based on a framework of the distribution permutation tests (DPT) (Fay and Shih, 1998; Shih and Fay, 1999). Specifically, we consider cases where the hazards are non-proportional, where the data are interval-censored, and where there is stratification, including the matched-pair case. Although we focus on the two-sample case here, it is straightforward to modify the method to handle K-sample tests and linear permutation tests (see Fay and Shih, 1998). The

DPT tests may be applied whenever the censoring mechanism can be assumed to be independent of the failure mechanism and of the treatment assignment. The advantage of the DPT approach is threefold. First, it presents a unifying approach for all the above situations. Second, when the DPT tests presented here are used on stratified data, they provide good power whether the strata effect is large or small. Thus, there is no need to decide a priori between a traditional stratified test, which gives better efficiency when there is a large strata effect, or an unstratified test, which gives better efficiency when there is little or no strata effect. Finally, exact DPT tests may be calculated for small sample sizes, but asymptotic methods are availible for large sample sizes. There are two disadvantages of the permutation approach; in some situations the assumptions on the censoring may not hold, and the approach cannot make adjustments for covariates as may be needed in some nonrandomized trials.

The DPT framework creates tests by permuting scores based on a functional of estimated distributions for right-, left-, or interval-censored data. The setup is flexible so that by choosing different functionals or estimated distributions new tests can be produced. We will focus on two functionals—the difference in means functional and the weighted Mann-Whitney functional. For stratified data, the estimated distribution function for each observation is based on a shrinkage estimator similar to the nonparametric empirical estimator of Ghosh, Lahiri, and Tiwari (1989), of which we will give the rationale and details later.

The remainder of the chapter is organized as follows. In Section 2, we review the DPT framework for censored, stratified data. In Section 3 we consider the two-sample case without stratification, in Section 4 we consider general stratified data, and in Section 5 we consider the special case of match-pair data. In Sections 3 to 5 we show how to apply the DPTs to each of these situations, and illustrate the methodology with real data. Finally, in Section 6 we reference some work for handling these types of data when the censoring assumptions of the permutation test do not hold.

2. DPT FRAMEWORK

Let X_{ij} and x_{ij} be the random variable and associated response for the jth response of the ith stratum, where $i = 1, \ldots, n$ and $j = 1, \ldots, m_i$. In later sections, we consider applications to special cases; in Section 3 we let $n = 1$ and in Section 5 we let $m_i = 2$ for all i. If the individual is censored, we do not observe x_{ij} but only know that it lies in some interval, say $(L_{ij}, R_{ij}]$. With a slight abuse of notation, we let $R_{ij} = \infty$ for right-censored data and $L_{ij} = \lim_{\varepsilon \to 0} R_{ij} - \varepsilon$ for data that are known, so we can write left-, right-, and interval-censored data in the form $x_{ij} \in (L_{ij}, R_{ij}]$. Thus, we write responses for the ith stratum as $\{y_{ij}\} \equiv \{(L_{ij}, R_{ij}]\}$. Let z_{ij} be the associated treatment assignment and assume that if $z_{ij} = a$ then X_{ij} comes from the distribution Ψ_{ia}, $a = 1, 2$. We assume that the censoring may vary with each stratum but not the treatment. We test the null hypothesis, H_0: $\Psi_{i1} = \Psi_{i2} = \Psi_i$, for all $i = 1, \ldots, n$, against the alternative H_1: $\Psi_{i1} \neq \Psi_{i2}$, for some i.

The DPT has a simple form. We create permutation tests based on a score for each subject. We define the score c_{ij} by

$$c_{ij} = \phi\left(F_{ij|\widehat{\Psi}_i}, \widehat{\Psi}_i\right) \tag{1}$$

where $\widehat{\Psi}_i$ is an estimated distribution for Ψ_i under the null hypothesis,

$$F_{ij|\widehat{\Psi}_i}(s) = \Pr\left[X_{ij} \leq s \mid y_{ij}, z_{ij} = a, \Psi_{ia} = \widehat{\Psi}_i\right]$$

$$= \begin{cases} 0 & \text{if } s < L_{ij} \\ \dfrac{\widehat{\Psi}_i(s) - \widehat{\Psi}_i(L_{ij})}{\widehat{\Psi}_i(R_{ij}) - \widehat{\Psi}_i(L_{ij})} & \text{if } L_{ij} \leq s \leq R_{ij} \\ 1 & \text{if } s > R_{ij} \end{cases}$$

which is the distribution for the jth response of the ith stratum under the null hypothesis given y_{ij} and $\Psi_i = \widehat{\Psi}_i$, and where $\phi(.\,,.)$ is a functional used to compare two distributions. In (1), ϕ is used to compare the individual distribution of a response with the distribution for its stratum. We consider two functionals:

Weighted Mann-Whitney (WMW) functional:

$$\phi_{WMW}(F, G) = \int w(s)G(s)\,dF(s) - \int w(s)F(s)\,dG(s)$$

Difference in means (DiM) functional:

$$\phi_{DiM}(F, G) = \int x\,dF(x) - \int y\,dG(y).$$

When the weight function $w(.) \equiv 1$, the WMW functional becomes the ordinary Mann-Whitney (MW) functional which can also be expressed by

$$\phi_{MW}(F, G) = 2\left\{\Pr(X > Y) + \frac{1}{2}\Pr(X = Y)\right\} - 1$$

where X and Y are the random variables associated with the distributions F and G, respectively.

With a functional chosen, the permutation test is based on the statistic

$$L_0 = \sum_i \sum_j (z_{ij} - \bar{z}_i)(c_{ij} - \bar{c}_i) \tag{2}$$

where $\bar{z}_i = \Sigma_j z_{ij}/m_i$ and $\bar{c}_i = \Sigma_j c_{ij}/m_i$. Under the null hypothesis, c_{ij}'s are exchangeable within each stratum and $E(L_0) = 0$, where the expectation is taken over the permutation distribution induced by the set of all $\prod_{i=1}^{n} m_i!$ possible permutations within each stratum of covariates to scores. The associated variance of L_0 is

$$V = \sum_i \frac{1}{m_i - 1} \left[\sum_j (c_{ij} - \bar{c}_i)^2 \right] \left[\sum_j (z_{ij} - \bar{z}_i)^2 \right].$$

The test statistic is $T = L_0^2/V$. When n and m_i's is are small, we create an exact permutation test. Under regularity conditions and the null hypothesis, as $n \to \infty$ or $\min_{1 \leq i \leq n}(m_i) \to \infty$, T is asymptotically distributed as χ^2 with 1 degree of freedom (Sen, 1985).

To understand how the DPT works, consider a simple case where $n = 1$ and x_{ij}'s are observed (i.e., we have two independent samples without censoring). If we use the empirical distribution for $\widehat{\Psi}_1$, the distribution of x_{1j} under H_0, then $F_{1j|\widehat{\Psi}_1}$ has point mass at x_{1j}. With the DiM functional, $c_{1j} = x_{1j} - \bar{x}_1$, where $\bar{x}_i = \Sigma_j x_{ij}/m_i$. The test statistic compares the mean difference in the two samples, and the permutations are done by permuting the treatment assignments. The test statistic $\sqrt{T}$ is similar to the conventional t-test but with the sample variance calculated about the overall mean.

Rank tests can also be generated using the DPT. For example, a generalization of the Wilcoxon rank sum test that fits the DPT uses the Mann-Whitney functional for ϕ. The Mann-Whitney scores c_{1j} under no censoring are linearly related to the midranks, which are the standard ranks that are averaged at tied values. Thus the test statistic compares the rank sum difference in the two samples, and the permutations are done by permuting the treatment assignments to the midranks.

The DPT framework is flexible. It creates different tests with different choices of ϕ and $\widehat{\Psi}_i$'s. In the sequel, we apply the DPTs with ϕ and $\widehat{\Psi}_i$ chosen to provide good power.

3. TWO INDEPENDENT SAMPLES

As mentioned earlier, for the case of two independent samples, the ordinary logrank test is commonly used and has full Pitman efficiency when the assumption of proportional hazards holds. However, the logrank test may lose efficiency when the assumption is violated. For example, when the difference of the two hazards decreases with time, the Wilcoxon statistic (Peto and Peto, 1972) is more efficient than the logrank test. When the two hazards cross, the logrank test may have more efficiency loss than alternative tests. Pepe and Fleming (1989) generalized the Z test to right-censored data by introducing the class of tests known as weighted Kaplan-Meier (WKM) statistics. Petroni and Wolfe (1994) generalized the WKM tests to interval-censored data. They call these tests IWD tests since the tests compare the integrated weighted difference between the survival estimators from the two samples. Numerical studies (Pepe and Fleming, 1989; Petroni and Wolfe, 1994) indicate that the IWD tests compare favorably with the logrank test even under the proportional hazards alternative, and may perform better than the logrank test under some crossing hazards alternatives.

The permutation form of the Wilcoxon, logrank, and Z test or t test (the permutation forms of the Z test and t test are equivalent) for censored data may be obtained from the DPTs with certain choices of the functionals and using a censored data estimator for Ψ_1. Unlike the IWD statistics which apply only to data with large samples, these permutation tests allow for exact tests for small sample sizes. In the following, we first consider estimation of Ψ_1, then consider the three functional choices.

3.1. Estimation of Ψ_1

When there is only one stratum, we use the nonparametric maximum likelihood estimate (NPMLE), $\tilde{\Psi}_1$, for $\hat{\Psi}_1$. If there is no censoring, then $\tilde{\Psi}_1$ is equal to the empirical distribution function and $F_{1j|\tilde{\Psi}_1}$ has point mass at x_{1j}. For right-censored data, $1 - \tilde{\Psi}_1$ is the usual Kaplan-Meier survival estimator. More generally, the NPMLE can be found iteratively by the self-consistent algorithm (Turnbull, 1976) a special case of the EM-algorithm (Dempster, Laird, and Rubin, 1977) or by the iterative convex minorant algorithm (Groeneboom and Wellner, 1992). We describe a simple self-consistent (or EM) algorithm to find $\tilde{\Psi}_1$. First, partition the response space into disjoint intervals, $(s_0, s_1], (s_1, s_2], \ldots, (s_{m-1}, s_m]$, such that $L_{ij} \in \{s_0, \ldots, s_{m-1}\}$ and $R_{ij} \in \{s_1, \ldots, s_m\}$. Given the bth estimate of $\Psi_1, \hat{\Psi}_1^{(b)}$, the E step of the EM algorithm assigns $F_{1j|\widehat{\Psi}_1^{(b)}}(s_k)$ for all $j = 1, \ldots, m_1$, and $k = 1, \ldots, m$. The M step is

$$\widehat{\Psi}_1^{(b+1)}(s_k) = m_1^{-1} \sum_j F_{1j|\widehat{\Psi}_1^{(b)}}(s_k) \qquad \text{for k} = 1, \ldots, \text{m}.$$

In practice, we use the self-consistent algorithm with some computational modifications (see Aragón and Eberly, 1992; and Gentleman and Geyer, 1994).

3.2. Tests

Wilcoxon Test

With no censoring, the Wilcoxon test may be derived from a score test on a shift in a logistic distribution based on the marginal likelihood of the ranks. The Wilcoxon test may be generalized to right-censored data, using either the marginal likelihood of the ranks (Prentice, 1978) or using the grouped continuous model (Peto and Peto, 1972). Both formulations give similar results and it is the latter formulation that produces the scores associated with the Mann-Whitney functional here. Fay and Shih (1998) show that the Mann-Whitney scores have the simple form

$$c_{1j} = \phi_{\mathrm{MW}}\left(F_{1j\,|\,\tilde{\Psi}_1}, \tilde{\Psi}_1\right) = \tilde{\Psi}_1(R_{1j}) + \tilde{\Psi}_1(L_{1j}) - 1.$$

The Wilcoxon test is efficient in detecting the early difference of the hazards (Fleming and Harrington, 1991).

Logrank Test

The logrank test may be derived as a score test from the proportional hazards model. As in the Wilcoxon case, when censoring occurs, two different forms of the test can be created depending on the assumed likelihood. For a detailed discussion on the two forms of the test as applied to both right-censored and interval-censored data see Fay (1999). In practice, both forms give similar results. Fay and Shih (1998) show that using the grouped continuous model and with a suitable choice of the weight function for the weighted Mann-Whitney functional, we can obtain a permutation form of the logrank test. The score has the expression

$$c_{1j} = \phi_{\mathrm{LR}}\left(F_{1j|\,\tilde{\Psi}_1}, \tilde{\Psi}_1\right) = \frac{\tilde{S}_1(R_{1j})\log\left[\tilde{S}_1(R_{1j})\right] - \tilde{S}_1(L_{1j})\log\left[\tilde{S}_1(L_{1j})\right]}{\tilde{S}_1(R_{1j}) - \tilde{S}_1(L_{1j})}$$

where we let $\tilde{S}_1(s) = 1 - \tilde{\Psi}_1(s)$ and we define $0 \log 0 = 0$.

Difference in Means Test

A permutation form of an unweighted IWD test may be obtained when the DPT with the DiM functional is applied to censored data. Inserting $F_{1j|\tilde{\Psi}_1}$ and $\tilde{\Psi}_1$ to the DiM functional, we obtain the score

$$c_{1j} = \sum_{k=1}^{m} s_k \left\{ \frac{\alpha_{1jk}}{\tilde{\Psi}_1(R_{1j}) - \tilde{\Psi}_1(L_{1j})} - 1 \right\} \{ \tilde{\Psi}_1(s_k) - \tilde{\Psi}_1(s_{k-1}) \}$$

where

$$\alpha_{ijk} = \begin{cases} 1 & \text{if } L_{ij} < s_k \leq R_{ij} \\ 0 & \text{otherwise.} \end{cases}$$

If $s_m = \infty$ and $\tilde{\Psi}(s_m) - \tilde{\Psi}(s_{m-1}) > 0$, then we let $s_m = s_{m-1}$ [but we do not change the value of $\tilde{\Psi}_1(s_m)$]. This modification is common for right-censored data (Efron 1967; James 1987). The IWD test usually gives lower weights to the smaller values of the survival function estimates because of their high variablity due to censoring. Because the DPTs are permutation tests and the instability does not affect the validity, we need not introduce weights to stabilize the test statistic. Fay and Shih (1998) show through simulations that the DPT with the DiM functional is more stable than the both an unweighted and a weighted IWD test.

3.3. Examples

We show two data examples below to emphasize the differences between the choices for the functional. In practice, only one test would be performed, and this test would be chosen prior to any data analysis and, ideally, prior to any data collection.

Example 1: Gastrointestinal Tumor Study

These data were previously analyzed by Stablein and Koutrouvelis (1985). The study reported on the results of a trial comparing chemotherapy versus combined chemotherapy and radiation therapy in the treatment of locally unresectable gastric cancer. There are 45 patients in each treatment group. Figure 1 displays the Kaplan-Meier survival curves. The two survival curves cross, suggesting that the DPT using the DiM functional may not be able to detect the difference, because the means, which are the areas under the survival curves, are similar. The crossing of the survival curves implies that the corresponding hazards also cross at some point before the survival

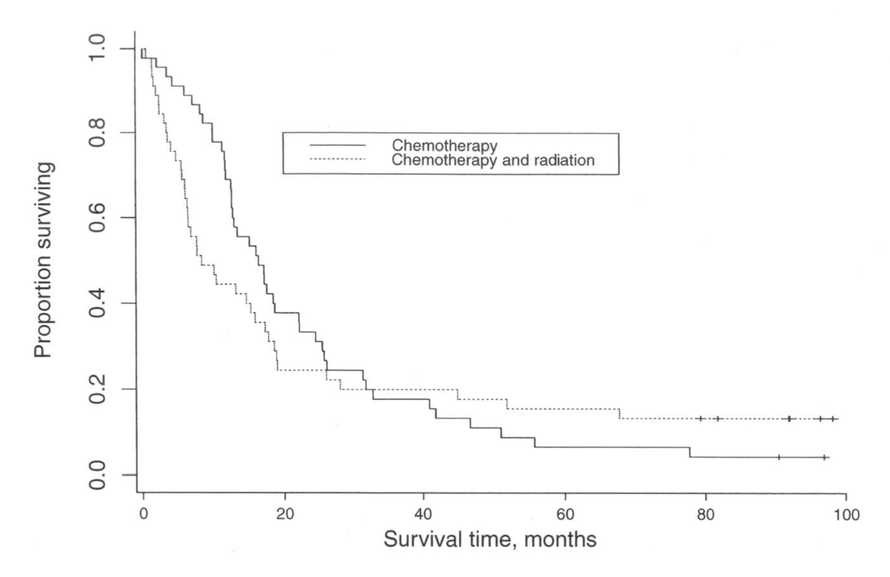

Figure 1 Kaplan-Meier estimate of the survival distribution for the gastrointestinal tumor study.

curves cross. Thus, the logrank test may not capture the difference in survival in the two treatment groups either. Figure 1 shows that a large difference in survival occurs during the early follow-up suggesting the Wilcoxon test is more suitable in detecting such a difference. The DPT using the DiM, MW, and logrank functionals result in asymptotic p values of .97, .05, and .66 respectively. Thus, only the DPT using the MW functional gives a significant result.

Example 2: Breast Cosmesis Study

For this data set, described in Finkelstein and Wolfe (1985), breast cancer patients were randomized to either radiation therapy with chemotherapy or radiation therapy alone. The outcome was time until the onset of breast retraction. A total of 94 patients were followed and were seen, on average, every 4–6 months. The frequency of visits decreased with increasing time from the completion of treatment. Forty percent of the patients had not experienced retraction by the time of their final visit and therefore were right-censored. The data are interval-censored because the time until occur-

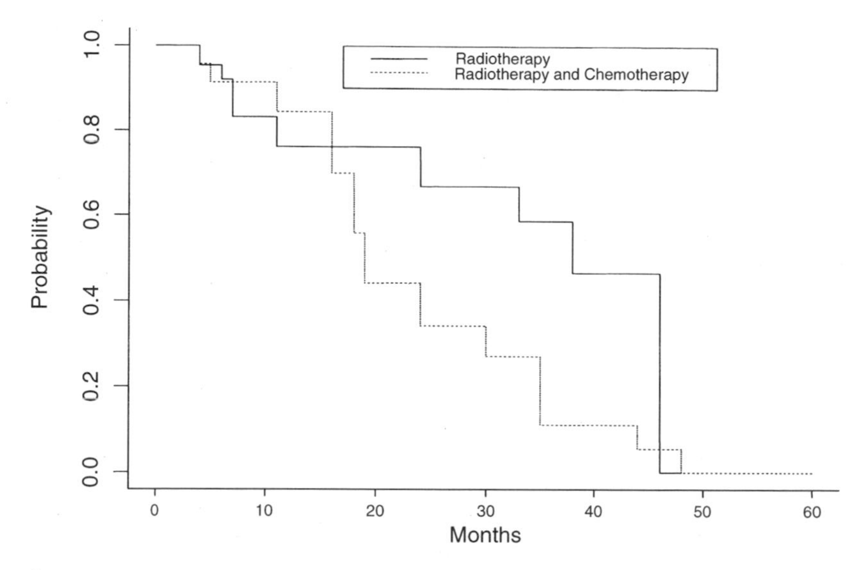

Figure 2 Self-consistent estimate of the survival distribution for the breast cosmesis study.

ence of breast retraction was not known exactly but only known to have occured between two visits. In addition, the time between visits was irregular and many patients missed visits. Figure 2 is a plot of the self-consistent survival estimates for each treatment. Although the two survival curves cross, the crossing occurs very early and thus wouldn't have much effect on the performance of any of these tests. The DPTs apply to the interval-censored data directly without requiring any modification. The DPT using the MW functional, WMW (logrank) functional, and the DiM functional yield asymptotic p values of .030, .007, and .019 respectively. Thus, the three tests all produce significant results.

4. STRATIFIED DATA

In clinical studies when survival changes with important prognostic factors, stratification on different level of those factors is often done either at the design stage to ensure treatment balance in each stratum, or at the analysis stage. The ordinary logrank test, ignoring strata effect, is conservative and is biased when there is treatment imbalance in each prognostic subgroup. The stratified logrank test, on the other hand, is unbiased and retains high efficiency as long as the number of strata is small. However, when the number of strata gets large, the stratified test can become very inefficient unless there is a large strata effect. Shih and Fay (1999) have developed a versatile test based on the DPT framework which combines the advantages of both the ordinary and stratified logrank tests. That is, when the number of observations in each stratum is large or when the within-strata variance is small relative to the between-strata variance, the test weights each stratum approximately equally and performs like the stratified logrank test. Conversely, when the within-strata variance is large relative to the between-strata variance, the test weights each stratum proportional to the stratum size and performs like the ordinary logrank test. For cases between these two extremes, the versatile test is a compromise between the ordinary logrank and stratified logrank tests. The attractive feature of the proposed method is that we do not need to choose in advance whether to do a stratified analysis or not and hope that the correct decision was made; the method automatically does this primarily based on the estimated within- and between-strata variances.

The DPT setup is the same as above, but now we choose an appropriate estimator for Ψ_i, $i = 1, \ldots, n$, when $n > 1$. Once chosen, this estimator is inserted in (1) to calculate the scores c_{ij} and then the test statistic (2).

4.1. Estimation of Ψ_i

We consider the following shrinkage estimator for Ψ_i, $i = 1, \ldots, n, n > 1$,

$$\widehat{\Psi}_i = w_i \tilde{\Psi}_i + (1 - w_i) \left\{ \frac{\sum_j w_j \tilde{\Psi}_j^*}{\sum_k w_k} \right\} \tag{3}$$

where $\tilde{\Psi}_i$ is the NPMLE for the ith stratum $\tilde{\Psi}_i^* = m_i^{-1} \sum_j F_{ij|\dot{\Psi}}$, $\dot{\Psi}$ is the NPMLE for all the data ignoring the strata, $w_i = m_i/(m_i + \hat{\tau})$, $\hat{\tau} = \hat{\sigma}^2/\hat{D}$ if $\hat{D} > 0$, and $\hat{\sigma}^2$ and $\hat{D}$ defined below, are the estimates of the within-cluster (i.e., strata) variance, σ^2, and between-cluster variance, D. When $\hat{D} \leq 0$, following Fay and Shih (1998), $\widehat{\Psi}_i$ is defined as $\widehat{\Psi}_i = \frac{\Sigma_j m_j \tilde{\Psi}_j^*}{\Sigma_k m_k} = \dot{\Psi}$. The above shrinkage estimator is slightly different from the one in Shih and Fay (1999) where $\tilde{\Psi}_j$ is used in place of $\tilde{\Psi}_j^*$. The two shrinkage estimators are identical for uncensored data, but are slightly different for censored data. For example, when $w_i \to 0$, (3) approaches $\dot{\Psi}$, but the estimator in Shih and Fay (1999) approaches $\sum_j m_j \tilde{\Psi}_j / \sum m_j$.

In the absence of censoring, the above estimator is the shrinkage estimator proposed by Ghosh, Lahiri, and Tiwari (1989), where $\tilde{\Psi}_i$ is the empirical distribution function for the ith stratum,

$$\hat{\sigma}^2 = \frac{\sum_{i=1}^{n} \sum_{j=1}^{m_i} \left(x_{ij} - \overline{x}_i\right)^2}{\sum (m_i - 1)}$$

$$\hat{D} = \frac{\left\{\sum m_i \left(\overline{x}_i - \overline{x}\right)^2\right\} - (n-1)\hat{\sigma}^2}{\sum m_i - \sum m_i^2 / \sum m_i}$$

where $\overline{x}_i$ is the mean of the ith strata and $\overline{x}$ is the overall mean. In the presence of censoring, since x_{ij} is not observed, $\hat{\sigma}^2$ and $\hat{D}$ are modified such that

$$\hat{\sigma}^2 = \frac{\sum_{i=1}^{n} \sum_{j=1}^{m_i} \mathrm{E}_{F_{ij|\dot{\Psi}}} \left(X_{ij} - \dot{\overline{x}}_i\right)^2}{\sum (m_i - 1)}$$

and

$$\hat{D} = \frac{\left\{\sum m_l (\dot{\overline{x}}_l - \dot{\overline{x}})^2\right\} - (n - 1)\hat{\sigma}^2}{\sum m_i - \sum m_i^2 / \sum m_i}$$

where $\dot{x}_{ij} = \mathrm{E}_{F_{ij|\dot{\Psi}}}(X_{ij}) = \sum_k s_k [F_{ij|\dot{\Psi}}(s_k) - F_{ij|\dot{\Psi}}(s_{k-1})]$, $\dot{\overline{x}}_l = m_i^{-1} \sum_j \dot{x}_{ij}$, and $\dot{\overline{x}} = (\sum m_i)^{-1} \sum_i \sum_j \dot{x}_{ij}$ and $\dot{\Psi}$ is the NPMLE for all the data ignoring the strata. We use Ψ instead of Ψ_i because when the number in each stratum is small, $\tilde{\Psi}_i$ shows little within stratum differences if the censoring intervals overlap.

The above estimates of σ^2 and D are not rank invariant. They would be used with tests using the difference in means functional. For rank tests, we transform the response to a function of the ranks by replacing $F_{ij|\dot{\Psi}}$ with F_{ij}^*, where $F_{ij}^*(s^*) = F_{ij|\dot{\Psi}}(s)$, $s^* = \phi_{MW}(\delta_s, |\dot{\Psi})$, and $\delta_s(x) = 1$ if $x \geq s$ and zero otherwise. When there is no censoring, the effect of the transformation is equivalent to replacing each x_{ij} with its midrank from the entire data ignoring strata.

Once the values for $\widehat{\Psi}_i$ are calculated, the calculation of the scores, c_{ij}, proceeds analogously to the calculations in Section 3. Thus, the logrank scores are

$$c_{ij} = \phi_{LR}\left(F_{ij|\widehat{\Psi}_i}, \widehat{\Psi}_i\right) = \frac{\hat{S}_i(R_{ij}) \log\left[\hat{S}_i(R_{ij})\right] - \hat{S}_i(L_{ij}) \log\left[\hat{S}_i(L_{ij})\right]}{\hat{S}_i(R_{ij}) - \hat{S}_i(L_{ij})} \tag{4}$$

where $\hat{S}_i(s) = 1 - \widehat{\Psi}_i(s)$, and the Mann-Whitney scores are

$$c_{ij} = \phi_{\text{MW}}\left(F_{ij|\widehat{\Psi}_i}, \widehat{\Psi}_i\right) = \widehat{\Psi}_i\left(R_{ij}\right) + \widehat{\Psi}_i\left(L_{ij}\right) - 1.$$

4.2. Features

An advantage of using $\widehat{\Psi}_i$ is that it induces the desired features of a versatile test. Consider a permutation form of the logrank test corresponding to the DPT with the WMW functional. If $\hat{\sigma}^2$ is small relative to $\hat{D}$ or m_i is large, then $w_i \to 1$, and $\widehat{\Psi}_i$ approaches the NPMLE $\tilde{\Psi}_1$. Thus L_0 is equal to the permutation form of a stratified logrank test. Conversely, if $\hat{\sigma}^2$ is large relative to $\hat{D}$, w_i is close to zero and $\widehat{\Psi}_i$ approaches $\dot{\Psi}$, the NPMLE for all the data ignoring strata. Consequently, the induced test is just a stratified permutation of an ordinary logrank test. That is, each score is calculated from all the data ignoring strata and then permutation is done within each stratum. We call this latter test the MC test because a similar test was proposed by Mantel and Ciminera (1979). (The only difference is that they use the other form of the logrank scores, see Section 3.2.)

We conducted a simulation study which compares the versatile test with three tests: permutation forms of the ordinary logrank test, stratified logrank test, and the MC permutation test. All simulations have 1000 replicates and test the equality of two treament effects. Each survival time has the following form: if $z_{ij} = a$, $a = 1, 2$, let Pr $(X_{ij} > x_{ij}) =$ (exp $(-\theta_a\beta_i x_{ij})$, where $\theta_1 = 1$, $\theta_2 = 2.4$. Let $\beta_i \equiv G(1/\omega,\omega)$, where $G(a, b)$ is a gamma distribution with mean ab and variance ab^2. We choose $\omega = 0$, .22, .86, 2 corresponding to values of 0, .01, .3, .5 respectively for Kendall's tau, where we define the distribution with $\omega = 0$ as a point mass at 1. The stratum size m_i is random were $m_i - 1$ follows a Poisson distribution with parameter $\gamma - 1$, such that $E(m_i) = \gamma$. In each stratum, half of the individuals receive one treatment. We introduce right-censoring which is uniformly distributed over (0, 1), producing 51, 53, 60, and 66% censoring for the four values of ω, respectively. We use the critical value based on the asymptotic permutation distribution.

Table 1 presents the simulated power. Overall, when there is no or only a small strata effect, the stratified logrank test has high efficiency loss unless the strata size is large. On the other hand, the ordinary logrank test retains high efficiency when the strata effect is small, but loses efficiency when the strata effect is large. The MC test and the versatile test are comparable for moderate strata effect, and the latter has higher power for a large strata effect. Both tests have the advantages of ordinary and

Table 1 Empirical Power at .05 Level with Uniform (0, 1) Right-Censoring and 1000 Replicates

$E(m_i)$, n	Strata effect ω	Ordinary LR	Stratified LR	MC	T
5, 20	0	84.4	71.3	82.0	81.9
	0.22	77.7	68.6	75.7	76.1
	0.86	61.9	63.4	67.0	69.3
	2.0	38.5	50.9	51.4	55.7
20, 5	0	83.4	78.6	81.7	81.7
	0.22	77.1	77.5	79.1	79.1
	0.86	60.2	70.6	67.4	71.8
	2.0	40.6	61.2	53.4	62.2
50, 2	0	85.4	84.1	85.4	85.2
	0.22	75.8	77.1	77.7	77.5
	0.86	63.7	73.5	70.1	73.8
	2.0	46.6	59.1	55.6	58.9

stratified logrank tests. That is, when the strata effect is small, they perform like the ordinary logrank test. And when the strata effect gets large, they perform like the stratified logrank test.

4.3. Example 3: Prostate Cancer Clinical Trial

This example concerns a VACURG (Veterans Administration Cooperative Urological Research Group) prostate treatment study. This study was the first of a series of multicenter randomized clinical trials to study treatments for newly diagnosed prostate cancer (see Byar and Corle, 1988 and references therein). Here, we reanalyze a subset of study I of those trials, where 299 patients were randomized to either radical prostatectomy and placebo, or radical prostatectomy and 5.0 mg diethylstilbestrol (DES) daily. The primary endpoint was death from any cause. Patients entered study I from 1960 until 1967, and here we have followup for patients until February 1995. We compare patients in the initial treatment groups, under an intent-to-treat analysis, noting that clinicians were free to change treatments at their discretion.

In these data, all patients had either stage I or stage II prostate cancer, defined prior to randomization. In these two stages the cancer is confined to the prostate, and the stages are differentiated by whether the tumor is detectable (stage II) or not (stage I) by rectal examination (standard staging for prostate cancer has changed since that time; see AJCC Cancer Staging Manual, 1997). Although stage I describes less severe cancer, the survival of the patients in stage I may be worse due to the differing methods of selecting patients in the two stages (Byar and Corle, 1988). For our analysis we use six strata, three age groups in each of the two stages, where we categorize age at randomization into three categories, < 65, 65–70, ≥ 70. This stratification and analysis is a reasonable one that could have been planned prior to the start of the study. The sample sizes in the 6 strata range from 29 to 54, and the values of $\hat{\sigma}^2$ and $\hat{D}$ are equal to .3295 and .0061, respectively. The resulting weights for the six strata range from .35 to .60. Since the protocol allowed modification of treatment after randomization, we expect the differences between treatments to become diluted as more time elapses from the randomization time. For this reason, we use the permutation form of the Peto-Prentice-Wilcoxon (PPW) test that emphasizes early differences. The resulting asymptotic p values for the ordinary PPW test, stratified PPW test, MC test, and the versatile test are .12, .12, .11, and .11, respectively.

5. MATCHED-PAIR DATA

In comparing the treatment effects, the two samples may be correlated either by design or by natural pairing. For example, in the Diabetic Retinopathy Study (Huster et al., 1989), patients with diabetic retinopathy in both eyes and visual acuity of 20/100 or better in both eyes were eligible for the study. One eye of each patient was randomly selected for treatment and the other eye was observed without treatment. Since each pair is considered a stratum, the versatile test described in the previous section applies. The purpose of this section is to relate the versatile test to many known tests for matched-pair survival data. In addition, we investigate a new test using the DPT with the DiM functional for matched-pair survival data.

5.1. Rank Tests

When the versatile test using the MW functional is applied to the matched-pair data with each stratum corresponding to a pair and $w_i = 1$ (i.e., no pooling over strata in estimating Ψ_i), the test is a sign test in the absence of censoring. When $w_i = 0$, it is similar to a permutation form of the paired Wilcoxon test by O'Brien and Fleming (1987). With the WMW functional corresponding to the logrank score and with $w_i = 1$, the versatile test is a stratified logrank test which also reduces to the sign test under no censoring, and with $w_i = 0$, it is similar to a permutation form of the paired logrank test by Mantel and Ciminera (1979). The simulation study (results not displayed) shows that with the WMW functional corresponding to the logrank test, the versatile test and the MC test have similar performance. Their power is similar to that of the ordinary logrank when the strata effect is small and higher than the stratified logrank test when the strata effect is large. Based on this simulation result and because of the simplicity, we recommend the use of the paired DPT test with $w_i = 0$ for matched-pair data (e.g., for proportional hazards, use the MC test).

5.2. Paired *t* Test

When there is no censoring, it can be shown that the versatile test with the DiM functional corresponds to the permutation paired *t* test regardless the values of w_i. This versatile test is the only test we know that compares the mean difference for paired censored data. Although the weighting makes no difference for uncensored data, it does for censored data because the paired difference in scores $c_{i1} - c_{i2} = \int x \, dF_{i1|\widehat{\Psi}_i} - \int y \, dF_{i2|\widehat{\Psi}_i}$ which generally depend on $\widehat{\Psi}_i$ and thus in turn on w_i.

We conducted a small simulation study which compares four DPT tests with the DiM functional. (1) a test that ignores pairing, paired tests with (2) $w_i = 1$, (3) $w_i = 0$, or (4) w_i estimated from the data (i.e., the "versatile test"). The simulation scheme is the same as the one specified in the previous section and there are 50 pairs in each replicate. The simulation results are displayed in Table 2. Similar to the simulation

Table 2 Empirical Power at .05 Level for DiM DPT Tests Applied to Paired Data with Uniform (0, 1) Right-Censoring and 1000 Replicates

Strata effect ω	Unpaired test	Paired test, $w_i = 1$	Paired test, $w_i = 0$	Paired test, w_i estimated
0	83.0	63.1	81.2	81.2
0.22	77.6	63.3	79.2	79.3
0.86	60.2	56.8	69.6	69.6
2.0	35.4	47.8	57.0	57.4

results for the rank tests, the versatile test performs similarly to the unpaired test when the strata effect is small and outperforms both the unpaired and paired test with $w_i = 1$ when the strata effect is large. Note that the versatile test and the paired test with $w_i = 0$ have similar performance. Thus, as for the rank test, the paired test with fixed weight of zero is recommended for practical use.

5.3. Example 4: Skin Graft Data

We apply the weight-zero paired test with the DiM functional and the logrank functional to data from a study on HLA matching and skin graft survival (Holt and Prentice, 1974; see also Kalbfleisch and Prentice, 1980, p. 190). The days of survival of closely matched and poorly matched skin grafts on the same person were recorded. There were in total of 11 patients. Four of the 22 observations are interval-censored, 2 right-censored, and the rest known exactly. Previous analyses have replaced the interval-censored observations with a point on the interior of the interval, but the DPT handles interval-censored observations in a straightforward way. The null hypothesis is that the closely matched and poorly-matched skin grafts have the same distribution. Using the DiM functional and logrank score gives exact p values of .010 and .012, respectively. Thus both tests produce statistically significant result, and show that closely matched skin grafts have better survival.

6. ALTERNATIVE METHODS

The class of permutation tests (DPT tests) described above provides a unifying approach to many types of survival data. For nonrandomized trials with covariates, regression methods may be more appropriate than the DPT tests to ensure that the apparent treatment effects are not related to the covariates (for right-censored data see, e.g., Kalbfleisch and Prentice, 1980; for proportional hazards models for interval-censored data see Satten, 1996 and Goggins et al., 1998). However, for randomized trials this adjustment is often not necessary nor desired.

When the assumption on the censoring does not hold, the DPT tests may not retain alpha level. When censoring is related to treatment and the data are right-censored, it has been suggested that the rank-based methods based on the score test may perform better than the permutation tests since the assumptions of the permutation tests do not hold (Kalbfleisch and Prentice, 1980). However, Janssen (1991) has shown that, in the nonstratified case at least, the permutation rank tests with unequal censoring between treatment groups are asymptotically equivalent to the likelihood approach. For the stratified case, Schoenfeld and Tsiatis (1987) developed a stratified logrank test for cases where the censoring depends on treatment. However, large sample sizes may be required to ensure that their test is close to alpha level (see Shih and Fay, 1999). The previously mentioned WKM test (Pepe and Fleming, 1989), a generalization of the Z test to right-censored data, should perform reasonably when censoring is related to treatment and sample sizes are large.

For paired right-censored data, Michalek and Mihalko (1980) offer an example where censoring is related to both treatment and the stratification variable, and they show how this can cause the Mantel-Ciminera test to give misleading results. When this violation of assumptions occurs, O'Brien and Fleming (1987) offered a modification to the MC-type tests (i.e., tests with $w_i = 0$ for paired right-censored data), which effectively eliminates from the analysis strata where there is censoring.

For interval-censored data, again the likelihood-based methods appear safer when there is unequal censoring between treatment groups (for the proportional hazards model see Satten, 1996, and Goggins et al., 1998; for more general rank methods see Self and Grossman, 1986 and Fay, 1999, for generalizations of the Z test see Petroni and Wolfe, 1994).

When censoring is not independent of failure time, then neither the permutation tests nor standard likelihood-based survival tests may be applied. In clinical trials, this may happen if patients are more likely to drop out of the study (and hence be censored) as they get sicker and are closer to death.

A type of survival data not discussed in this chapter is clustered failure time data where all individuals within a cluster receive the same treatment. Cai and Shen (2000) describe how permutation tests may be formed for this type of data. They study several test statistics, weighted logrank statistics (e.g., the logrank and Wilcoxon tests), as well as supremum versions of those statistics. These statistics are the standard ones that ignore clustering, and Cai and Shen (2000) estimate the permutation distribution associated with the test statistics by taking Monte Carlo samples from the $\binom{n}{n_1}$ possible permutations of clusters to treatments, where here n is the total number of clusters and n_1 is the number of clusters getting the first treatment. We can write their Wilcoxon-type test statistic in our notation. The test statistic is

$$L_0^* = \sum_i \sum_j (z_{ij} - \bar{z})(c_{ij} - \bar{c}) = \sum_i \sum_j z_{ij} c_{ij} = \sum_i z_{i1} m_i \bar{c}_i$$

where the i index here denote clusters not strata, $\bar{c} = \left(\sum_i m_i\right)^{-1}\left(\sum_i \sum_j c_{ij}\right) = 0$, $\bar{z} = \left(\sum_i m_i\right)^{-1}\left(\sum_i \sum_j z_{ij}\right)$, for the Wilcoxon-type test we use the the Mann-Whitney functional, and Ψ_i is estimated with $\dot{\Psi}$. [To show the equivalence of the two notations see Fay (1999) and Fleming and Harrington (1991, pp. 256–257], and note that when Ψ_i is estimated with $\dot{\Psi}$ then $\bar{c} = 0$ for any of the functionals discussed in this chapter.] A logrank-type test can be formed similarly but it is a slightly different form than Cai and Shen's test (see Section 3.2). We can extend Cai and Shen's work by using the DiM functional to get a difference in means test. Further, a permutational central limit theorem may be applied to permutations done this way; the variance in this situation is

$$V^* = \frac{1}{n-1}\left\{\sum_i (m_i \bar{c}_i)^2\right\}\left\{\sum_i \left(z_{i1} - \frac{\sum_h z_{h1}}{n}\right)^2\right\}$$

and L_0^{*2}/V^* is asymptotically distributed as χ^2 with 1 degree of freedom (see Sen, 1985 for details).

ACKNOWLEDGMENT

We thank Don Corle for providing the data for Example 3.

REFERENCES

American Joint Committee on Cancer. (1997). AJCC cancer staging manual. Philadelphia, PA: Lippincott-Raven Publishers.

Aragón, J., Eberly, D. (1992). On convergence of convex minorant algorithms for distribution estimation with interval-censored data. Journal of Computational and Graphical Statistics 1:129–140.

Byar, D. P., Corle, D. K. (1988). Hormone therapy for prostate cancer: results of the veterans administration cooperative urological research group studies. NCI Monographs 7:165–170.

Cai, J., Shen, Y. (2000). Permutation tests for comparing marginal survival functions with clustered failure time data. Statistics in Medicine 19:2963–2973.

Dempster, A. P., Laird, N. M., Rubin, D. B. (1977). Maximum likelihood from incomplete data via the EM algorithm (with discussion). Journal of the Royal Statistical Society, Series B 39:1–38.

Efron, B. (1967). The two sample problem with censored data. Proceedings of the 5th Berkeley Symposium 4:831–853.

Fay, M. P., Shih, J. H. (1998). Permutation tests using estimated distribution functions. Journal of the American Statistical Association 93:387–396.

Fay, M. P. (1999). Comparing several score tests for interval censored data. Statistics in Medicine 18:273–285.

Finkelstein, D. M., Wolfe, R. A. (1985). A semiparametric model for regression analysis of interval-censored failure time data. Biometrics 41:933–945.

Fleming, T. R., Harrington, D. P. (1991). Counting Processes and Survival Analysis. New York: Wiley.

Gentleman, R., Geyer, C. J. (1994). Maximum likelihood for interval censored Data: consistency and computation. Biometrika 81:618–623.

Ghosh, M., Lahiri, P., Tiwari, R. C. (1989). Nonparametric empirical Bayes estimation of the distribution function and the mean. Communications in Statistics—Theory and Methods 18(1):121–146.

Goggins, W. B., Finkelstein, D. M., Schoenfeld, D. A., Zaslavsky, A. M. (1998). A Markov chain Monte Carlo EM algorithm for analyzing interval-censored data under the cox proportional hazard model. Biometrics 54:1498–1507 (Journal of Chronic Diseases 31, 445–454).

Groeneboom, P., Wellner, J. A. (1992). Information Bounds and Nonparametric Maximum Likelihood Estimation. Boston: Birkhäuser-Verlag.

Holt, J. D., Prentice, R. L. (1974). Survival analysis in twin studies and matched pair experiments. Biometrika 65:159–166.

Huster, W. J., Brookmeyer, R., Self, S. G. (1989). Modeling paired survival data with covariates. Biometrics 45:145–156.

James, I. R. (1987). Tests for location with k samples and censored data. Biometrika 74:599–607.

Janssen, A. (1991). Conditional rank tests for randomly censored data. Annals of Statistics 19:1434–1456.

Kalbfleisch, J. D., Prentice, R. (1980). The Statistical Analysis of Failure Time Data. New York: Wiley.

Mantel, N. (1966). Evaluation of survival data and two new rank statistics arising in its consideration. Cancer Chemo. Rep. 50:163–170.

Mantel, N., Ciminera, J. L. (1979). Mantel-Haenszel analysis of litter-matched time-to-response data with modification for recovery of interlitter information. Cancer Research 37:3863–3868.

Michalek, J. E., Mihalko, D. (1983). On the use of logrank scores in the analysis of litter-matched data on time to tumor appearance. Statistics in Medicine 2:315–321.

O'Brien, P. C., Fleming, T. R. (1987). A paired Prentice-Wilcoxon test for censored paired data. Biometrics 43:169–180.

Pepe, M. S., Fleming, T. R. (1989). Weighted Kaplan-Meier statistics: A class of distance tests for censored survival data. Biometrics 45:497–507.

Peto, R., Peto, J. (1972). Asymptotically efficient rank invariant test procedures (with discussion). Journal of the Royal Statistical Society, Series A 135, part 2:185–207.

Petroni, G. R., Wolfe, R. A. (1994). A two-sample test for stochastic ordering with interval-censored data. Biometrics 50:77–87.

Prentice, R. L. (1978). Linear rank tests with right censored data. Biometrika 65:167–179.

Satten, G. A. (1996). Rankbased inference in the proportional hazards model for interval censored data. Biometrika 83:355–370.

Schoenfeld, D. A., Tsiatis, A. A. (1987). A modified log rank test for highly stratified data. Biometrika 74:167–175.

Self, S. G., Grossman, E. A. (1986). Linear rank tests for interval-censored data with application to PCB. Biometrics 42:521–530.

Sen, P. K. (1985). Permutational central limit theorems. In: Kotz, S., Johnson, N. L. (Eds.), Encyclopedia of Statistical Sciences Vol. 6. New York: Wiley.

Shih, J. H. (1999). A class of permutation tests for stratfied survival data. Biometrics 55:1156–1161.

Stablein, D. M., Koutrouvelis, I. A. (1985). A two-sample test sensitive to crossing hazards in uncensored and singly censored data. Biometrics 41:643–652.

Turnbull, B. W (1976). The empirical distribution function with arbitrarily grouped, censored, and truncated data. Journal of the Royal Statistical Society (Series B) 38:290–295.

9

Bayesian Reporting of Clinical Trials

Simon Weeden and Mahesh Parmar
Medical Research Council Clinical Trials Unit, London, England

Laurence S. Freedman
Bar-Ilan University, Ramat Gan, Israel

1. INTRODUCTION

Over the last 10 years many articles have been written about the use of Bayesian statistical methods for designing, monitoring, analyzing, and interpreting the results of randomized clinical trials. Spiegelhalter and colleagues provided a summary and synthesis of such work (Spiegelhalter, Freedman, and Parmar, 1994), but extensions and applications for particular circumstances continue to appear (Parmar, Ungerleider, and Simon, 1996; Thall, Simon, and Estey, 1996; Abrams, Ashby, and Errington, 1996; Simon and Freedman, 1997; Stangl and Greenhouse, 1998; Parmar et al., 2001).

Despite these developments, very few reports of clinical trials analyzed exclusively by Bayesian methods appear in the medical literature. The main reason for this is probably due to the anticipation of authors that they will encounter extra resistance from referees to such a "novel" form of analysis. Every investigator writes a report in the hope that it will be accepted by his/her journal of choice, and after the arduous and often long process of a clinical trial, the investigator wishes to minimize the difficulties of the publication process. Thus conventional methods of analysis are the natural choice.

However, behind this very real barrier there lie some other difficult issues relating to the form of presentation of a Bayesian analysis of a clinical trial. As will be explained in more detail, Bayesian methods use prior clinical opinion in a formal manner. How should we explain this in a succinct way in a clinical paper? How should we describe the clinical opinion that has been used in the trial? How should we present results illustrating different interpretations of the results according to a clinician's own starting position? How do we preserve the "objective" nature of the trial results in the light of the introduction of all this subjectivism?

These matters have been discussed in a theoretical manner by several authors (Spiegelhalter et al., 1994; Hughes, 1993; Greenhouse and Wasserman, 1995; Carlin and Sargent, 1996). In this paper we propose a solution by way of example. We present a Bayesian version of a clinical report of a randomized trial of two chemotherapy schedules for operable osteosarcoma, a malignant disease of the bone, which occurs in children, teenagers, and adults. We choose this trial particularly because a survey of clinical opinion regarding the expectations of the treatments was conducted before its start, and this provides the basis for the prior clinical opinion that is used in the Bayesian analysis. The conventional version of the trial report was published in 1997 (Souhami et al., 1997). The main novelty in the presentation is the introduction of an "Interpretation" section between the Results and the Discussion. In this section we present a sensitivity analysis in which we consider the impact of different prior opinions on the interpretation of the data. The hope in this type of analysis is to show that the conclusions are robust to a wide range of "starting positions". Of course, if they are not, this is also important to know. Besides this section the reader may not notice much difference from the conventional type of paper (aside from the lack of the often overused *p* value, and a somewhat extended Statistical Methods section which will be needed at first to explain the new methodology). If that is the case, then we may have succeeded in our aim of finding a way of slotting in a new and informative type of analysis which will help to clarify the clinical information and interpretation of the paper.

2. RANDOMIZED TRIAL OF TWO REGIMENS OF CHEMOTHERAPY IN OPERABLE OSTEOSARCOMA: A BAYESIAN PERSPECTIVE ON A TRIAL OF THE EUROPEAN OSTEOSARCOMA INTERGROUP

We have compared in a randomized trial the effects of a multidrug 44-week chemotherapy regimen, based on the T10 protocol, with a two-drug (cisplatin and doxorubicin) 18-week regimen for the treatment of operable limb osteosarcoma. The primary endpoint was length of survival after randomization. Of 407 patients, 391 were eligible and have been followed for at least 4 years (median 5.6 years). Toxicity was qualitatively similar, but 94% of the 199 patients on two-drug treatment completed their course compared with 51% of the 192 patients on multidrug treatment. Overall survival at 5 years was 54% in the multidrug arm and 56% in the two-drug arm. The hazard-ratio estimate was 0.94 (95% CI 0.69–1.27, where HR $<$ 1 indicates a benefit to two-drug therapy). In a pretrial survey clinicians indicated that to prefer multidrug treatment they would require an absolute increase of about 10% in overall 5-year survival. The results of the trial indicate that such an increase is highly unlikely. Bayesian analysis demonstrates that this conclusion is robust to a wide variety of "starting positions" of skepticism or enthusiasm with regard to the likely benefit of the multidrug treatment.

2.1. Background

Although the survival of patients with operable osteosarcoma is improved by chemotherapy (Eilber et al., 1987; Link et al., 1986), the optimum duration of treatment and the relative contributions of the constituent drugs have not been assessed in randomized trials. Randomized comparisons of treatment present formidable difficulties in this rare disease, which each year affects only 1 in 200,000 of the population. The European Osteosarcoma Intergroup (EOI) was formed in 1982 in order to perform randomized studies of sufficient size to allow investigation of important aspects of treatment. EOI consists of the Bone Sarcoma Working Party of the UK Medical Research Council (MRC), the UK Children's Cancer Study Group (UKCCSG), the Société Internationale d'Oncologie Paedriatrique (SIOP), and the European Organisation for Research and Treatment of Cancer (EORTC) Soft Tissue and Bone Sarcoma Group.

In the first EOI trial (Bramwell et al., 1992) 307 patients with osteosarcoma were randomized to one of two regimens of chemotherapy. In that trial a regimen of cisplatin (CDDP) and doxorubicin (DOX), given pre- and postoperatively for a total of 6 cycles to patients with operable nonmetastatic osteosarcoma, produced a 5-year survival rate of 64% and a 5-year progression-free survival (PFS) rate of 57%. These results were comparable with those reported from a collaborative West German study in pediatric osteosarcoma (Winkler et al., 1984), in which the chemotherapy was based on the T10 regimen introduced by Rosen et al (Rosen et al., 1982). A modification of the T10 regimen was also used in Link's study (Link et al., 1986), in which 36 patients were randomized after surgery to either early chemotherapy or chemotherapy at relapse. The results showed an advantage in PFS for the early use of chemotherapy.

The T10 regimen has been the basis of much osteosarcoma chemotherapy and an update of the results of this and other similar regimens used at the Memorial Sloan Kettering Cancer Center showed that 65% of 279 patients were alive and disease free at 8 years (Meyers et al., 1992). Their results are among the best reported in this disease.

Nonrandomized studies of treatment do not allow an unbiased comparison of treatment outcomes. For this reason, after completion of the previous trial (Bramwell et al., 1982), the EOI embarked on a formal comparison of a 44-week multidrug T10-based regimen (multidrug) with the 18-week CDDP and DOX (two-drug) regimen, which was the more effective of the two treatments previously compared. This paper reports the results of the trial. We use a Bayesian framework of analysis that allows interpretation of the results both from the usual "objective" viewpoint and also incorporating the prior opinions of participating clinicians. Using this analysis framework we are able to show how the observed results would affect these opinions.

2.2. Patients and Methods

Patients

The details of this trial are only summarized in this paper as they have previously been reported elsewhere (Souhami et al., 1997). Patients were eligible for this trial if they were ≤40 years, had histologically diagnosed osteosarcoma of the extremity, no evidence of metastatic disease, and normal renal and cardiac function. Patients were excluded if they had received previous chemotherapy or had a previous malignancy. A member of the pathology panel of the EOI reviewed histological diagnosis. The accepted interval between diagnostic biopsy and randomization was 35 days. Preliminary staging included plain radiological examination of the tumor, isotope bone scan, chest X-ray, and CT scan of the thorax. CT and MRI scans of the primary tumor were performed according to local practice.

Chemotherapy

The details of drug administration were as follows:

Two-drug: DOX 25 mg/m^2 days 1–3, CDDP 100 mg/m^2 day 1. Each cycle administered at 21-day intervals for 6 cycles. Surgery was planned for week 9 (day 63) after 3 preoperative cycles. Two weeks after surgery the first of 3 postoperative cycles was scheduled. Details of administration have been described elsewhere (Bramwell et al., 1992).

Multidrug: Preoperative treatment consisted of vincristine (VCR) 1.5 mg/m^2 (max. 2 mg) and high dose methotrexate (HDMTX) 8 g/m^2 (12 g/m^2 below 12 years of age) on days 0, 8, 35, 42, and DOX 25 mg/m^2 dl–3 on days 15–17. Folinic acid 12 mg/m^2 intravenously or 15 mg/m^2 orally commencing at 24 hr given every 6 hr × 10 doses, the dose being adjusted according to 24 and 48 hr serum concentrations. Surgery was scheduled at week 7 (day 49). Postoperatively patients received the first cycle of BCD (Bleomycin 15 mg/m^2, Cyclophosphamide 600 mg/m^2, and Dactinomycin 0.6 mg/m^2 each on days 1 and 2) on week 9. Further cycles of VCR and HDMTX were given on weeks 12, 13, 17, and 18, and a further cycle of DOX on week 14 (all at the same preoperative dose). On week 20 the regimen changed to DOX 30 mg/m^2 days 1 and 2 and CDDP 120 mg/m^2 day 1. This was given on weeks 20, 23, 29, 32, 38, and 41. Further cycles of BCD were given on weeks 26, 35, and 44.

For both regimens recommended dose modifications were based on blood counts (all counts 10^9L) obtained between 9 and 14 days and at 21 days. Reductions were based on the lower of these two counts and applied to all subsequent cycles. The scheme was as follows: Total white blood count (WBC) > 2.0, platelets > 50—100% dose; WBC > 1.0 and < 2.0, platelets > 25 and < 50—85% dose; WBC < 1.0, platelets < 25—70% dose. If the total WBC was < 3.0 or granulocyte count < 1.0 at scheduled time of next treatment, this treatment was delayed 1 week.

Surgery

At the time of randomization the projected surgical procedure was recorded. In the multidrug regimen surgery was planned for week 7, 1 week after the fourth course of HDMTX. In the two-drug arm surgery was at week 9, 3 weeks after the third cycle of CDDP and DOX. The decision about whether to perform an amputation or limb sparing surgery (usually endoprosthetic replacement) was made by the individual clinical teams.

Response Assessment

Clinical response was defined as a definite reduction of swelling and pain following preoperative chemotherapy and was assessed by the responsible clinician. Radiological criteria of response were not used. During the period of this trial MRI scans were not generally available for response assessment. Those patients in whom response was not assessed are regarded as nonresponders.

Histopathological response was based on the resection specimen. Good response was defined as at least 90% necrosis of the tumor and poor response any degree less than this. Pathology was reviewed centrally at diagnosis and in assessment of response.

Treatment at Relapse

Local recurrence was treated according to the judgment of the participating clinicians and consisted of local resection or amputation sometimes combined with radiotherapy. Pulmonary and other metastases were managed according to the clinical circumstances and treatments consisted of second-line chemotherapy, thoracotomy, or palliative care.

Statistical Methodology—Sample Size

The multidrug schedule was anticipated to result in, at best, a survival rate of 70% at 5 years. The two-drug regimen was associated with a 5-year survival rate of approximately 55%. The sample size was determined to give at least a 80% chance of rejecting the null hypothesis of no difference between the treatments (on the basis of the 95% credible interval for the treatment difference not including zero, using an uninformative prior distribution) when the true difference in 5-year survival rates is 15%. This 15% difference corresponds to a hazard ratio (HR) of 1.68 (where $HR > 1$ implies a survival advantage to multidrug treatment). The target recruitment to achieve this was 400 patients (Machin et al., 1997).

Statistical Methodology—Analysis

The analysis of this trial has been performed on an intention to treat basis including as many eligible patients as possible for each endpoint. The statistical analyses were conducted using the SPSS and SAS statistical packages. Survival curves were calculated using the Kaplan-Meier method. The Mantel-Cox version of the logrank statistic was calculated to provide the likelihood portion of the Bayesian analysis (see below). Estimated hazard ratios are used to compare treatments (Parmar and Machin, 1995). Survival was calculated from date of randomization and progression-free survival (PFS) from date of surgery as inadequate surgery is thought to be a cause of disease progression.

We employ Bayesian methods to analyze the data from this trial. The use of Bayesian methodology in the design, monitoring, and analysis of clinical trials have been described in detail in the statistical literature (Spiegelhalter et al., 1994; Spiegelhalter, Freedman, and Parmar, 1993; Parmar, Spiegelhalter, and Freedman, 1994; Fayers, Ashby, and Parmar, 1997).

A Bayesian approach to trial analysis allows external evidence to be formally incorporated into the reporting of a trial. Usually trial reports introduce such evidence informally in the Discussion section, the aim being to put the results in some kind of clinical context. In this paper an extra Interpretation section is placed between the Results and Discussion to contain the Bayesian perspective. In the Interpretation section, attention is focused on the impact that the trial results will have on the opinion of participating clinicians.

The crucial issue in performing a Bayesian analysis is appropriate specification of the *prior distribution*, which is a statistical formulation of the prestudy beliefs. When deciding on a prior distribution, many options are available: the uninformative prior, which represents a lack of clinical opinion about the potential treatment difference; the skeptical prior, which considers only a small probability that the alternative hypothesis (in this case that multidrug therapy offers a significant survival advantage) is true; the clinical prior, which formalizes the opinion of individuals who are reasonably well informed of the nature of the treatments on trial; and the enthusiastic prior, which takes the treatment difference specified in the alternative hypothesis to be the best guess of the true treatment difference. We will consider all these priors in relation to the analysis of the primary endpoint, survival time, and we will thereby examine the robustness of our conclusions from the trial to a variety of different "starting points."

While the trial was still in the design stage, information was collected on clinicians' opinions of the likely efficacy of the new treatment, via a carefully structured interview (Freedman and Spiegelhalter, 1983). Seven clinicians planning to take part in the trial were interviewed and asked to indicate what weight of belief they would give to probable differences in 5-year survival between the two treatments. These could thus be expressed as probability distributions representing the likely treatment difference. Converted to the log hazard ratio (LHR) scale they form the clinical prior distributions for the Bayesian analysis. The reason for converting to the LHR scale is because it is approximately normally distributed with variance $4/n$, where n is the number of observed events (Tsiatis, 1981).

The clinicians were also asked to mark on a given scale the absolute improvement required in the 5-year survival rate to offset the extra difficulty, cost and possible extra toxicity of the multidrug regimen. Following early discussions it was assumed that if the absolute improvement in 5-year survival with multidrug therapy was 0% then they would use the two-drug regimen and if the improvement was 20% they would presumably adopt the multidrug regimen. Somewhere between these values there would be a changeover point, or a range of points (termed the range of equivalence), where it is difficult to decide between the two chemotherapy schedules. After the trial was closed, the log hazard ratio for the difference between the treatments was calculated. The probability of obtaining this value of the LHR for different values of the treatment difference was calculated and is known as the *likelihood*.

Finally, the *posterior distribution* was calculated, which is simply the prior distribution modified as a consequence of the observed results, expressed via the likelihood. As the prior and likelihood distributions are all approximately normally distributed, combining them to form the posterior distribution is straightforward. When a clinical prior is used, the posterior distribution provides an estimate of the clinician's belief if realistic allowance is made for the information obtained from the trial. It is this posterior distribution that provides the necessary information for judging the opinion of each clinician on the efficacy of the new treatment. All endpoints besides survival were analyzed assuming noninformative prior distributions. Such analysis corresponds to the usual frequentist analysis. Results are given as estimates with credible intervals (CIs) which are the Bayesian equivalent of confidence intervals when a noninformative prior distribution is assumed.

Prior Beliefs

The prior beliefs of the participating clinicians are shown in Table 1, along with range of equivalence and median expected improvement in 5-year survival. These distributions are represented graphically in Figure 1. The histograms of opinions are superimposed with a normal distribution obtained from these opinions. The normal distribution is actually fitted on the log hazard ratio (LHR) scale, using their median expected improvement compared to the baseline 5-year survival rate of 55%,

Table 1 Pretrial Prior Beliefs of Seven Clinicians Interested in Participating in the Trial

Clinician	Range of equivalence	Absolute 5-year survival advantage (%) of two-drug over multidrug									Median expected improvement (%)
		−20–−15	−15–−10	−10–−5	−5–0	0–5	5–10	10–15	15–20	20–25	
1	0–5	0	1	12	20	26	21	13	6	1	3
2	5–5	1	4	12	22	28	18	9	5	1	0
3	0–7	0	0	1	9	15	26	29	19	1	10
4	5–10	1	5	18	26	30	19	1	0	0	4
5	5–12	0	1	4	15	35	31	13	1	0	6
6	10–15	0	0	5	10	25	50	8	2	0	2
7	5–10	1	14	32	33	14	5	1	0	0	−5
Mean	4–9	0	4	12	19	25	24	11	5	0	3%

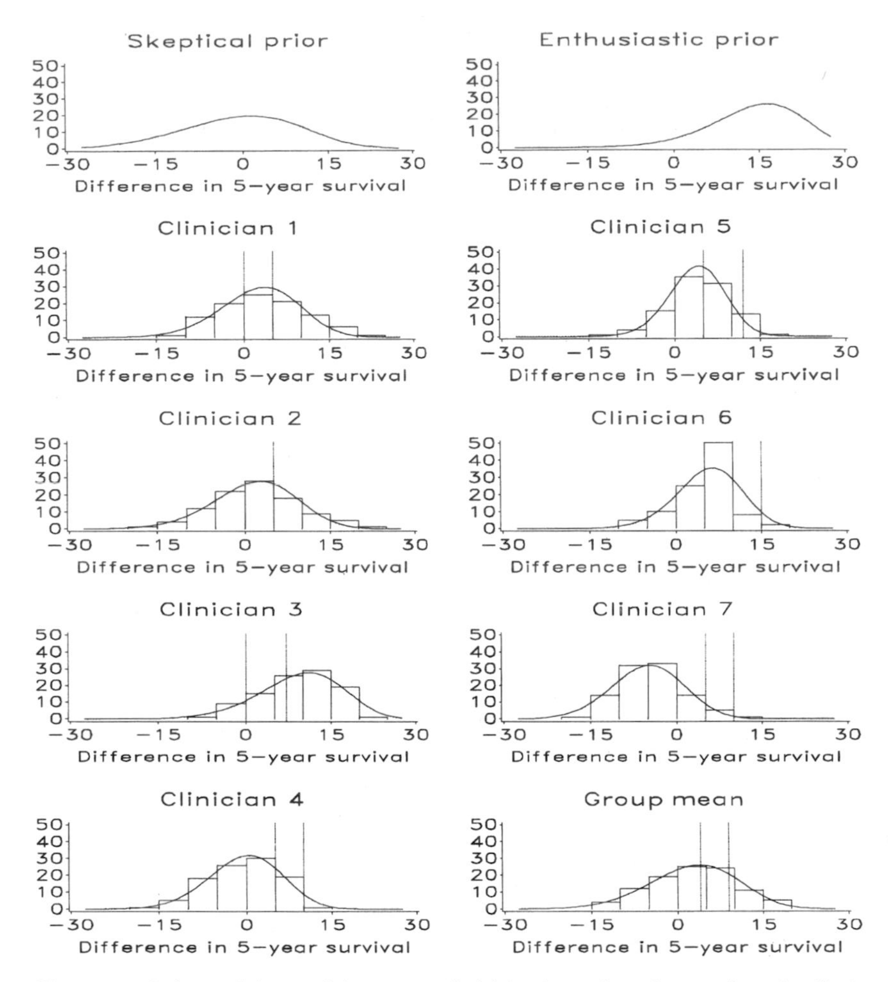

Figure 1 Prior opinions of the seven clinicians interviewed regarding the likely difference between two-drug and multidrug chemotherapy, plus the skeptical and enthusiastic prior distributions. Vertical lines represent the boundaries of the range of equivalence. Superimposed on the histograms are fitted normal distributions (see text for details).

and the probability they accord to observing a treatment difference of less than zero.

The skeptical and enthusiastic prior distributions are also shown on Figure 2. The skeptical prior was calculated by assuming that there is no difference between the two treatments and that the probability of the difference in 5-year survival being more than 15% in favor of multidrug (the alternative hypothesis) is 0.05. The enthusiastic prior distribution was calculated by assuming the alternative hypothesis to be true; i.e., multidrug therapy offers a 5-year survival advantage of 15%. It is assumed to have the same precision as the skeptical prior.

The prior opinions of the seven participating clinicians on the log hazard ratio (LHR) scale are shown in Figure 2. The ranges of equivalence are also converted to the LHR scale, assuming a baseline 5-year survival rate of 55%, and are shown on the graphs. These distributions will form the clinical prior distributions for the Bayesian analysis.

It can be seen that there is much variation in the clinicians' prior opinions regarding the relative efficacy of multidrug chemotherapy. Clinician 3, for example, believed that the new treatment would improve 5-year survival by 10% whereas clinician 7 predicted it would most likely be worse than the two-drug regimen. It can be seen that clinician 3's opinions were most similar to the enthusiastic prior, whereas clinician 7's opinions were more negative than those represented by the skeptical prior.

There was also considerable variety in the ranges of equivalence recorded by the seven clinicians. Some (clinician 1 and 3) would consider using multidrug treatment if it offered a benefit in 5-year survival of greater than zero, whereas clinician 2 would not consider adopting it if it did not improve 5-year survival by 10% or more.

Looking at the group means on Figures 1 and 2, it is worth noting that the lower bound of the range of equivalence is close to the median expected improvement on multidrug chemotherapy. This provides an argument for the ethical basis for randomization, since in general the participating clinicians are unsure whether the new treatment will prove to be clinically worthwhile. It has been previously stated that the variance of the prior on the LHR scale is approximately equal to $4/n$, where n is the number of deaths to have occurred. Thus the distribution of the group mean of the clinicians' opinions can be considered equivalent to having conducted a trial in which a total of 69 deaths have occurred with equal follow-up in the two arms. This is in contrast to the trial design which anticipated 124 deaths.

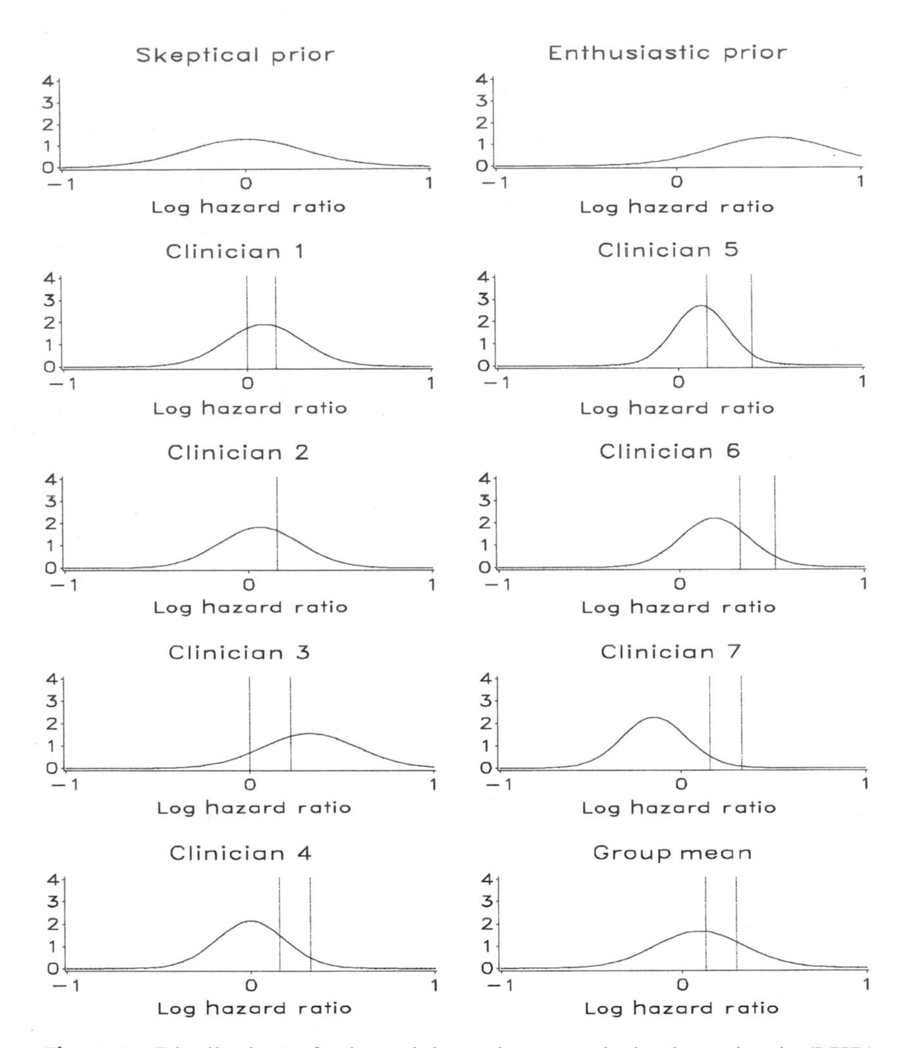

Figure 2 Distributions of prior opinions, shown on the log hazard ratio (LHR) scale. Vertical lines represent the boundaries of the range of equivalence.

2.3. Results

Patient Characteristics

Between September 1, 1986 and January 31, 1993, 407 patients with operable nonmetastatic limb osteosarcoma were entered into the trial. Of the patients randomized 139 (69 two-drug, 70 multidrug) came from the MRC, 139 (71, 68) came from the UKCCSG, 54 (28, 26) from the EORTC, 44 (22, 22) from CSG, 14 (7, 7) from Brazil, 13 (6, 7) from SIOP, and 4 (2, 2) from New Zealand. Of these patients, 15 (3.7%) were ineligible for the following reasons: incorrect pathology 9 (4 two-drug and 5 multidrug); metastases or previous chemotherapy 4 (1, 3); nonlimb tumors 2 (1, 1). In addition, for one patient randomized to multidrug the date of randomization is known and no further information was obtained. This left 391 eligible patients who have been followed for a minimum of 4.5 years with median duration of follow-up 5.6 years.

The characteristics of eligible patients in the two treatment groups are shown in Table 2. The two arms were well balanced with respect to each of the characteristics. Approximately half (56%) of the patients were less than 17 years old; tumors of the femur (55%), tibia (26%), and humerus (13%) were most prevalent, and a large majority (67%) had common histology.

Compliance with Protocol

In the two-drug arm 164 (84%) patients underwent surgery after the third cycle of treatment as specified in the protocol. Of the remainder, 20 (10%) had their operation earlier and 12 (6%) later than that specified by the protocol. In the multidrug arm 133 (72%) patients had surgery after the fifth cycle as specified by the protocol, 42 (23%) had surgery earlier, and 10 (5%) later.

The median time to surgery was 75 days for the two-drug treatment and 57 days for multidrug. The difference between these medians of 18 days is a little longer than the planned 2-week difference but it is clear that the majority of patients underwent surgery at or very near the planned time. Of those who did not have surgery, two died (one in each treatment arm), before it could be performed, two were lost to follow-up (both receiving multidrug), one developed pulmonary metastases while on treatment (multidrug); for two (one on each arm), the parents refused any further treatment, one patient moved and was lost to follow-up after

Table 2 Characteristics of Eligible Patients by Treatment

	Two-drug		Multidrug		Total	
	N	%	*N*	%	*N*	%
Age						
≤11	43	22	25	13	68	17
12–16	72	36	80	42	152	39
≥17	84	42	87	45	171	44
Sex						
Male	131	66	130	68	261	67
Female	68	34	62	32	130	33
Site of tumor						
Femur	113	57	102	53	215	55
Tibia	50	25	51	27	101	26
Humerus	24	12	25	13	49	13
Fibula	9	5	10	5	19	5
Radius	3	2	0	0	3	1
Ulna	0	0	3	2	3	1
Calcaneus	0	0	1	1	1	0
Histology						
Common	133	67	128	67	261	67
Chondroblastic	25	13	19	10	44	11
Fibroblastic	23	12	20	10	43	11
Osteoclast rich	4	2	4	2	8	2
Telangiectatic	4	2	6	3	10	3
Anaplastic	4	2	12	6	16	4
Small cell	2	1	0	0	2	1
Osteoblastic	4	2	3	2	7	2
Total	199		192		391	

three cycles of chemotherapy (two-drug), and surgery was not done for an unspecified reason in one patient who went on to complete 19 cycles (multidrug).

The distribution of the (total) number of cycles actually received by patients was summarized in Table 3. There was considerably more variability in the total number of cycles administered in the multidrug regimen. In this regimen 97 patients (51%) received 18 or more cycles, 125 (65%) 15 cycles or more, and 141 (73%) more than 12 cycles. The reasons for failure to complete the assigned chemotherapy are given in Table 4. The numbers discontinuing treatment were very similar in the

Table 3 Total Number of Chemotherapy Cycles Received

	Two-drug			Multidrug		
	Cycles	*N*	%	Cycles	*N*	%
No chemotherapy	0	0	0	0	3	2
Before surgery						
Phase I	1–3	21	11	1–5	23	12
After surgery						
Phase II	4–6	178	89	6–11	25	13
Phase III	—	—	—	12–14	16	8
Phase IV	—	—	—	15–17	28	15
Phase V	—	—	—	18–20	97	51
Total		199			192	

two-drug group and in the multidrug group during the first six cycles; however, after cycle 6 of the multidrug regimen the most common reasons for discontinuing treatment were toxic effects or patient refusal.

Toxic Effects

Both regimens produced considerable toxicity, the main components of which are given in Table 5. The most severe toxicities were associated

Table 4 Reasons for Terminating Protocol Chemotherapy

			Multidrug			
Reason for terminating treatment	Two-drug		First six cycles		After cycle 6	
	N	%	*N*	%	*N*	%
Treatment completed	167	84	—	—	72	37
Progression	14	7	10	5	22	11
Toxic effects	10	5	5	3	30	16
Refusal	3	2	3	2	24	12
Postoperative complications	2	1	0	0	3	2
Change from protocol schedule	2	1	6	3	14	7
Lost to follow-up	1	1	1	1	2	1
Total	199				192	

Table 5 Serious (WHO Grade 3 or 4) Toxic Effects During Treatment

	Two-drug		Multidrug			
			First six cycles		After cycle 6	
	N	%	*N*	%	*N*	%
Leucopenia	150	75	35	19	124	73
Thrombocytopenia	91	46	5	3	48	28
Nausea and vomiting	148	74	85	85	112	66
Mucositis	40	20	11	6	23	14
Alopecia	171	86	104	57	153	90
Cardiac rhythm disturbance	0	0	1	1	4	2
Infection	42	21	6	3	31	18
Renal impairment	3	2	1	1	5	3
Liver	1	1	35	19	20	12
Hearing loss	0	0	0	0	3	2
Skin effects	1	1	1	1	3	2
Neurotoxicity	1	1	1	1	1	1
Pulmonary	0	0	1	1	1	1

with the cisplatin/doxorubicin cycles of treatment in both arms. Severe nausea and vomiting, thrombocytopenia, leucopenia, mucositis, and infection were common. Liver function abnormalities were common after high-dose methotrexate in the multidrug arm, but were not so prevalent during later cycles. Severely impaired renal function was rare (2%). There were no deaths from cardiac toxic effects. Chemotherapy toxicity was a major reason for dose reduction and delay, and for discontinuation of chemotherapy.

Surgery

The surgical procedures planned at diagnosis for each patient, and the procedure eventually carried out, are shown by treatment arm in Table 6. 138 (69%) in the two-drug arm and 129 (67%) in the multidrug arm actually underwent the surgery planned at diagnosis. Of 40 patients in the two-drug arm who were planned to undergo amputation, this was performed in only 22 while 17 were able to have a limb sparing procedure. In the multidrug arm 13 of 41 were spared the planned amputation. Conversely, of 141 patients scheduled for conservative surgery in the

Table 6 Planned and Actual Surgery Received

	Intended surgery						
Actual surgery	Amputation	Prosthesis	Rotation	Other conservative	Allograft	Unknown	Total
Two-drug							
Amputation	22	19	1	1	0	2	45
Prosthesis	9	106	0	3	0	—	118
Rotation	3	1	2	0	0	—	6
Other conservative	5	13	0	8	1	—	27
Allograft	0	0	0	0	0	—	0
None	1	2	0	0	0	—	3
Total	40	141	3	12	1	2	199
Multidrug							
Amputation	27	24	1	3	0	1	56
Prosthesis	5	95	0	2	0	—	102
Rotation	0	1	0	0	0	—	1
Other conservative	8	6	1	7	2	—	24
Allograft	0	2	0	0	0		2
None	1	6	0	0	0	—	7
Total	41	134	2	12	2	1	192

two-drug arm, 19 (13%) had to have an amputation, while in the multidrug arm the figures were 24 (18%) of 134

Clinical Response

It was not possible to obtain data on response for eight patients (one two-drug, seven multidrug). The response rates in the two-drug and multidrug were 117/198 (59%) and 85/185 (46%), respectively, with an odds ratio of 2.02 (95% credible interval (CI) 1.34–3.07) in favor of the two-drug arm. Although the response rate differed according to type of histology (for example, the highest response rates were observed in those with fibroblastic tumors), the odds ratio for comparing the two treatments was unaffected after adjustment for histology.

Histopathological Response

268 (69%) tumors were available for detailed analysis. The histopathological response rate was similar in the two arms: 41 (30%) of 137 tumors

showed a good response in the two-drug group compared with 37 (29%) of 129 in the multidrug group (OR = 1.10, 95% CI 0.66-1.88).

Progression-Free Survival

Progression-free survival is shown in Figure 3 and was very similar in the two arms with an estimated value at 3 years after surgery of 47% (95% CI 42–52) and at 5 years after surgery of 44% (95% CI 39–49%). There was a high rate of tumor progression in the first year; 117 (56%) of the 208 relapses or deaths occurred during that time. The hazard ratio (two-drug/multidrug) for risk of progression or death was 1.01 (95% CI 0.77–1.33).

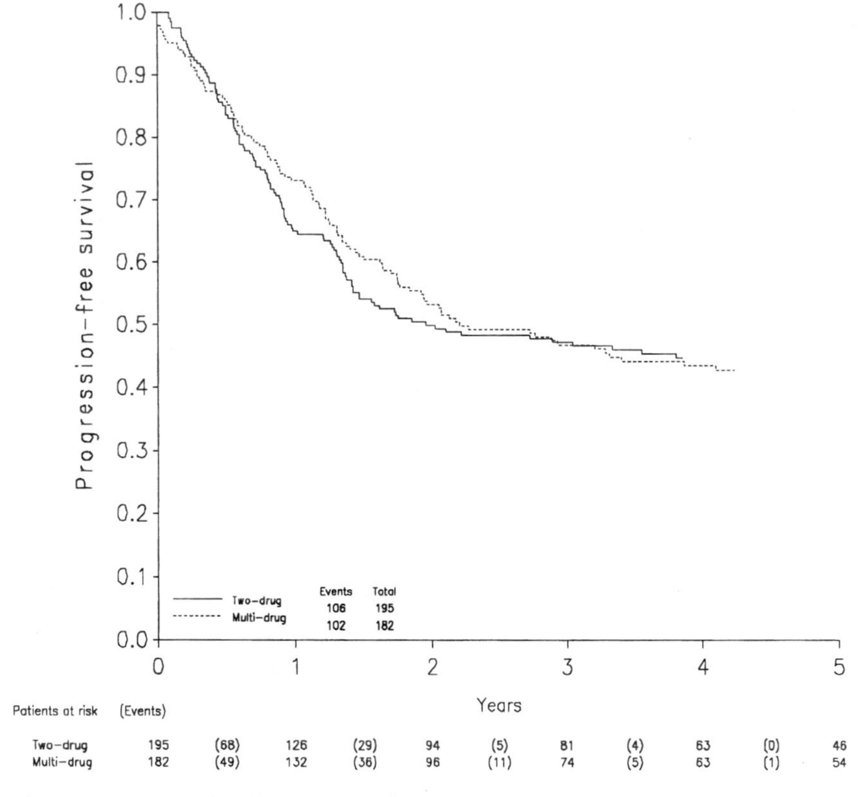

Figure 3 Progression-free survival by treatment group.

Survival

The analysis in this section assumes a noninformative prior distribution. Other prior distributions are considered in the Interpretation section that follows. The hazard ratio for risk of death was 0.94 (95% CI 0.69–1.27) in favor of the two-drug arm, representing a 2% (95% CI −8–12%) absolute difference in 5-year survival from 54% for the multidrug arm to 56% for the two-drug arm (Figure 4). Adjustment of the treatment comparison for age, sex, tumor site, and initial pathology by means of Cox regression models made little difference to the estimate of the hazard ratio. Preoperative histopathological response appears to be a major prognostic indicator for survival (Figure 5), although this result should be

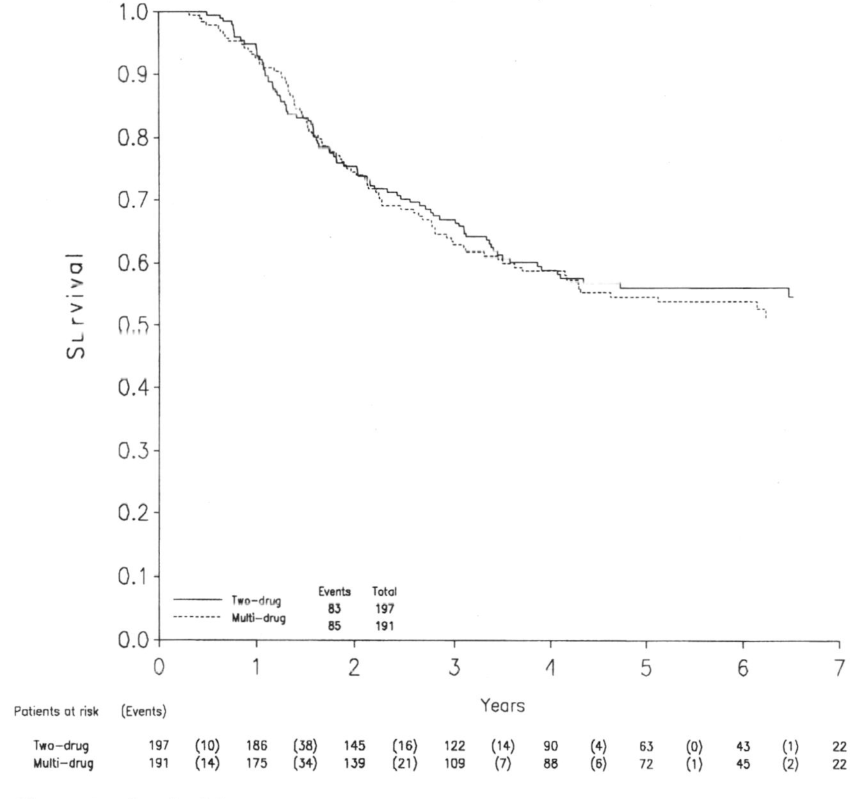

Figure 4 Survival by treatment group.

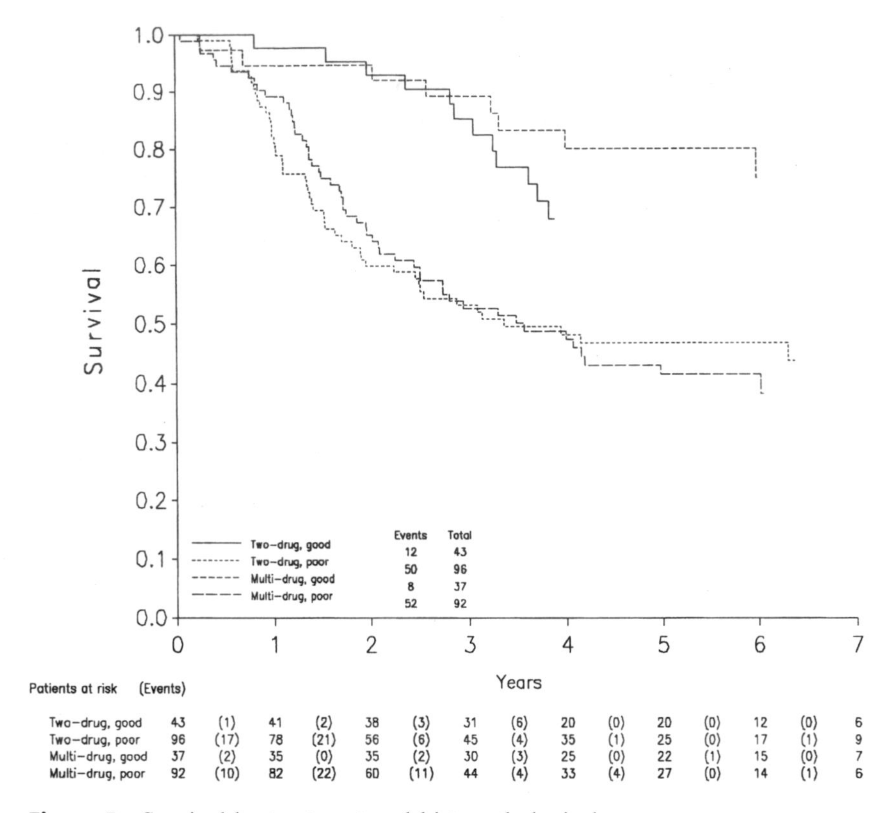

Figure 5 Survival by treatment and histopathological response.

treated with caution as histological response was determined after randomization. There was no evidence that the hazard ratio was different in groups with good histological response and those with a poor response. The hazard ratio for treatment was 1.44 (95% CI 0.60–3.46) in the good responders and 1.05 (95% CI 0.71–1.54) in the poor responders.

2.4. Interpretation

Assuming an uninformative prior distribution, the hazard ratio for survival comparing two-drug therapy to multidrug therapy is 0.94 (95% CI 0.69–1.27) in favor of two-drug therapy. This represents a 6% reduction in the risk of death with the two-drug regimen. A total of 168 deaths occurred in this trial. These results can be expressed in the form of a normal distribution with mean log(0.94) and variance 4/168. This distribution is called the likelihood and is shown on the log hazard ratio scale in Figure 6.

The likelihood was combined with the various prior distributions (Figure 2) to form posterior distributions, shown in Figure 7. These posterior distributions represent the prior opinions taking into account the results of the trial. It is worth noting that these estimates of treatment difference are considerably more precise than those expressed in the prior distributions. This is the consequence of prior opinions being updated by evidence from the results of a randomized trial.

From the skeptical posterior distribution, the probability of there being any benefit to multidrug therapy is 36%, and the probability of observing an absolute benefit in 5-year survival of 5% or more is 7%, so a skeptic is likely to feel that their initial caution was justified. An enthusiast's posterior probability of there being benefit to the multidrug treatment would be 64%, but they would still have only a 22% probability of a benefit of 5% or more.

The participating clinicians would only consider using the multidrug treatment if the difference in 5-year survival was greater than the lower bound of their range of equivalence, and would adopt it routinely if the survival difference was greater than the upper bound. The posterior probabilities that the real treatment difference is greater than the lower

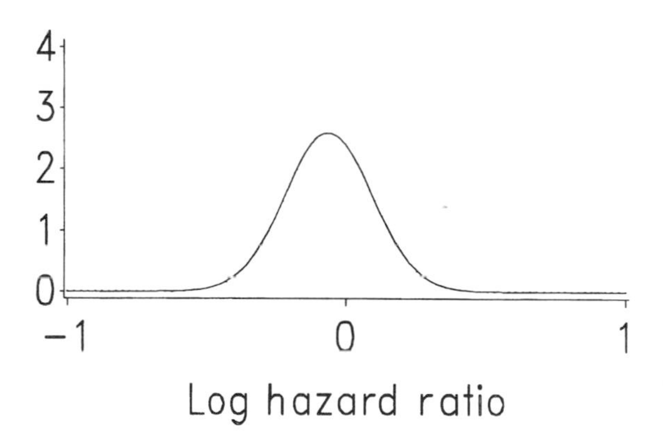

Figure 6 Likelihood distribution of the observed data on the log hazard ratio (LHR) scale.

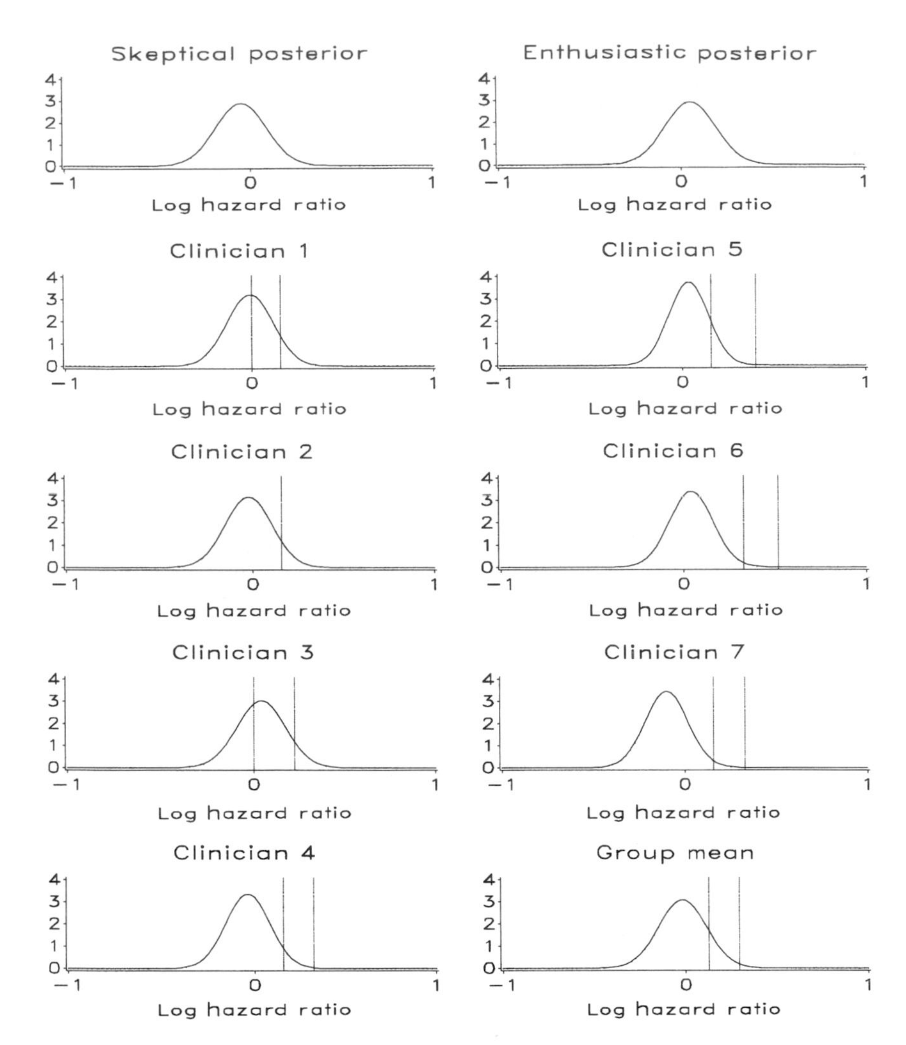

Figure 7 Posterior distributions, including the opinions of the seven participating clinicians modified by the results of the trial. Vertical lines represent the boundaries of the range of equivalence.

and upper bounds of the range of equivalence for each clinician are shown in Table 7. These probabilities vary considerably depending on the outlook of the clinician involved.

Clinician 3, who was the most enthusiastic about the new treatment, may require the most convincing that there was little difference observed between the treatments. Combining his or her prior opinion with the data suggested that his or her probability of the multidrug regimen being clinically worthwhile was 63%. However, the posterior probability of the LHR exceeding the upper bound of the range of equivalence was only 9% and thus even clinician 3 would be unlikely to adopt multidrug therapy on the basis of these results. Clinician 7, who did not believe that multidrug therapy would offer any survival benefit, would feel further vindicated by the result of the trial. According to that individual's posterior distribution, there is only a 1% chance that the multidrug regimen is likely to be clinically worthwhile. The maximum posterior probability over the seven participating clinicians that the effect of multidrug treatment exceeds their upper limit of the range of equivalence, and therefore is clearly indicated, was only 0.09.

The group mean posterior distribution, which summarizes average clinical opinion on the trial, suggests that multidrug therapy offers insufficient survival benefit to warrant usage. The probability of the LHR exceeding the minimum clinically worthwhile benefit (4% benefit to multidrug) was 14%, and the probability of exceeding the upper bound of the range of equivalence (9% benefit) was 1%.

Table 7 Probability That the Log Hazard Ratio Is Greater Than the Boundaries of the Range of Equivalence for Each Clinician

	Range of equivalence	*P* (LHR > lower bound)	*P* (LHR > upper bound)	*P* (LHR lies in range of equivalence)
Clinician 1	0–5	0.48	0.09	0.39
Clinician 2	5–5	0.08	0.08	0.00
Clinician 3	0–7	0.63	0.09	0.54
Clinician 4	5–10	0.05	<0.01	0.05
Clinician 5	5–12	0.13	<0.01	0.13
Clinician 6	10–15	0.01	<0.01	0.01
Clinician 7	5–10	0.01	<0.01	0.01
Group mean	4–9	0.14	0.01	0.13

2.5. Discussion*

In rare tumors such as osteosarcoma, nonrandomized studies are useful to show whether new treatments are feasible and effective. However, major differences in treatment policy must be assessed by randomized trials. One such major difference, between the complex and lengthy T10 protocol and the shorter and simpler two-drug regimen, was the subject of our randomized trial.

The reported results of Rosen using the T10 protocol in a nonrandomized study (Rosen et al., 1982) were so much better than the results reported from studies of simpler chemotherapy regimens [e.g., the first EOI study (Bramwell et al., 1992)], that a randomized comparison was demanded to settle the issue.

This trial found no evidence of a difference in progression-free or overall survival in favor of the T10 protocol. The hazard ratio estimated from the trial was 0.94, representing a 2% absolute reduction in the 5-year survival rate (i.e., a reduction from 56 to 54%). However, values of the hazard ratio from 0.69 up to 1.27 are feasible, equivalent to anything from a 12% decrease to an 8% increase in the 5-year survival rate due to multidrug treatment.

The social consequences of very lengthy chemotherapy regimens are quite severe in patients of this age group, many of whom are attending school or university courses. There is a substantial advantage to a treatment that takes only 18 weeks. The cost of drugs was substantially greater for the multidrug regimen (about $9000) than for the two-drug regimen (about $3000), and the bed occupancy rate was higher. Both regimens were associated with considerable toxicity for the duration of treatment. For these reasons, participating clinicians felt that to be clearly preferable multidrug therapy needed to increase the 5-year survival rate by about 10% (see Table 1). The results of the trial indicate that such an increase is highly unlikely.

Our Bayesian analysis demonstrates that this conclusion is robust to a wide variety of "starting positions" with regard to the likely benefit of the multidrug treatment. Table 7 shows that after the trial the posterior probability that multidrug treatment is clearly preferable to two-drug

* Author's note: The original trial report (Souhami et al., 1997) provides a full discussion of the results of this trial, and although the rest of the paper follows exactly the lines of an intended medical publication, in this section we will reproduce only some of their more general points and will add some extra points that result from the use of a Bayesian analysis.

treatment was less than 0.1 for all the participating clinicians, despite their starting from varying positions of skepticism or enthusiasm.

Despite this conclusive result, the cure rate for ostcosarcoma is still unsatisfactory and further progress is necessary. The European Osteosarcoma Intergroup has shown that cisplatin and doxorubicin can be intensified further with the use of hemopoietic growth factors such as granulocyte-colony stimulating factor (Ornadel et al., 1994), and this approach is the basis of the new treatment being tested in their current randomized trial. Since we have shown in our trial that shorter periods of intensive treatment are as effective for osteosarcoma, dose intensification becomes a feasible option. Other drugs, such as ifosfamide, have activity in osteosarcoma, but no randomized comparison of the efficacy of regimens including this drug have been reported. Future trials should aim to discover more effective ways of combining these agents.

3. EPILOGUE

In this chapter we have attempted to show by example how to report a clinical trial analyzed using Bayesian methods. The advantage of such an approach in the present example is undoubtedly the sensitivity analysis in the Interpretation section, which supports the conclusions drawn in the Discussion and demonstrates their robustness. The availability of prior clinical opinion in this trial no doubt strengthens the sensitivity analysis. However, sensitivity analysis can be conducted without the elicitation of prior opinion as shown in the calculation of the 'skeptical' and 'enthusiastic' posterior distributions, and can be used in a similar manner to support or qualify the conclusions from a trial.

Bayesian analysis carries other advantages, particularly for trial monitoring, and for the analysis of trials that terminate early for some reason. Those advantages are not seen in this particular trial which continued until its recruitment goals were met and until all patients were followed for an adequate period. It might be instructive to repeat the present exercise for such an example.

The approach outlined in this chapter is not the only way that Bayesian methods can be used to analyze clinical trials. In a pair of recent papers, Goodman argues that the p value approach to hypothesis testing is fundamentally flawed (Goodman, 1999a) and advocates basing inference on the likelihood, or Bayes factor (Goodman, 1999b). The rationale for this is to emphasize that Bayesian methods do have a solid, data-based core and are not simply based on subjective opinion. However, the Bayes factor in itself is not necessarily easy to interpret, and the advantage of our method is that it provides a context for the trial results which can be easily understood by the intended audience.

One of the criticisms that could be levelled at this paper is that the sections explaining the methodology and analysis of the trial are too long. We accept this argument, but feel it is necessary to give a detailed and hopefully understandable explanation of techniques that are still unfamiliar to a nonstatistical audience. If Bayesian methods become more popular they will require as little explanation as Kaplan-Meier curves, the logrank test and Cox proportional hazards models in current trial reports.

The same criticism could be made of the Interpretation section. We would argue that a full explanation of how the trial results would influence participants who hold a wide range of opinions is one of the advantages of these methods. It is also likely that the addition of the Interpretation section will lead to a proportionate reduction in the length of the Discussion section, which can be fully devoted to examining the wider implications of the trial results.

We hope that the example we present in this chapter will help to convince investigators that it is quite possible to present a report of a clinical trial analyzed by Bayesian methods in a manner that will be acceptable and even welcomed by the clinical community, or at least will encourage them to try!

ACKNOWLEDGMENTS

We would like to thank the chairman of the European Osteosarcoma Intergroup, Professor Alan Craft, and the coordinator of this study, Professor Robert Souhami, for permission to use data and ideas from their 1997 paper to produce our "medical paper."

REFERENCES

Abrams, K., Ashby, D., Errington, D. (1996). A Bayesian approach to Weibull survival models—application to a cancer clinical trial. Lifetime Data Analysis 2:159–174.

Bramwell, V. H. C., Burgers, M., Sneath, R., Souhami, R., van Oosterom, A. T.,

Voute, P. A., Rouesse, J., Spooner, D., Craft, A. W., Somers, R., Pringle, J., Malcolm, A. J., van der Eijken, J., Thomas, D., Uscinska, B., Machin, D., van Glabbeke, M. (1992). A comparison of two short intensive chemotherapy regimens in operable osteosarcoma of limbs in children and young adults: The first study of the European Osteosarcoma Intergroup. Journal of Clinical Oncology 10:1579–1591.

Carlin, B. P., Sargent, D. J. (1996). Robust Bayesian approaches for clinical trials monitoring. Statistics in Medicine 15:1093–1106.

Eilber, F., Giuliano, A., Eckardt, J., Patterson, K., Moseley, S., Goodnight, J. (1987). Adjuvant chemotherapy for osteosarcoma: a randomized prospective trial. Journal of Clinical Oncology 5:21–26.

Fayers, P. M., Ashby, D., Parmar, M. K. B. (1997). Tutorial in Biostatistics: Bayesian data monitoring in clinical trials. Statistics in Medicine 16:1413–1430.

Freedman, L. S., Spiegelhalter, D. J. (1983). The assessment of subjective opinion and its use in relation to stopping rules for clinical trials. The Statistician 33:153–160.

Goodman, S. N. (1999a). Towards Evidence-Based Medical Statistics. 1: The P Value Fallacy. Annals of Internal Medicine 130:995–1004.

Goodman, S. N. (1999b). Towards Evidence-Based Medical Statistics. 2: The Bayes Factor. Annals of Internal Medicine 130:1005–1013.

Greenhouse, J. B., Wasserman, L. (1995). Robust Bayesian methods for monitoring clinical trials. Statistics in Medicine 14:1379–1391.

Hughes, M. D. (1993). Reporting Bayesian analysis of clinical trials. Statistics in Medicine 12:1651–1663.

Link, M. P., Goorin, A. M., Miser, A. W., Green, A. A., Pratt, C. B., Belasco, J. B., Pritchard, J., Malpas, J. S., Baker, A. R., Kirkpatrick, J. A., et al. The effect of adjuvant chemotherapy on relapse-free survival in patients with osteosarcoma of the extremity. New England Journal of Medicine 314:1600–1606.

Machin, D., Campbell, M., Fayers, P., Pinol, A. (1997). Sample Size Tables for Clinical Studies. 2nd ed. Oxford: Blackwell Science.

Meyers, P. A., Heller, G., Healey, J., Huvos, A., Lane, J., Marcove, R., Applewhite, A., Vlamis, V., Rosen, G. (1992). Chemotherapy for non-metastatic osteogenic sarcoma: The Memorial Sloan-Kettering experience. Journal of Clinical Oncology 10:5–15.

Ornadel, D., Souhami, R. L., Whelan, J., Nooy, M., de Elvira, C. R., Pringle, J., Lewis, I., Steward, W. P., George, R., Bridgewater, J., Wierzbicki, R., Craft, A. W. (1994). Doxorubicin and cisplatin with granulocyte colony stimulating factor as adjuvant therapy for osteosarcoma: Phase II trial of the European Osteosarcoma Intergroup. Journal of Clinical Oncology 12:1842–1847.

Parmar, M. K. B., Machin, D. (1995). Survival Analysis: A Practical Approach. Chichester, England: Wiley.

Parmar, M. K. B., Spiegelhalter, D. J., Freedman, L. S. (1994). The CHART trials: Bayesian design and monitoring in practice. Statistics in Medicine 13:1297–1312.

Parmar, M. K. B., Ungerleider, R. S., Simon, R. (1996). Assessing whether to perform a confirmatory randomized clinical trial. Journal of the National Cancer Institute 88:1645–1651.

Parmar, M. K. B., Griffiths, G. O., Spiegelhalter, D. J., Souhami, R. L., Altman, O. G., van der Scheven, E. (2001). Monitoring of large randomised clinical trials: a new approach with Bayesian methods. Lancet 358:375–381.

Rosen, G., Caparros, B., Huvos, A. G., Kosloff, C., Nirenberg, A., Cacavio, A., Marcove, R. C., Lane, J. M., Mehta, B., Urban, C. (1982). Preoperative chemotherapy for osteogenic sarcoma: selection of postoperative adjuvant chemotherapy based on the response of the primary tumor to preoperative chemotherapy. Cancer 49:1221–1230.

Simon, R., Freedman, L. S. (1997). Bayesian design and analysis of 2 × 2 factorial clinical trials. Biometrics 53:456–464.

Souhami, R. L., Craft, A. W., Van der Eijken, J. W., Nooij, M., Spooner, D., Bramwell, V. H. C., Wierzbicki, R., Malcolm, A. J., Kirkpatrick, A., Uscinska, B. M., Van Glabbeke, M., Machin, D. (1997). Randomized trial of two regimens of chemotherapy in operable osteosarcoma: a study of the European Osteosarcoma Intergroup. Lancet 350:911–917.

Spiegelhalter, D. J., Freedman, L. S., Parmar, M. K. B. (1993). Applying Bayesian ideas in drug development and clinical trials. Statistics in Medicine 12: 1501–1511.

Spiegelhalter, D. J., Freedman, L. S., Parmar, M. K. B. (1994). Bayesian approaches to randomized trials. Journal of the Royal Statistical Society A 157:357–416.

Stangl, D. K., Greenhouse, J. B. (1998). Assessing placebo response using Bayesian hierarchical survival models. Lifetime Data Analysis 4:5–28.

Thall, P. F., Simon, R. M., Estey, E. H. (1996). New statistical strategy for monitoring safety and efficacy in single-arm clinical trials. Journal of Clinical Oncology 14:296–303.

Tsiatis, A. A. (1981). The asymptotic joint distribution of the efficient scores test for the proportional hazards model over time. Biometrika 68:311–315.

Winkler, K., Beron, G., Kotz, R., Salzer-Kuntschik, M., Beck, J., Beck, W., Brandeis, W., Ebell, W., Erttmann, R., Gobel, U., et al. Neoadjuvant chemotherapy for osteogenic sarcoma: results of a cooperative German/Austrian study. Journal of Clinical Oncology 2:617–624.

10

Methods Incorporating Compliance in Treatment Evaluation

Juni Palmgren
Stockholm University and Karolinska Institutet, Stockholm, Sweden

Els Goetghebeur
University of Ghent, Ghent, Belgium

1. INTRODUCTION

As pointed out by Neyman (1923) and Fisher (1925), randomization is a cornerstone of scientific experimentation. Traditional theories of inference based on randomization formally require that all experimental units comply with their assigned treatment. However, in studies involving human subjects, noncompliance is common and the compliance pattern may differ between treatment arms. The standard approach is to rely on the randomization distribution as if compliance had been perfect, and thus to compare response distributions by assignment, ignoring information on compliance (Lee et al., 1991). This is often referred to as the intent-to-treat analysis. The intent-to-treat analysis does not, however, measure biologic efficacy, but rather programmatic effectiveness, which depends on the biologic action as well as on the compliance with the treatment regimen. As the number of noncompliers increases, effectiveness will decrease regardless of the biologic efficacy of the treatment.

Treatment effectiveness and treatment efficacy address distinct scientific questions, both of which are important. Biologic efficacy is, however, more likely to be reproducible in different populations and subgroups. Similarly, potential effect modification is better assessed on the efficacy scale, since factors that modify the treatment effect may also influence compliance. While the intent-to-treat analysis is usually straightforward, acceptable approaches for estimating efficacy have been lacking. It is reasonable to assume that the treatment protocol presents a different challenge for compliance than the control protocol, and those who adhere to the protocol in the different treatment arms are not as a rule comparable. This results in serious potential for selection bias if individuals who complete the treatment regimen are compared with controls who complete the control regimen.

The causal framework of Rubin (1978) and Holland (1986) provides new tools for evaluating average treatment efficacy. Models are specified in terms of potential responses and potential receipt of the experimental treatment, and a randomization-based inference procedure is used. In order to avoid selection bias comparison is made to the subgroup in the placebo arm that corresponds to the treatment compliers and not to the subgroup of placebo compliers. Although the individual treatment compliers in the placebo arm cannot be identified, their average response can be compared to the average response among similar treatment compliers in the treated arm. The efficacy so estimated pertains to the subgroup of compliers, and extrapolation to the full population under study requires additional model assumptions. Additional model assumptions are also needed if non-compliance is measured on an ordered categorical or continuous scale.

Our aim is to give a flavor of the recent development of methodology for estimating treatment efficacy when faced with nonrandom noncompliance. We focus on model specification for the two-group parallel trial, with one treatment arm and one placebo arm. Basic concepts are illustrated using the Efron and Feldman (1991) data from the Lipid Research Clinics Coronary Primary Prevention Trial (LRC-CPPT). This was a placebo-controlled double-blind randomized clinical trial assessing the efficacy of cholestyramine for lowering cholesterol level and thereby reducing coronary heart disease. The Lipid Research Clinic Program (1984) describes the complete study. Efron and Feldman estimated the efficacy of treatment received by making a strong assumption for noncompliance: They assumed corresponding compliance quantiles in the treated and in the control arm to have similar average treatment-free response distributions. As argued by Albert and DeMets (1994) this nonselection assumption has considerable impact on the inferences drawn.

In Section 2 we dichotomize the nominal dose of cholestyramine received for the purpose of illustrating null versus full compliance. Those on the lower relative dose are treated as null compliers and those on the higher relative dose as full compliers. Following Angrist, Imbens, and Rubin (1996) we define a set of potential outcomes and present the concept of Local Average Treatment Effect (LATE), i.e., the average effect of treatment received on cholesterol reduction in the subgroup of compliers. Angrist, Imbens, and Rubin also emphasize that the randomization indicator serves as a so-called instrumental variable, a well-known tool for handling errors that are correlated with the explanatory variable in linear econometric models. In Section 3 we dichotomize the response (cholesterol reduction) and recapture the procedure proposed by Sommer and Zeger (1991) and Zeger (1998) for estimating biologic efficacy for a binary response with null versus full compliance. We extend the argument to ordered categorical compliance by elaborating on the Goetghebeur and Molenberghs (1996) analysis of the cholestyramine data. They present efficacy estimates for partial dose in the subgroup of partial treatment compliers and for full dose in the subgroup of full treatment compliers.

When data on compliance with experimental treatment are more detailed a parametric structural model may be used, which links the compliance information to the potential response data. The structural model may further include compliance-covariate interaction terms, which describe differential efficacy in subgroups determined by values of measured covariates. In Section 4 we present the main features of the structural mean model used by Goetghebeur and Lapp (1997) for assessing blood pressure reduction for 300 hypertensive patients randomized to treatment or placebo. The blood pressure was measured on a continuous scale, and compliance to treatment was assessed by the medical event monitoring system (MEMS) producing essentially continuous relative dose information. While the structural mean models handle responses measured on a continuous scale, structural failure time models are useful for responses measured on a time-to-event scale. In Section 5 we refer to several applications of structural failure time models, and in Section 6 we sketch current directions for the development of models and procedures for nonrandom noncompliance.

Inferences for the models discussed throughout this chapter rely heavily on the randomization distribution: conditional on any subspace spanned by covariates measured before randomization, the expected distribution for any pre-randomization characteristic should be identical in the two trial arms. Two constructs are used as prerandomization characteristics: the potential *treatment compliance* and the potential *treatment-free response*. These two constructs are assumed to exist as inherent features of the individual prior to randomization. Treatment compliance is subsequently observed for those randomized to the treated arm, but for those in the placebo arm it remains a latent construct. Treatment-free response is observed for those who receive no treatment, and for others it may be computed from a more or less complex structural model. For the models in Section 3 we formulate a multinomial likelihood with the cell probabilities parameterized to reflect similarity for treatment compliance and for treatment-free response, respectively, in the two trial arms. For the structural models in Sections 4 and 5 we set up estimating equations that correspond to test statistics for testing equality of features of the distributions for the expected treatment-free response in the two trial arms.

In the treated arm the compliance subgroups may differ in terms of measured covariates. We argue throughout that conditioning on covariates that simultaneously predict treatment compliance and placebo response improves the precision for estimating efficacy.

2. POTENTIAL OUTCOMES AND "CAUSAL" EFFECTS

2.1. Potential Outcomes

Figure 1 illustrates the observed cholesterol reduction for 337 patients in the Lipid Research Clinics Coronary Prevention Trial (LRC-CPPT) as a function of percentage of prescribed dose actually taken of cholestyramine and placebo, respectively. Smoothed curves are fit to the scatterplots.

The data in Figure 1 were analyzed by Efron and Feldman (1991), who treated cholesterol reduction and dose as continuous variables and focused on a linear model for the average reduction as function of dose and other covariates. For the same data Zeger (1998) used a dichotomized dose scale and response scale, and Goetghebeur and Molenberghs (1996) used an ordered categorical dose scale.

It is clear from Figure 1 that the percentage of the dose actually taken varies between the two treatment arms, with a tendency for higher percentages in the placebo arm. Figure 1 also shows a steeper rise in cholesterol reduction in the treated group as function of percentage of prescribed dose. Although randomization guarantees overall comparability between the treated and the control arm, it is likely that individuals are differently distributed over the compliance axes in a fashion which may directly or indirectly be associated with cholesterol reduction. If selection of this kind is present, it would be seriously misleading to draw conclusions

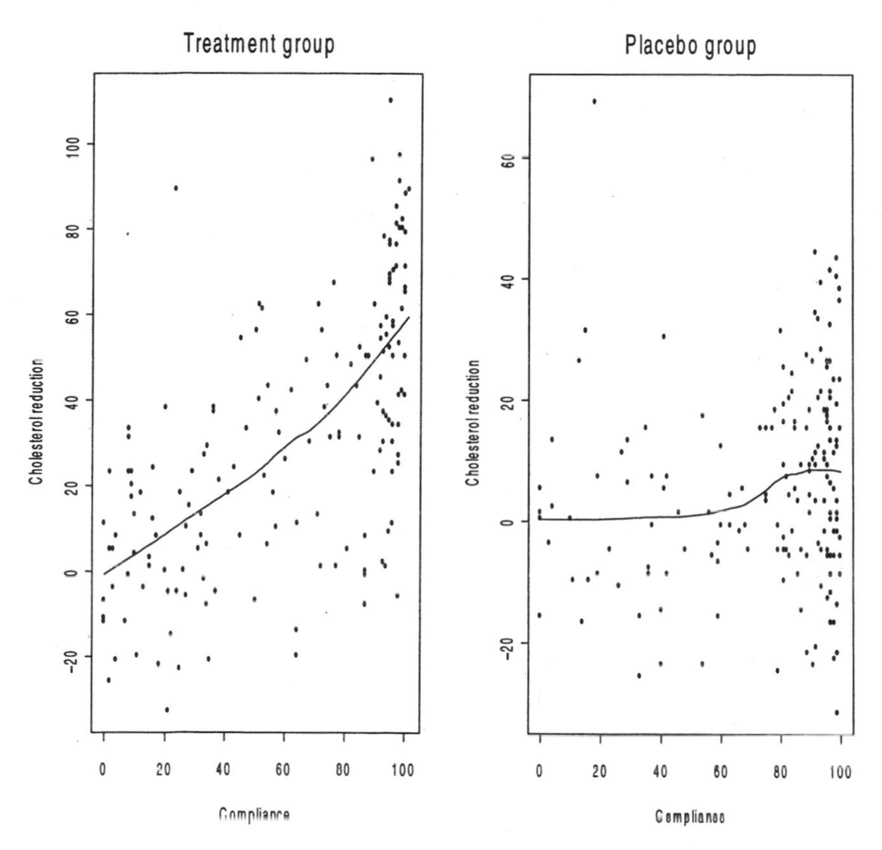

Figure 1 Observed compliance-response relationship in the LRC-CPPT trial.

concerning efficacy from comparing the trend in cholesterol reduction for the two panels in Figure 1.

Here we treat cholesterol reduction as a continuous response variable, while the percentage of the nominal dose actually received is dichotomized at 60%. Those below the cut point are treated as noncompliers and those above the cutpoint as full compliers. This crude approximation serves the purpose of illustrating the *null* versus *full* compliance pattern. Let $R_i = 1$ and $R_i = 0$ indicate the assignment of individual i to the cholestyramine arm or to the control arm, respectively. For given assignment R_i, the individual receives a dose of cholestyramine as indicated by

$D_i(R_i) = 0$ ($\leq 60\%$ of nominal dose) or 1 ($>60\%$), and then experiences a cholesterol reduction of $Y_i\{R_i, D_i(R_i)\}$ units. Note that $D_i(R_i)$ refers to the dose received of the *experimental treatment* in the respective arms, and that the percentage of nominal *placebo dose* will not be used in the model specification. If the experimental treatment is not available in the placebo arm, then $D_i(0) = 0$ for all i. We refer to $D_i(R_i)$ and $Y_i\{R_i, D_i(R_i)\}$, for $R_i =$ 0 or 1, as potential outcomes. The potential outcomes that get observed for any given individual i depends on the random assignment of treatment. If individual i is assigned to experimental treatment, then $D_i(1)$ and $Y_i\{1, D_i(1)\}$ are observed, and if assigned to placebo, then $D_i(0)$ and $Y_i\{0, D_i(0)\}$ are observed. Throughout we assume that $D_i(R_i)$ and $Y_i\{R_i, D_i(R_i)\}$ depend only on R_i, the treatment assigned to individual i, and not on the treatment assignment to other individuals under study. In the causal literature this independence assumption is called the *stable unit treatment value assumption* (Angrist, Imbens, and Rubin, 1996).

The double argument for the cholesterol reduction is useful for making explicit the so-called exclusion restriction: $Y_i\{R_i, D_i(R_i)\} = Y_i\{D_i(R_i)\}$ (Angrist, Imbens, and Rubin 1996). This restriction states that any effect of R_i on $Y_i\{R_i, D_i(R_i)\}$ must be via the effect of $D_i(R_i)$. The treatment assignment is thus assumed conditionally independent of the response, given the dose of the experimental treatment that was actually received. This exclusion restriction is plausible if the study was appropriately blinded, in which case the random assignment per se is not expected to affect the response. Under the exclusion restriction any comparison of $Y_i\{D_i(1)\}$ with $Y_i\{D_i(0)\}$, i.e., the potential response for an individual i if allocated to the treatment arm versus if allocated to the placebo arm, will depend solely on the experimental treatment received in the respective arms.

In studies with prolonged follow-up, postrandomization treatment changes for reasons other than non-compliance may occur. Distinctions between direct and indirect effects of treatment are discussed by Greenland and Robins (1994) and by White and Pocock (1996). They are also taken up in Chapter 12 by Babiker and Walker on AIDS models.

2.2. Local Average Treatment Efficacy (LATE)

In Table 1 the difference in cholesterol reduction between the treated arm and the control arm for an individual i is cross-classified according to the value of the potential treatment compliance variable $D_i(1)$ when assigned to the treatment arm, and $D_i(0)$ when assigned to placebo.

Table 1 Treatment Arm Difference in Cholesterol Reduction $Y_i(1, D_i(1)) - Y_i(0, D_i(0))$, for an Individual i Classified by $D_i(1)$ and $D_i(0)$

	$D_i(0)$	
	0	1
$D_i(1)$ 0	$Y_i(1, 0) - Y_i(0, 0) = 0$ Never taker	$Y_i(1, 0) - Y_i(0, 1) = -(Y_i(1) - Y_i(0))$ Defier
1	$Y_i(1, 1) - Y_i(0, 0) = Y_i(1) - Y_i(0)$ Complier	$Y_i(1, 1) - Y_i(0, 1) = 0$ Always taker

The category corresponding to $D_i(0) = D_i(1) = 0$ in Table 1 defines an individual who would never take the treatment, regardless of treatment assignment. If the experimental treatment is available also in the placebo arm, then the category $D_i(0) = D_i(1) = 1$ defines an "always taker." Under the exclusion restriction the never takers and the always takers contribute nothing to an aggregated group difference in cholesterol reduction when comparing the two trial arms. Following Angrist, Imbens, and Rubin (1996) we summarize the entries in Table 1 as $Y_i\{1, D_i(1)\} - Y_i\{0, D_i(0)\} = Y_i\{D_i(1)\} - Y_i\{D_i(0)\}$, and for $D_i(0) = D_i(1)$ this difference is zero. For the category $D_i(1) = 1$, $D_i(0) = 0$, i.e., for the *compliers*, the difference $Y_i\{D_i(1)\} - Y_i\{D_i(0)\}$ is written $Y_i(1) - Y_i(0)$, and for the category $D_i(1) = 0$, $D_i(0) = 1$, the *defiers*, i.e., those who always do the reverse of what their assignment requires, the difference is $-\{Y_i(1) - Y_i(0)\}$.

Referring to Table 1, the difference in cholesterol reduction for an individual i as function of treatment arm allocation can be written in the form

$$
\begin{aligned}
Y_i\{1, D_i(1)\} - Y_i\{0, D_i(0)\} &= Y_i\{D_i(1)\} - Y_i\{D_i(0)\} \\
&= [Y_i(1)D_i(1) + Y_i(0)\{1 - D_i(1)\}] - [Y_i(1)D_i(0) \\
&\quad + Y_i(0)\{1 - D_i(0)\}] = \{Y_i(1) - Y_i(0)\}\{D_i(1) - D_i(0)\}.
\end{aligned} \tag{1}
$$

Before taking expectations the *strong monotonicity* assumption of Imbens and Angrist (1994) is invoked, which states that $D_i(1) \geq D_i(0)$ for all i, with inequality for at least one i. This monotonicity assumption excludes the existence of defiers, and the proportion of compliers $Pr\{D_i(1) - D_i(0) = 1\}$ equals the expected value $E\{D_i(1) - D_i(0)\}$, with $E\{D_i(1) - D_i(0)\} > 0$. When averaging both sides of the expression in (1), the always takers and the never takers contribute nothing, and by excluding the existence of defiers, the average difference in response between treatment arms 'as assigned' has the form

$$
\begin{aligned}
&E[Y_i\{1, D_i(1)\} - Y_i\{0, D_i(0)\}] \\
&\quad = E[\{Y_i(1) - Y_i(0)\}\{D_i(1) - D_i(0)\}] \\
&\quad = E\{Y_i(1) - Y_i(0) \mid D_i(1) - D_i(0) = 1\}Pr\{D_i(1) - D_i(0) = 1\} \\
&\quad = E\{Y_i(1) - Y_i(0) \mid D_i(1) - D_i(0) = 1\}E\{D_i(1) - D_i(0)\}
\end{aligned}
$$

and we can write the average difference in response among the compliers as

$$
\begin{aligned}
&E\{Y_i(1) - Y_i(0) \mid D_i(1) - D_i(0) = 1\} \\
&\quad = \frac{E[Y_i\{1, D_i(1)\} - Y_i\{0, D_i(0)\}]}{E\{D_i(1) - D_i(0)\}}.
\end{aligned}
\tag{2}
$$

By virtue of the random assignment, the numerator in (2) is equal to $E(Y_{j1}) - E(Y_{j0})$, and the denominator is equal to $E(D_{j1}) - E(D_{j0})$, with j_k indexing individuals assigned to arm k, for $k = 0, 1$. An estimate of the right-hand side of (2) is obtained by dividing the difference in mean response between the two treatment arms by the difference in the average experimental treatment received between the two treatment arms. An estimator for the biologic treatment efficacy among compliers can thus be computed from observable data, by dividing the intention-to-treat estimator of treatment effectiveness with the treatment arm difference in the proportion taking the experimental substance. Imbens and Angrist (1994) call this the Local Average Treatment Effect (LATE). Although this average efficacy measure is estimable, it is in general not possible to identify the latent subgroup of compliers (cf. Table 1) to which the effect pertains. This is particularly true if the experimental treatment is available also in the placebo arm, in which case the observed group of treatment compliers is a mixture of true compliers and always takers. If the experimental treatment is not available in the placebo arm, then the column $D_i(0) = 1$ in Table 1 vanishes, and the compliers are identified from the observed entries in the treated arm.

In the LRC-CPPT-trial cholestyramine was not available for those randomized to placebo, i.e., $D_i(0) = 0$ for all i, and thus neither "defiers" nor "always takers" were possible. Those observed to comply with the assignment to cholestyramine in the treated arm are all "compliers" and those observed not to comply with the assignment to experimental treatment are all "never takers." For the cholestyramine data the intent-to-treat effectiveness, i.e., the difference in cholesterol reduction between the treated arm and the control arm "as assigned" is estimated to $E(Y_{j1}) - E(Y_{j0}) = 20.79$ units. The treatment arm difference in the propotion taking at least 60% of the prescribed dose of experimental treatment is $E(D_{j1}) - E(D_{j0}) = E(D_{j1}) = 88/165 = 0.53$, and thus an estimate of the Local Average Treatment Efficacy (LATE) is $20.79/0.53 = 39.23$ units for the compliant subgroup. Here the biologic efficacy is by definition greater than the intent-to-treat effectiveness of treatment.

As emphasized by Angrist, Imbens, and Rubin, an analogue to the LATE estimator in (2) may be derived from a simple structural linear equation model (Haavelmo, 1943; Goldberger, 1972). The randomization indicator R_i plays the role of an exogenous *instrumental variable*. An instrumental variable is useful for disentangling "causal" effects when the regression of response on exposure has residual errors which are correlated with exposure. The instrumental variable is defined to be associated with exposure, but conditionally independent of response given exposure. If such a variable is available, then an appropriate set of structural equations allows estimation of the causal effect of exposure on response. Use of instrumental variables in econometric modeling is hampered by the difficulty in finding real world instruments that fulfill the required conditions. In the compliance setting the randomization indicator R_i does by definition fulfill the conditions for an instrument, provided treatment allocation has been both random and appropriately blinded. The assumption of random as well as blinded treatment allocation constitutes the key which allows causal questions to be asked when faced with nonrandom noncompliance in clinical trials.

3. STRUCTURAL MODELS FOR BINARY RESPONSES

3.1. "Null" versus "Full" Compliance

Table 2 summarizes the information in Figure 1 by dichotomizing cholesterol reduction using 20 units as the cutpoint, and by retaining the null versus full compliance, with 60% as the cutpoint for the percentage of the prescribed dose actually taken. Note that the placebo compliance rate in the placebo arms is $126/172 = 73\%$, which is considerably larger than the treatment compliance rate in the treated arm, which is $88/165 = 53\%$. The possibility of nonrandom noncompliance is apparent. Table 3 summarizes the structure of the observed data that will be used for assessing efficacy.

Table 2 Cross-Classification of Cholesterol Reduction ($Y = 1$ if at least 20 units; $Y = 0$ otherwise), Treatment Arm Assignment ($R = 1$ for treated arm; $R = 0$ for control arm) and Compliance (≤60%; >60%)

		Placebo ($R = 0$)			Treatment ($R = 1$)		
		Placebo compliance			Treatment compliance		
		≤60%	>60%		≤60%	>60%	
Y	0	42	98	140	50	16	66
	1	4	28	32	27	72	99
		46	126	172	77	88	165

In Table 3 placebo compliance categories are replaced by latent unobserved treatment compliance categories in the placebo arm. The selection problem for compliance is thus avoided since by definition the compliance categories in the two arms in Table 3 are comparable.

The observed data in Table 3 follow a multinomial distribution with four cells in the treated arm, and a binomial distribution in the placebo arm. We write $\Pr\{D_i(1) = 1 \mid R_i = 1\} = \Pr\{D_i(1) = 1 \mid R_i = 0\} = \delta$ and $\Pr\{Y_i(0) = 1 \mid D_i(1) = 0, R_i = 0\} = \Pr\{Y_i(1) = 1 \mid D_i(1) = 0, R_i = 1\} = \alpha_0$, to reflect that the distributions for expected treatment compliance and expected treatment-free response are similar in the two trial arms, due to randomization. We further write $\Pr\{Y_i(0) = 1 \mid D_i(1) = 1, R_i = 0\} = \alpha_1$ for the response probability in the subgroup of potential treatment compliers in the placebo arm. The corresponding

Table 3 Data in Table 2 Used for Estimation of Efficacy Among Compliers

		Placebo ($R = 0$)			Treatment ($R = 1$)		
		Treatment compliance			Treatment compliance		
		$D = 0$	$D = 1$		$D = 0$	$D = 1$	
Y	0	$m_{00} = ?$	$m_{01} = ?$	$m_{0+} = 140$	$n_{00} = 50$	$n_{01} = 16$	$n_{0+} = 66$
	1	$m_{10} = ?$	$m_{11} = ?$	$m_{1+} = 32$	$n_{10} = 27$	$n_{11} = 72$	$n_{1+} = 99$
		$m_{+0} = ?$	$m_{+1} = ?$	$m_{++} = 172$	$n_{+0} = 77$	$n_{+1} = 88$	$n_{++} = 165$

response probability in the treated arm is $\Pr\{Y_i(1) = 1 \mid D_i(1) = 1, R_i = 1\}$, and the risk of interest γ is defined as the ratio

$$\gamma = \frac{\Pr\{Y_i(1) = 1 \mid D_i(1) = 1, R_i = 1\}}{\Pr\{Y_i(0) = 1 \mid D_i(1) = 1, R_i = 0\}}.$$

Table 4 presents the multinomial cell probabilities for the observed and latent counts in Table 3. The risk parameter γ simply captures the excess risk in the subgroup $D_i(1) = 1$ due to experimental treatment actually received in the treated arm. The treated arm has 3 degrees of freedom and the placebo arm one degree of freedom for joint estimation of δ, α_0, α_1, and γ. The model is thus saturated with four parameters, all of which are identifiable. Using the notation for the observed counts in Table 3 and for the expected counts in Table 4, we write the log likelihood function $l = l^P + l^T$, with l^T the contribution from the multinomial in the treated arm

$$l^T = n_{00} \log\{(1 - \delta)(1 - \alpha_0)\} + n_{01} \log\{\delta(1 - \gamma\alpha_1)\}$$
$$+ n_{10} \log\{(1 - \delta)\alpha_0\} + n_{11} \log(\delta\gamma\alpha_1)$$

and l^P the contribution from the binomial in the placebo arm

$$l^P = m_{0+} \log\{(1 - \delta)(1 - \alpha_0) + \delta(1 - \alpha_1)\} + m_{1+} \log\{(1 - \delta)\alpha_0$$
$$+ \delta\alpha_1\}.$$

Table 4 Expected Cell Probabilities for the Cross-Classification in Table 3, Assuming Similar Placebo Response and Treatment Compliance in the Two Treatment Arms. (The relative risk γ captures the treatment efficacy among compliers.)

		Placebo ($R = 0$)		Treatment ($R = 1$)	
		Treatment compliance		Treatment compliance	
		$D = 0$	$D = 1$	$D = 0$	$D = 1$
Y	0	$(1 - \delta)(1 - \alpha_0)$	$\delta(1 - \alpha_1)$	$(1 - \delta)(1 - \alpha_0)$	$\delta(1 - \gamma\alpha_1)$
	1	$(1 - \delta)\alpha_0$	$\delta\alpha_1$	$(1 - \delta)\alpha_0$	$\delta\gamma\alpha_1$
		$1 - \delta$	δ	$1 - \delta$	δ

The maximum likelihood estimators have the form

$$\hat{\alpha}_0 = \frac{n_{10}}{n_{00} + n_{10}} \qquad \hat{\delta} = \frac{n_{01} + n_{11}}{n_{++}}$$

$$\hat{\alpha}_1 = \frac{\hat{m}_{11}}{\hat{m}_{11} + \hat{m}_{01}} \qquad \hat{\gamma} = \frac{n_{11}}{n_{11} + n_{01}} \hat{\alpha}_1^{-1}$$

with $\hat{m}_{11} = m_{1+} - \frac{m_{++}}{n_{++}} n_{10}$ and $\hat{m}_{01} = m_{0+} - \frac{m_{++}}{n_{++}} n_{00}$. The estimated expected cell counts for the cholestyramine data are given in Table 5, and the corresponding estimates are $\hat{\alpha}_0 = 0.35$, $\hat{\alpha}_1 = 0.042$, $\hat{\delta} = 0.53$, and $\hat{\gamma} = 19.5$.

A straightforward extension of the above model is obtained by conditioning on baseline covariates. For a vector of given baseline covariate values Z, the expected counts have a similar structure as in Table 4, parameterized in terms of $\alpha_0(Z)$, $\alpha_1(Z)$, $\delta(Z)$, and $\gamma(Z)$. Different subsets of Z may be used for the different parameters. A rich set of restrictions on the parameter space may thus be tested using standard methods for likelihood inference. For a product of binomial and multinomial likelihoods, where the cell probabilities are nonlinear functions of the parameters of interest, it is convenient to use the relation to a likelihood of independent Poisson counts. The restrictions needed for the estimated expected Poisson counts to be equivalent to the expected product multinomial counts are inherent in the parameterization of Table 4 (Palmgren and Ekholm, 1987). Baseline covariates of interest include the set of predictors for treatment compliance and for placebo response, denoted Z_1 and Z_2, respectively. To form a master set of

Table 5 Estimated Expected Cell Counts for the Multinomial Data Structure in Table 3, with Parameterization as in Table 4

		Placebo ($R = 0$)			Treatment ($R = 1$)		
		Treatment compliance			Treatment compliance		
		$D = 0$	$D = 1$		$D = 0$	$D = 1$	
Y	0	$\hat{m}_{00} = 52.12$	$\hat{m}_{01} = 87.88$	$m_{0+} = 140$	$n_{00} = 50$	$n_{01} = 16$	$n_{0+} = 66$
	1	$\hat{m}_{10} = 28.15$	$\hat{m}_{11} = 3.85$	$m_{1+} = 32$	$n_{10} = 27$	$n_{11} = 72$	$n_{1+} = 99$
		$\hat{m}_{+0} = 80.27$	$\hat{m}_{+1} = 91.73$	$m_{++} = 172$	$n_{+0} = 77$	$n_{+1} = 88$	$n_{++} = 165$

baseline covariates Z, the union of Z_1 and Z_2 may be supplemented by covariates argued from biologic plausibility. A parsimonious model for efficacy $\gamma(Z)$ is the main target. By specifying treatment compliance in terms of $\delta(Z_1)$, and placebo response in terms of $\alpha_0(Z_2)$ and $\alpha_1(Z_2)$, the precision for estimating $\gamma(Z)$ may be substantially increased. This is likely to be the case even when $\gamma(Z)$ is modeled using covariates that are not included in the sets Z_1 and Z_2. For modeling $\gamma(Z)$ one may thus start by conditioning on a rich set of covariates Z_1 and Z_2 to form $\delta(Z_1)$, $\alpha_0(Z_2)$, and $\alpha_1(Z_2)$, and then proceed to search for a parsimonious model for $\gamma(Z)$. Standard likelihood based tools may be used to assess goodness of fit for the overall model.

3.2. Null, Partial, and Full Compliance

In Table 6 the cholestyramine data is presented with dichotomized response and the compliance in three categories defined by the cutpoints 20 and 60% for percentage experimental and placebo dose, respectively. As before, we are not interested in the placebo compliance categories, and the structure for the observed data used for modeling is given in Table 7.

The three treatment compliance categories in Table 7 are referred to as null, partial, and full compliance. The null compliance in the treated arm translates to receiving no experimental treatment, and the full compliance to receiving 100% of the nominal dose. This is at best a

Table 6 Cross-Classification of Cholesterol Reduction ($Y = 1$ if at least 20 units; $Y = 0$ otherwise), Treatment Arm Assignment ($R = 1$ for treated arm; $R = 0$ for control arm) and Ordered Compliance (≤20%; 20–60%; >60%)

		Placebo ($R = 0$)				Treatment ($R = 1$)			
		Placebo compliance				Treatment compliance			
		≤60%	20–60%	>60%		≤60%	20–60%	>60%	
Y	0	14	28	98	140	24	26	16	66
	1	3	1	28	32	8	19	72	99
		17	29	126	172	32	45	88	165

Table 7 Data in Table 6 Used for Estimation of Partial Efficacy Among Partial Compliers and Full Efficacy Among Full Compliers

		Placebo ($R = 0$)				Treatment ($R = 1$)			
		Treatment compliance				Treatment compliance			
		$D=0$	$D=1$	$D=2$		$D=0$	$D=1$	$D=2$	
Y	0	$m_{00}=?$	$m_{01}=?$	$m_{02}=?$	$m_{0+}=140$	$n_{00}=24$	$n_{01}=26$	$n_{02}=16$	$n_{0+}=66$
	1	$m_{10}=?$	$m_{11}=?$	$m_{12}=?$	$m_{1+}=32$	$n_{10}=8$	$n_{11}=19$	$n_{12}=72$	$n_{1+}=99$
		$m_{+0}=?$	$m_{+1}=?$	$m_{+2}=?$	$m_{++}=172$	$n_{+0}=32$	$n_{+1}=45$	$n_{+2}=88$	$n_{++}=165$

crude approximation for the cholestyramine trial, but serves the purpose of illustrating the model. The observed data follow a multinomial distribution with six cells for the treated arm, and a binomial distribution for the placebo arm. By virtue of the randomization, the distributions for the expected treatment compliance and for the expected treatment free response are again assumed similar in the two trial arms. This is reflected in the parameterization $\Pr\{D_i(1) = k \mid R_i = 1\} = \Pr\{D_i(1) = k \mid R_i = 0\} = \delta_k$, with $\Sigma_{k=0}^{2} \delta_k = 1$, and $\Pr\{Y_i(0) = 1 \mid D_i(1) = 0, R_i = 0\} = \Pr\{Y_i(1) = 1 \mid D_i(1) = 0, R_i = 1\} = \alpha_0$. We further write $\Pr\{Y_i(0) = 1 \mid D_i(1) = k, R_i = 0\} = \alpha_k$ and $\Pr\{Y_i(1) = 1 \mid D_i(1) = k, R_i = 1\} = \gamma_k \alpha_k$, for $k = 0, 1, 2$. The two risk parameters of interest are

$$\gamma_k = \frac{pr\{Y_i(1) = 1 \mid D_i(1) = k, R_i = 1\}}{pr\{Y_i(0) = 1 \mid D_i(1) = k, R_i = 0\}} \quad k = 1, 2.$$

Note that since treatment-free response is assumed equal in the two treatment arms, $\gamma_0 = 1$ by definition, and γ_1 and γ_2 reflect respectively the partial treatment efficacy in the group of partial compliers, and full treatment efficacy in the group of full compliers. Expressions for the expected cell probabilities for the data structure in Table 7 are given in Table 8.

In the treated arm the multinomial distribution has 5 degrees of freedom and in the placebo arm the binomial distribution has 1 degree of freedom, resulting in a total of 6 degrees of freedom for estimating the seven parameters α_0, α_1, α_2, δ_1, δ_2, γ_1, and γ_2 ($\gamma_0 = 0$, $\delta_0 = 1 - \delta_1 - \delta_2$). The model is overparameterized and at least one additional restriction is

Table 8 Expected Cell Probabilities for the Cross-Classification in Table 7 (The distribution of placebo response and treatment compliance is similar in the two treatment arms, with $\delta_0 + \delta_1 + \delta_2 = 1$. The relative risk parameters γ_1 and γ_2 capture the treatment efficacy among partial and full compliers, respectively.)

		Placebo ($R = 0$)			Treatment ($R = 1$)		
		Treatment compliance			Treatment compliance		
		$D = 0$	$D = 1$	$D = 2$	$D = 0$	$D = 1$	$D = 2$
Y	0	$\delta_0(1-\alpha_0)$	$\delta_1(1-\alpha_1)$	$\delta_2(1-\alpha_2)$	$\delta_0(1-\alpha_0)$	$\delta_1(1-\gamma_1\alpha_1)$	$\delta_2(1-\gamma_2\alpha_2)$
	1	$\delta_0\alpha_0$	$\delta_1\alpha_1$	$\delta_2\alpha_2$	$\delta_0\alpha_0$	$\delta_1\gamma_1\alpha_1$	$\delta_2\gamma_2\alpha_2$
		δ_0	δ_1	δ_2	δ_0	δ_1	δ_2

needed for identification. Goetghebeur and Molenberghs (1996) suggest a model in which the two parameters γ_1 and γ_2 are kept distinct, and instead a set of intuitively reasonable, but rather complex second-order parametric restrictions are put on the association between the treatment compliance and the response. This approach is feasible for the three ordered categories, null, partial and full compliance, but when a more refined compliance scale is used, the Goetghebeur and Molenberghs essentially nonparametric relative risk model becomes intractable.

An alternative to the Goetghebeur and Molenberghs model for the ordered categorical null, partial, and full compliance is to give the compliance categories numerical scores, $k = 0, 1, 2$, and to use a linear model of the form $\gamma_k = \beta' D(1)$, with $D(1) = k$. The structural parameter β captures how a change in the level of experimental treatment received affects the risk. As argued earlier, it will be efficient for the estimation of the structural parameter to stratify the data according to baseline covariates Z which predict both placebo response and treatment compliance. Furthermore, differential treatment efficacy over subgroups can be incorporated by adding effect modification by baseline covariates to the structural model. The extended model takes the form $\gamma_k = \beta' D(1) + \tau' D(1) * Z$, with $D(1) * Z$ the interaction term. These linear restrictions on the γ parameters allow for a smooth conceptual transition from models presented for the binary and ordered categorical compliance scales to structural models for compliance measured on a continuous scale. The latter approach is discussed in Sections 4 and 5 and the dual role of baseline covariates as *conditioning* *covariates in the estimation model* and *effect modifiers in the structural model* is further elaborated upon.

4. STRUCTURAL MEAN MODELS

4.1. The Model and Semiparametric Estimation

Continuous measures of exposure raise the problem of estimating the average effect of treatment over very detailed exposure levels. The approach in Section 3 leads naturally to a structural mean model for inference regarding partial efficacy in this setting. Let $D(R)$ be a possibly continuous and multidimensional measure of exposure to experimental treatment following assignment R, with $D = 0$ indicating no exposure. As before, both $D(1)$ and $D(0)$ are considered potential exposures, by design equally distributed over randomized arms. In the special case where subjects on the control arm have no access to experimental therapy, $D(0) = 0$, different values of D are seen only on the treatment arm.

A linear structural model assuming the expected difference between potential outcomes with and without treatment to be constant over subgroups with different Z values is

$$E\{Y(1) - \beta' D(1) \mid Z, D(1)\} = E\{Y(0) \mid Z, D(1)\}. \tag{3}$$

In words, after subtracting $\beta' d$ from observed outcomes in the treatment arm subset $[Z = z, D(1) = d]$ one recaptures expected treatment-free outcome for this subset. More generally, $E\{Y(1) - Y(0) \mid Z, D(1)\}$ may depend on Z as well as $D(1)$, and a linear model respecting the zero dose constraint can, for instance, take the form

$$\begin{aligned} &E\{Y(1) - \beta' D(1) - \tau'(D(1) * Z) \mid Z, D(1)\} \\ &\quad = E\{Y(0) \mid Z, D(1)\} \end{aligned} \tag{4}$$

where $D(1) * Z$ refers to interaction terms between dose and baseline covariates. Estimation for models (3) and (4) is not fundamentally different. For ease of expression we develop the argument for the simpler model (3) and refer to extensions in the discussion (cf. also Fischer-Lapp and Goetghebeur, 1999).

Equation (3) does not enable straightforward least squares or likelihood estimation. Although for given β the left-hand side is observable in the treatment arm, the placebo arm carries no direct information on the association between observed $(Y(0),Z)$ and the corresponding latent $D(1)$. Since the assumption of random noncompliance is not made, one cannot rely on $E\{Y(0)|Z, D(1)\} = E\{Y(0)|Z\}$, but unbiased estimating equations follow from an equation implied by (3):

$$E\{Y(1) - \beta' D(1) \mid Z\} = E\{Y(0) \mid Z\}. \tag{5}$$

For any choice of Z dependent weights, the weighted average of the left-hand side of (5) equals the similarly weighted average of the right-hand side:

$$E^w[E\{Y(1) - \beta' D(1) \mid Z\}] = E^w[E\{Y(0) \mid Z\}] \tag{6}$$

where E^w indicates the weighted mean. Due to randomization unbiased estimates of the left- and right-hand sides of (6) can be derived from the treatment and control arm, respectively. For fixed weights this leads to unbiased linear estimating equations for β which are easy to solve. The corresponding estimator $\hat{\beta}$ is consistent and asymptotically unbiased under mild regularity conditions, with covariance matrix estimated by the sandwich estimator. This estimator $\hat{\beta}$ relies heavily on the randomization assumption and can be seen as a dose-specific intent-to-treat estimator.

4.2. Efficiency

Efficiency is an issue in this semiparametric setting with no direct assumptions on the selectivity of compliance. Consider the extreme situation where no baseline covariates are measured. With just a single equation (5), structural models with more than one unknown parameter are unidentified. In the special case of a single structural parameter however, equation $E\{Y(1) - \beta D(1)\} = E\{Y(0)\}$ imposes no restrictions on the observed data and can be solved by the (inefficient) instrumental variable estimator described in Section 3. A good choice of weights in Eqs. (6) leads to more efficient parameter estimates when the stricter assumption (5) holds. Optimal weights have been derived for general structural nested mean models by Robins (1994). Goetghebeur and Lapp (1997) suggest estimation of those weights in placebo-controlled trials using predictions of placebo outcome and treatment compliance from baseline covariates. The better those predictions, the more precise the treatment effect estimates. The clear message for design is that good baseline predictors for compliance as well as for treatment-free response should be recorded to increase information on dose-specific intent-to-treat estimators. Sometimes, compliance measures taken over a run-in period during which all subjects are given the same treatment yield good predictors for treatment compliance. Some have argued against run-in periods on placebo, however, claiming it is incompatible with the informed consent obligation. Creative run-in designs which avoid the certainty of placebo for the entire run-in period may provide an alternative that does not hamper accrual and resolves ethical concerns.

4.3. Implementation: An Example

That useful results can be obtained is illustrated by the blood pressure example previously analyzed by Goetghebeur and Lapp (1997). A new treatment is compared with placebo in a double blind randomized blood pressure reduction trial, assigning patients to take one tablet daily. Drug intake is electronically monitored over the experimental study period which follows a run-in on placebo. The dosing experience is subsequently summarized in a scalar $D(1)$ representing the percentage of prescribed experimental drug which is taken. The experimental treatment is not available on the control arm; hence $D(0) = 0$. The response measure of interest is change in blood pressure over the experimental study period (negative is good). An intent-to-treat analysis shows a highly significant difference between mean response on placebo, −3.54 mmHg (s.e. 1.49), and on treatment, −11.04 mmHg (s.e. 0.95). Table 9 shows the fit of three structural mean models with structural predictors: 1. $\{D(1)\}$, 2. $\{I\{D(1) > 0\}, D(1)\}$, 3. $\{D(1), D(1) * W\}$, where $I\{D(1) > 0\}$ indicates whether any experimental drug was taken versus none at all and W represents body weight minus its sample average. The effect is modeled conditionally on baseline predictors Z which include sex, height, weight, several run-in blood pressures and

Table 9 Estimated Structural Mean Models for Blood Pressure Reduction, with $D(1)$ the Percentage of Prescribed Dose of Active Drug, W the Centered Body Weight, and $I\{D(1) > 0\}$ an Indicator for Any Drug Taken or Not

Model	Structural effects	$\hat{\beta}_S$	$se(\hat{\beta}_S)$
1.	$D(1)$	−7.41	1.84
2.	$I(D(1) > 0)$	15.90	13.38
	$D(1)$	−24.83	14.88
3.	$D(1)$	−7.61	1.73
	$D(1)^* W$	0.36	0.14

their interaction with sex and height. This analysis is based on 54 available patients in the treatment arm and 51 in the placebo arm.

Model 1 estimates a linear dose effect quite precisely, but model 2 requires more information to formally distinguish between a constant effect of dose within the observed range and a linear effect. The fit suggests, however, that more variation in outcome is explained by the linear dose effect. Diagnostic plots constructed after fitting model 1 suggested an interaction effect with baseline covariate W, centered body weight. Model 3 confirms a significant interaction: heavier people achieve less reduction at the same dose level.

In general, once an identifiable structural mean model has been proposed, estimation is relatively straightforward. Implementation is achieved through just a few lines of code in Splus or SAS, for instance. However, without further assumptions on the selection mechanism, limited information makes parsimony for the structural model paramount. The challenge in practice thus lies in proposing meaningful structural models and in interpreting parameters correctly. The key question is: What aspect of drug exposure drives the treatment effect and how? Depending on the drug, different biologically plausible candidates present themselves. Besides percentage of prescribed drug taken, compliance summaries may contain length and duration of drug holidays and other covariates related to timing and dose of drug actually taken.

5. STRUCTURAL DISTRIBUTION MODELS

Besides the mean difference, other contrasts between the distributions of $Y(1)$ and $Y(0)$ can be modeled. One then relies on the randomization assumption to demand equality of the $(Y(1), Y(0), Z)$ distribution between arms rather than mere equality of means. Particularly for right censored response data, comparing estimated distributions via Kaplan-Meier curves rather than via means is a natural approach. Structural failure time models based on accelerated failure time models were introduced by Robins and Tsiatis (1991). Mark and Robins (1993) use these to estimate the effect of smoking cessation in the MRFIT study which randomizes over a life style intervention targeting multiple risk factors. Greenland and Robins (1994) compared high and low dose AZT in a trial which did randomize over the high and low dose, but where differential administration of a third drug (PCP prophylaxis) over the two arms had taken place post randomization. White et al. (1999) and White and Goetghebeur

(1998) examine the effect of treatment changes in randomized trials with long-term follow-up (see also Chapter 12). Recently, Korhonen, Laird and Palmgren (1999) and Korhonen and Palmgren (2001) have used the structural accelerated failure time model to assess the effect of beta-carotene supplementation on right-censored times to death from all causes in the ATBC Study. Along the same lines, Korhonen et al. 2000 estimate the effect of one dose of vitamin A on subsequent 4-month mortality in children under 6 months of age in a randomized, double-blind, placebo-controlled community trial in Nepal (West et al., 1995). Cluster randomization is an added complexity in this vitamin A trial.

6. DISCUSSION

Naive interpretation of intent-to-treat estimators ignoring actual exposure breeds poorly informed decisions (Goetghebeur and Shapiro, 1996). Incorporating exposure explicitly in an analysis bridges the gap between "biological" and "statistical" models. This cannot be done, however, without some additional assumptions. Recent approaches avoid the extreme assumption of completely nonselective noncompliance. Rather, randomization-based estimators are constructed for models cast in terms of potential outcomes (latent variables). This chapter has introduced the basic principle behind these estimators.

More general models than the ones presented here can be cast in this framework and have been usefully implemented in clinical trials. When active treatment is received on several (all) arms of the trial, estimating equations are derived from equalities between arms of potential treatment-free distributions, none of which need to be directly observed on any one arm (Greenland and Robins, 1994). Repeated outcomes and sequentially randomized designs can be analyzed by structural nested mean models or marginal structural models (Robins, Greenland, and Hu, 1999; Robins, 1999). Also, Bayesian approaches were built on the causal formulation; see for instance, Imbens and Rubin (1997) and Hirano et al. (2000). Besides the hopes generated by all these tools, there are also hazards as pointed out by Pocock and Abdalla (1998).

Diagnostic tools for latent variable models are necessarily limited in power. The model assumptions are sometimes subtle and must be well understood. It is not generally recognized for instance, that once structural (mean) models have been estimated, the (average) selection mechanism is identified, for instance in model (5), by regressing $Y(2) - \hat{\beta}D(1)$

on $D(1)$ in the treatment arm. Sensitivity of conclusions to untestable assumptions must be explored. Another important concern in practice regards data quality. Urquhart and De Klerk (1998) point out that good measures of compliance are hard to get and Dunn (1999) emphasizes that analyses treating compliance as an explanatory variable should account for this.

It is reassuring that the structural analyses discussed here protect the α-level when testing the null hypothesis of no difference between randomized arms. However, the corresponding estimators rely in part on modeling assumptions. For this reason, the traditional intent-to-treat analysis will continue to hold a key position.

In summary, while structural estimators are potentially more meaningful, they are also more complex. It will take time to educate statisticians and clinicians alike to better understand their role. There is a need for more practical experience and further theoretical development for instance in the realm of design and sample size calculation, analysis of equivalence studies, analysis of repeated outcome measures, the study of dynamic treatment regimes (involving sequentially randomized designs to study treatment changes over time as a function of observed effects and covariate evolutions), sensitivity analysis with respect to various model assumptions, etc. In our view, the recent developments show exciting prospects for subject matter scientists as well as statisticians. When handled with care, the new tools will lead to deeper insight into the nature of drug action in patient populations.

REFERENCES

Albert, J. M., DeMets, D. L. (1994). On a model-based approach to estimating efficacy in clinical trials. Statistics in Medicine 13:2323–2335.

Angrist, J. D., Imbens, G. W., Rubin, D. B. (1996). Identification of causal effects using instrumental variables. With rejoinder. Journal of the American Statistical Association 91:444–471.

Dunn, G. (1999). The problem of measurement error in modelling the effect of compliance in a randomized trial. Statistics in Medicine 21:2863–2877.

Efron, B., Feldman, D. (1991). Compliance as an explanatory variable in clinical trials. Journal of the American Statistical Association 86:9–26.

Fischer-Lapp, K., Goetghebeur, E. (1999). Practical properties of structural mean models for the analysis of noncompliance data. Controlled Clinical Trials 20:531–546.

Fisher, R. A. (1925). Statistical Methods for Research Workers. London: Olivier and Boyd.

Goetghebeur, E., Lapp, K. (1997). The effect of treatment compliance in a placebo-controlled trial: regression with unpaired data. Applied Statistics 46:351–364.

Goetghebeur, E., Molenberghs, G. (1996). Causal inference in a placebo controlled clinical trial with binary outcome and ordered compliance. Journal of the American Statistical Association 91:928–934.

Goetghebeur, E. J. T., Shapiro, S. H. (1996). Analyzing non-compliance in clinical trials: Ethical imperative or mission impossible? Statistics in Medicine 15:2813–2826.

Goldberger, A. S. (1972). Structural equation methods in the social sciences. Econometrica 40:979–1001.

Greenland, S., Robins, J. (1994). Adjusting for differential rates of PCP prophylaxis in high versus low dose AZT treatment arms in an AIDS randomized trial. Journal of the American Statistical Association 89:737–749.

Haavelmo, T. (1943). Statistical implications of a system of simultaneous estimating equations. Econometrica 11:1–12.

Hirano, K., Imbens, G. W., Rubin, D. B., Zhou, X. -H. (2000). Assessing the effect of an influenza vaccine in an encouragement design. Biostatistics 1:69–88.

Holland, P. W. (1986). Statistics and causal inference. Journal of the American Statistical Association 81:945–970.

Imbens, G. W., Angrist, J. (1994). Identification and estimation of local average treatment effects. Econometrica 62:467–476.

Imbens, G. W., Rubin, D. B. (1997). Bayesian inference for causal effects in randomized experiments with noncompliance. Annals of Statistics 25:305–327.

Korhonen, P. A., Laird, N. M., Palmgren, J. (1999). Correcting for non-compliance in randomized trials: An application to the ATBC Study. Statistics in Medicine 18:2879–2897.

Korhonen, P. A., Palmgren, J. (2002). Effect modification in a randomized trial under non-ignorable non-compliance. Applied Statistics 51:115–133.

Korhonen, P., Loeys, T., Goetghebeur, E., Palmgren, J. (2000). Vitamin A and infant mortality: beyond intention-to-treat in a randomized trial. Lifetime Data Analysis 6:107–121.

Lee, Y. J., Ellenberg, J. H., Hirtz, D. G., Nelson, K. B. (1991). Analysis of clinical trials by treatment actually received—Is it really an option? Statistics in medicine 10:1595–1605.

The Lipid Research Clinic Program (1984). The Lipid Research Clinics Coronary Primary Prevention Trial results, parts I and II. Journal of the American Medical Association 251:351–374.

Mark, S. D., Robins, J. M. (1993). A method for the analysis of randomized trials with compliance information—An application of the multiple risk factor intervention trial. Controlled clinical trials 14:79–97.

Neyman, J. (1923). On the application of probability theory to agricultural experiments. Essay on principles. Section 9. 1923. [Translated in Statistical Science 5, 465–480.]

Palmgren, J., Ekholm, A. (1987). Exponential family nonlinear models for categorical data with errors of observation. Applied Stochastic Models and Data Analysis 13:111–124.

Pocock, S. J., Abdalla, M. (1998). The hope and the hazards of using compliance data in randomized controlled trials. Statistics in Medicine 17:303–317.

Robins, J. M. (1994). Correcting for non-compliance in randomized trials using structural nested mean models. Communications in Statistics—Theory and Methods 23:2379–2412.

Robins, J. M. (1999). Marginal structural models versus structural nested mean models as tools for causal inference. In: Halloran, M.E., Berry, D., eds. Statistical Models in Epidemiology: The Environment and Clinical Trials. IMA. Vol. 16. New York: Springer-Verlag, pp. 95–134.

Robins, J. M., Greenland, S., Hu, F. -C. (1999). Estimation of the causal effect of a time-varying exposure on the marginal mean of a repeated binary outcome. Journal of the American Statistical Association 94:708–712.

Robins, J. M., Tsiatis, A. A. (1991). Correcting for noncompliance in randomized trials using rank preserving structural failure time models. Communication in Statistics—Theory and Methods 20:2609–2631.

Rubin, D. B. (1978). Bayesian inference for causal effects: The role of randomization. The Annals of Statistics 7:34–58.

Sommer, A., Zeger, S. L. (1991). On estimating efficacy from clinical trials. Statistics in Medicine 10:45–52.

Urquhart, J., De Klerk, E. (1998). Contending paradigms for the interpretation of data on patient compliance with therapeutic drug regimens. Statistics in Medicine 17:251–267.

West, K. P., Katz, J., Shrestha, S. R., LEclerq, S. C., Khatry, S. K., Pradhan, E. K., Adhikari, R., Wu, L. S. F., Pokhrel, R. P., Sommer, A. (1995). Mortality of infants less than 6 months of age supplemented with Vitamin A—A randomized double-masked trial in Nepal. American Journal of Clinical Nutrition 62:143–148.

White, I. R., Babiker, A. G., Walker, S., Darbyshire, J. H. (1999). Randomization-based methods for correcting for treatment changes: Examples from the Concorde trial. Statistics in Medicine 18:2617–2634.

White, I. R., Goetghebeur, E. J. T. (1998). Clinical trials comparing two treatment arm policies: which aspects of the treatment policies make a difference? Statistics in Medicine 17:319–340.

White, I. R., Pocock, S. J. (1996). Statistical reporting of clinical trials with individual changes from allocated treatment. Statistics in Medicine 115:249–262.

Zeger, S. (1998). Adjustment for noncompliance. In: Armitage, P., Colton, T., eds. Encyclopedia of Biostatistics. Vol. 4. New York: Wiley, pp. 3006–3009.

11

Analysis of Longitudinal Data with Missingness*

Paul S. Albert
National Cancer Institute, National Institutes of Health, Bethesda, Maryland, U.S.A.

Margaret C. Wu[†]
National Heart, Lung, and Blood Institute, National Institutes of Health, Bethesda, Maryland, U.S.A.

1. INTRODUCTION

The defining feature of a longitudinal clinical trial is that individuals are measured repeatedly across time. This is in contrast to many clinical trials in which observations are taken at baseline and then perhaps at one follow-up time. In this chapter, we will make the distinction between longitudinal analysis in which individuals are followed over time and multiple measurements are made, and survival analysis, in which individuals are followed and their time to event or censoring is analyzed. Our focus will be on discussing issues in missing data for longitudinal clinical trials in which the outcome is measured repeatedly at follow-up visits.

---

* The portions of this chapter written by Margaret Wu were written in her private capacity. The views expressed in the chapter do not necessarily represent the views of NIH, DHHS, nor the United States.

[†] Retired.

We will discuss three clinical trials in which the primary outcome is observed repeatedly in a longitudinal setting and the repeated outcomes are occasionally missing due to missed visits or censoring due to death or loss to follow-up (to be referred to as dropout). The scientific focus in all these studies is on evaluating the effect of treatment over time. These clinical trials will serve as motivation for methodological issues relating to analyzing longitudinal data in clinical trials with missingness. These examples are:

1. The Intermittent Positive Pressure Breathing (IPPB) Trial (Intermittent Positive Pressure Trial Group, 1983). This was a randomized clinical trial that evaluated the effect of an intervention (IPPB) as compared with standard compressor nebulizer therapy on pulmonary function over time in 985 patients with obstructive pulmonary disease. The primary response was forced expiratory volume in 1 second (FEV_1) measured at baseline and at 3 month intervals over a 3 year period postrandomization (13 scheduled visits including baseline). The outcomes are continuous with many missing observations due to missed scheduled visits or dropout due to death and loss to follow-up. Approximately 23% of the patients died before the end of the study and 13.5% dropped out because they moved away or refused to return for follow-up visits. In addition, almost all subjects have at least one missed scheduled visit either before the occurrence of death or the end of the study.
2. A three-arm randomized clinical trial to compare buprenorphine with two doses of methadone for reducing opiate use in a group of 162 addicts (Johnson et al., 1992). Sample sizes were 53, 55, and 54 patients in the buprenorphine, methadone 20 mg, and methadone 40 mg groups, respectively. The outcomes of this trial were a series of repeated binary responses of whether an individual failed a urine test at each of three visits per week (on Monday, Wednesday, and Friday) over a 17 week period. These repeated responses are often missing due to missed visits or withdrawal from the study. More than 50% of the patients withdrew from the study before the end of the follow-up period. A substantial number of patients occasionally missed visits but remained in the study.
3. A randomized trial of felbmate versus placebo for treating intractable partial epilepsy (Theodore et al., 1995). The study randomized 40 patients and the outcomes were repeated daily seizure counts over a 3 day titration period and a 14 day follow-

up period. Approximately one-half of the patients withdrew from the study prematurely. An inspection of average seizure frequency by dropout time suggested that seizure frequency was positively related to dropout time and that this relationship might be different in the two treatment groups.

There are many other examples of clinical trials in which the outcome is measured longitudinally. In Chapter 12, Babiker and Walker discuss the issue of analyzing repeated biological markers subject to informative censoring in an AIDS clinical trial. Other examples include cancer clinical trials in which quality-of-life assessments are measured repeatedly over follow-up and may be subject to different informative censoring mechanisms in the treatment and control arms.

Before discussing methodology for analyzing longitudinal data with missingness, we will briefly review the literature on longitudinal data. This review is presented in Section 2. Section 3 discusses terminology, and Section 4 discusses the implications of various type types of missingness on standard methodology for analyzing longitudinal data. General approaches for analyzing longitudinal data with missingness are outlined in Section 5. We will analyze our motivating examples in Sections 6 to 8. Conclusions follow in Section 9.

2. METHODOLOGY FOR ANALYZING LONGITUDINAL DATA

A review of methodology for analyzing longitudinal data in clinical trials is presented by Albert (1999). This section summarizes much of that review. Methods for longitudinal data can be separated into three broad categories: (1) simple univariate analyses of summary measures where the longitudinal outcome are summarized by a single variable for each subject, (2) methods for continuous longitudinal data, (3) and methods for discrete longitudinal data.

2.1. Simple Univariate Analyses of Summary Measures

When the treatment comparisons reduce to comparing the average responses over follow-up time, a simple approach is to summarize each person's longitudinal observations and compare these univariate measures across treatment groups (Pocock, 1983). These comparisons can be done with univariate statistical techniques (i.e., two-sample t tests or Wilcoxon rank sum tests) since there is only one summary measure per person and observations on different subjects are independent. For the epilepsy clinical trial data, a comparison of average daily seizure frequency between treatment groups was performed (Theodore et al., 1995). In the analysis of the IPPB trial (Intermittent Positive Pressure Trial Group, 1983), the progression of lung function over time was compared by testing differences in the average individually estimated slopes between treatment groups. In the opiate clinical trial, the average individual proportions of positive urine tests were compared across treatment arms (Johnson et al., 1992). Univariate comparisons of means or slopes can be an attractive alternative to complex modeling approaches. However, for highly imbalanced data caused by missing observations, as in the three previous examples, this simple comparison can be highly inefficient. This is demonstrated in Albert (1999) using IPPB clinical trial data. It is shown that an analysis based on comparing individually estimated slopes between treatment groups is substantially less efficient than an analysis based on a longitudinal model. We present this example in detail in Section 6.

2.2. Longitudinal Methods for Gaussian Data

Various methodologies exist for analyzing longitudinal Gaussian data. Traditional multivariate techniques (Morrison, 1976) such as the Hotelling's T^2, the multivariate analog of the t test for testing whether mean vectors are different in two samples, and profile analysis, a method for testing for parallelism and differences between two mean vectors in multivariate data, can be used to analyze continuous longitudinal data when observations are taken at the same time points on all subjects and there are no missing data. This is rarely true in longitudinal clinical trials where observations are not taken at the same time points on all subjects and data are often missing.

Alternatively, random effects models can be used to analyze longitudinal data. They provide a framework for analyzing longitudinal clinical trials data in which there is a sizable amount of missing observations (either due to missed visits, loss to follow-up, or death). In the IPPB trial, for example, scheduled follow-up visits at 3 month intervals were often missed or delayed and a large percentage of patient observations were censored due to death or dropout; only 77 out of 985 patients (8%) had complete equally spaced follow-up measurements.

The random effects model is typically formulated in two stages. Conditional on each subject's random effects, the model for the first stage is

$$Y_{ij} = \mathbf{X}_{\mathbf{ij}}'\boldsymbol{\beta} + \mathbf{Z}_{\mathbf{ij}}'\boldsymbol{\gamma}_{\mathbf{i}} + \varepsilon_{ij} \tag{1}$$

where $\mathbf{X_{ij}}$ and $\mathbf{Z_{ij}}$ are p and q element vectors of fixed and random effects covariates, respectively, and ε_{ij} are considered independent Gaussian with mean 0 and variance σ_ε^2, or can have an autoregressive moving average (ARMA) correlation structure. In the second stage, the random effects $\boldsymbol{\gamma}_{\mathbf{i}}$ are assumed to have a multivariate normal distribution with covariance matrix $\mathbf{D}$. The parameter vectors $\boldsymbol{\beta}$ and $\boldsymbol{\gamma}_{\mathbf{i}}$ measure the effect of fixed and random effect covariates on the mean responses. In a clinical trial, fixed effects covariates may include treatment group, time, treatment by time interaction, or baseline characteristics, while only the intercept and time effects are included as random effects covariates. Tests of treatment effects are usually constructed by testing for the significance of fixed effect covariates corresponding to treatment. Laird and Ware (1982) discuss an estimation procedure which allows for highly irregularly spaced observations where ε_{ij} are independent. Chi and Reinsel (1989) discuss estimation when the ε_{ij}'s follow an autogressive process.

2.3. Longitudinal Methods for Discrete Data

Many longitudinal clinical trials collect repeated outcomes which are not Gaussian. The epilepsy and opiate clinical trials are examples in which the repeated responses are seizure counts and binary opiate-use responses at repeated times post-randomization. Broadly speaking, models for discrete longitudinal data can be separated into three categories: marginal, random effects, and transition models.

Marginal models focus on estimating the effect of a set of covariates on the average response in a population. Liang and Zeger's (1986) generalized estimating equation (GEE) approach is the seminal work in this area. They extend the generalized linear and quasi-likelihood models (McCullagh and Nelder, 1989), regression models for discrete and continuous outcomes, to the longitudinal setting. Denote μ_{ij} as the mean of the jth response on the ith subject. In the terminology of generalized linear models, the mean can be related to a set of covariates through a link function, h, where $h(\mu_{ij}) = h(E(y_{ij})) = \mathbf{X}_{\mathbf{ij}}'\boldsymbol{\beta}$. The relationship between the variance and mean is specified as $\text{Var}(Y_{ij}) = \phi g(\mu_{ij})$ and the correlations on observations taken on the same subject are modeled by the function Corr(Y_{ij}, Y_{ij}) = $\rho(\alpha)$, where the parameter vector α characterizes this function. The approach is attractive in that both continuous and discrete response variables can be modeled by choosing h and g in an appropriate way. For Gaussian longitudinal data like FEV_1 in the IPPB trial, $h(\mu_{ij}) = \mu_{ij}$ and $g(\mu_{ij}) = 1$. For binary longitudinal data as in the opiate clinical trial, h and g may be chosen as $h(\mu_{ij}) = \text{logit}(\mu_{ij})$ and $g(\mu_{ij}) = \mu_{ij}(1 - \mu_{ij})$. For repeated count data like in our epilepsy clinical trial, $h(\mu_{ij}) = \log(\mu_{ij})$ and $g(\mu_{ij}) = \mu_{ij}$. The appeal of the GEE approach is that although a model for the correlation and variance structure of the longitudinal observations must be specified, inferences are not sensitive to the assumed model. Liang and Zeger propose the use of a robust variance estimator which produces the correct asymptotic inference even when the correlation structure is misspecified. Diggle, Liang, and Zeger (1993) apply the GEE approach to analyze an epilepsy clinical trial where the outcome is repeated seizure counts.

Random effects models have been proposed for modeling discrete longitudinal data (Zeger, Liang, and Albert, 1988, among others). Patient-to-patient variability is modeled by adding random effects as linear predictors in the regression terms in a generalized linear model. These random effects models generalize the standard random effects models for Gaussian data and are often referred to as generalized linear mixed models. As in the linear mixed models discussed in the previous section, generalized linear mixed models can be viewed in two stages. In the first stage, the mean response for the ith person is $\mu_{ij} = h(Y_{ij}|\boldsymbol{\gamma}_i) = \mathbf{X}'_{ij}\boldsymbol{\beta} + \mathbf{Z}'_{ij}\boldsymbol{\gamma}_i$, and the conditional variance is specified as $\text{var}(Y_{ij}) = \phi g(\mu_{ij})$. In the second stage, a distribution for the random effects is assumed to be normal with mean $\mathbf{0}$ and variance $\mathbf{D}$. The generalized linear mixed model encompasses a wide range of random effects models. The linear mixed model, obtained with $h(\mu_{ij}) = \mu_{ij}$, can be used to analyze the IPPB trial data. A random effects model for logistic regression, obtained with $h(\mu_{ij}) = \text{logit}(\mu_{ij})$ and $g(\mu_{ij}) = \mu_{ij}(1 - \mu_{ij})$, can be used to analyze the opiate clinical trial data. Likewise, a random effects model for count data, obtained with $h(\mu_{ij}) = \log(\mu_{ij})$ and $g(\mu_{ij}) = \mu_{ij}$, can be used to analyze the epilepsy trial data. These models have been discussed by a number of authors (Zeger, Liang, and Albert, 1988; Zeger and Karim, 1991; Breslow and Clayton, 1993, among others). Covariates such as treatment group can be interpreted as the effect of treatment on an individual's average response. This is in contrast to marginal models where the effect of covariates is on the population averaged mean response. For this reason, Lindsey and Lambert (1997) have argued that random effects models are more appropriate than marginal models for analyzing data in longitudinal clinical trials.

A third approach for analyzing longitudinal discrete data is transitional models. They examine the effect of covariates on the transition patterns in binary or categorical longitudinal data. Specifically, for binary data, as in our opiate trial, these models reduce to lagging previous observations in a logistic regression,

$$\operatorname{logit} P(Y_{it} = 1 | Y_{it-1}, Y_{it-2}, \ldots, Y_{it-q}) = \mathbf{X}_{\mathbf{it}}'\boldsymbol{\beta} + \sum_{k=1}^{q} \theta_k Y_{it-k} \tag{2}$$

where q is the order of the Markov dependence (Cox, 1970). This model has been used to analyze the opiate trial data by Follmann (1994) and by Albert (2000). Transitional models have been generalized to generalized linear model outcomes by Zeger and Qaqish (1988), and to ordinal data by Diggle, Liang, and Zeger (1993).

3. MISSINGNESS IN LONGITUDINAL CLINICAL TRIALS: TERMINOLOGY

There is a distinction between two types of missingness in longitudinal studies: dropout and intermittently missed observations. Dropout refers to the case when an individual ceases to participate in the study due to loss to follow-up or death. Dropout occurs for both reasons in our examples. Dropout in the opiate trial occurs when patients refuse to participate (i.e., return for scheduled visits) after being randomized in the study. Patients in the epilepsy clinical trial drop out when they withdraw from the study and leave the hospital. Patients in the IPPB trial drop out because of death or refusal to return for follow-up visits. Intermittent missingness occurs when individuals miss particular follow-up visits, but do not withdraw from the study. In the opiate clinical trial, many subjects miss particular visits and then return for additional follow-up visits. In the IPPB data, many observations are missed, followed by subjects returning and then dropping out from the study due to death or withdrawal from the study. Missing data mechanisms in which patients do not return after having missed an observation are called monotonically missing mechanisms. Similarly, missing data mechanisms in which patients return after having missed an observation are called non-monotonic missing data mechanisms.

Missing data can be missing for various reasons which may relate to the actual longitudinal responses. Little and Rubin (1987) classify missing data into three categories. First, data are missing completely at random (MCAR) if the missing data mechanism is independent of both the observed and actual missing values. Second, data are said to be missing at random (MAR) if the occurrence of missing data relates to the values of the observed responses, but not on the values of the missing observations. Last, data are missing nonrandomly if the probability of missing depends on the actual value of the missed observation. Little and Rubin (1987) have coined the phrase *ignorable missingness* to describe MCAR and MAR missing data mechanisms and *nonignorable missingness* to describe nonrandomly missing data mechanisms in which the probability of missingness depends on the actual value of the missed responses. The terms ignorable and nonignorable missingness refer to the fact that likelihood-based methodology is insensitive to ignorable missing data mechanisms, but will be biased when missing data are nonignorable.

In longitudinal clinical trials, a special type of nonignorable missingness called *informative missingness* is used to describe a missing data mechanism in which the distribution for both the repeated response and the missing process are linked by common random effects. Models that induce informative missingness are called shared random effects models (Wu and Carroll, 1988; Follmann and Wu, 1995). These models are discussed in detail in Section 5.3.

4. IMPLICATIONS OF MISSING DATA ON LONGITUDINAL METHODOLOGY

Most methods for the analysis of longitudinal data make valid inference with MCAR data. For MAR data, as was previously mentioned, likelihood-based methods are valid. However, moment-based methods, such as GEE, are biased. This point has been mentioned by various authors, including Liang and Zeger (1986) in their original paper on GEE. Rotnitzky and Wypij (1994) quantify this bias for GEE. Thus, recent methodology for analyzing longitudinal data with missingness has focused on MAR data for GEE and nonignorable missingness for likelihood based procedures. We discuss these methodologies in Section 5.

5. MISSING DATA IN LONGITUDINAL CLINICAL TRIALS: GENERAL APPROACHES

5.1. Analyses on Summary Measures

There have been various general approaches proposed for analyzing longitudinal clinical trials data with missingness. We begin by discussing simple summary measures across groups. Dawson and Lagakos (1993) propose an approach which involves summarizing each individual's longitudinal outcome into a single summary measure, and then propose a non-parametric test which stratifies over the missing data patterns. This approach is shown to have the correct type I error rate under a wide range of ignorable missing data patterns. The approach does, however, make the restrictive assumption that there are only a few missing data patterns and does not have the correct type I error rate when missingness is nonignorable. Unstratified comparisons of summary measurements (e.g., the comparison of individual summary measures across treatment groups) have the advantage of allowing for large numbers of missing data patterns and have the correct type I error rate under certain types of nonignorable missingness. The disadvantage of unstratified tests, as mentioned by Dawson (1994), is that they have substantially less power than stratified tests. In the IPPB study, for example, interest focuses on comparisons of rate of change in FEV_1 across treatment groups. There are too many missing data patterns in this relatively long sequence to perform a stratified test. Unstratified tests that compare summary measures between treatment groups can be done by estimating each individual slope and comparing these slopes across treatment groups. The IPPB data was originally analyzed in this way. Similarly, the original analysis in the epilepsy clinical trial was a comparison between average individual seizure frequency between treatment arms. Wu and Carroll (1988) show that such an unstratified comparison produces unbiased estimation of treatment effects even under certain types of nonignorable missing data mechanisms. They point out, however, that tests based on these unstratified comparisons can have low power, particularly in situations like the IPPB data where there is very large variation across individuals in the number of available observations. Wu and Carroll (1988) propose a modeling strategy for informative missing data which does not suffer from this low power which will be discussed in Section 5.3.

Follmann, Wu, and Geller (1994) propose approaches for testing treatment efficacy in clinical trials with repeated binary measurements with missing data. The methods they discuss include (1) rank tests between treatment groups where the unit of analysis is each subject's average observed binary response, (2) a combined test of missingness and efficacy using a multivariate rank test (O'Brien, 1984), where the units of analysis are the subject's average observed binary response along with the subject's estimated proportion of missed visits, and (3) simple imputation where missed responses are replaced with positive responses (this method makes the assumption that missed visits if they had been observed would have resulted in positive opiate tests).

5.2. Selection Versus Pattern Mixture Models

Two very general classes of models have been proposed for modeling longitudinal data with nonignorable missingness. Little (1995) discusses the distinction between selection models and pattern mixture models for modeling longitudinal data with missingness. Denote $\mathbf{Y_i} = (y_{i1}, y_{i2}, \ldots, y_{in})'$ as the complete data vector for the ith subject, $\mathbf{M_i}$ as a vector of indicator variables which represent the missing data status, and $\mathbf{X_i}$ as a vector of covariates which could include a treatment indicator as well as baseline or time-dependent covariates. For both classes of models, maximum-likelihood estimation involves parameterizing the joint density of the complete data and missing data indicator vector, $f(\mathbf{Y_i}, \mathbf{M_i})$. For selection models,

$$f(\mathbf{Y_i}, \mathbf{M_i} \mid \mathbf{X_i}) = g(\mathbf{Y_i} \mid \mathbf{X_i}) h(\mathbf{M_i} \mid \mathbf{Y_i}, \mathbf{X_i}). \tag{3}$$

Estimation follows by maximizing the joint density of the observed data and the missing data vetor, $f(\mathbf{Y_i^o}, \mathbf{M_i}) = \sum(\mathbf{Y_i^o}, \mathbf{Y_i^m}, \mathbf{M_i})$, where $\mathbf{Y_i^o}$ and $\mathbf{Y_i^m}$ are vectors of observed and missed observations, respectively, and the summation is taken over all possible occurrences of the binary missed observations.

In selection models, the complete data distribution of the $\mathbf{Y_i}$'s is parameterized separately from the missing data mechanism conditional on the complete-data vector. Parameters in this formulation have a natural interpretation. Parameters for $g(\mathbf{Y_i}|\mathbf{X_i})$ address the scientific question of interest, namely, the effect of treatment on the complete-data vector $\mathbf{Y_i}$. Parameters for $h(\mathbf{M_i}|\mathbf{Y_i}, \mathbf{X_i})$ characterize the nonignorable missing data mechanism.

Various authors have proposed selection models in which the missing data mechanism depends on the repeated responses $\mathbf{Y_i}$, either observed or missing. Diggle and Kenward (1994) propose a model for continuous Gaussian data with nonignorable dropout. They parameterize g as a multivariate Gaussian and h as a logistic regression which characterizes the probability of dropping out at the jth time point. Specifically, the probability of dropout is modeled as

$$\text{logit } P(i\text{th subject drops out at time } j) = \beta_0 + \beta_1 y_{ij} + \sum_{k=1}^{q} \beta_k y_{ij-k}. \tag{4}$$

For these dropout models, testing whether $\beta_1 = 0$ would be a test of whether dropout was non-ignorable. Testing whether $\beta_1 = \beta_2 = \cdots = \beta_q = 0$ would be a test of whether dropout was completely at random. Molenberghs et al. (1997) extend this model to repeated ordinal data and propose an E-M algorithm for parameter estimation. Troxel et al. (1998) proposes methodology for analyzing repeated continuous data with non-montone missingness (e.g., intermittent missingness). This methodology is well suited for a situation where we have short sequences of continuous data on each subject. In the spirit of these models, Albert (2000) propose a transitional model for binary data subject to nonignorable missingness. This work extends work by Conaway (1993) to allow for long sequences of repeated binary data with both nonignorable dropout and intermittent missing data as in our opiate dependence trial. In (3), g is a transitional model as in (2), and the dropout mechanism h is modeled as a three state Markov chain (states corresponding to the binary response observed, intermittently missed, or dropout) which depends on the current value of the binary response. An E-M algorithm is implemented for parameter estimation.

For pattern mixture models, the joint probability of $\mathbf{Y}_i$ and $\mathbf{M}_i$ given $\mathbf{X}_i$ is decomposed as

$$f(\mathbf{Y}_i, \mathbf{M}_i \mid \mathbf{X}_i) = g(\mathbf{Y}_i \mid \mathbf{M}_i, \mathbf{X}_i)h(\mathbf{M}_i \mid \mathbf{X}_i) \tag{5}$$

where h parameterizes the missing data pattern and g the complete-data distribution conditional on the missing data pattern. For example, Little and Wang (1996) propose a pattern mixture model for dropout in which g is a multivariate normal whose parameters are indexed by dropout time, and h is a multinomial which characterizes the marginal distributions of dropout times. Inferences about treatment effect can be made by comparing the parameters of g across treatment groups (i.e., an analysis which stratifies by dropout time) or by comparing functions of the marginal complete-data likelihood by *averaging* the g over the missing data pattern. In the case of a saturated model, this approach reduces to an unweighted analysis.

5.3. Shared Random Effects Models and Informative Missingness

In longitudinal clinical trials, repeated measures are often highly variable over time. Rather than modeling the missing data mechanism directly as a function of $\mathbf{Y_i}$, as in the selection models discussed in the previous section, Wu and Carroll (1988) exploit the fact that we have repeated responses on each individual to model the missing data mechanism in terms of features of an individual's underlying response process. They propose methodology in which informative dropout is accounted for by introducing random effects that are shared between the model for the longitudinal observations and the dropout mechanism. Thus, the missing data mechanism depends on an individual's underlying response process as opposed to the actual responses. Let d_i denote the dropout time for the ith subject. The joint distribution of $(\mathbf{Y_i}, d_i, \boldsymbol{\beta}_\mathbf{i} \mid \mathbf{X_i})$ can be factored as

$$f(\mathbf{Y_i}, d_i, \boldsymbol{\beta}_\mathbf{i} \mid \mathbf{X_i}) = g(\mathbf{Y_i} \mid \mathbf{X_i}, \boldsymbol{\beta}_\mathbf{i})k(\boldsymbol{\beta}_\mathbf{i} \mid \mathbf{X_i})h(d_i \mid \mathbf{X_i}, \mathbf{Y_i}, \boldsymbol{\beta}_\mathbf{i}) \tag{6}$$

where $h(d_i \mid \mathbf{X_i}, \mathbf{Y_i}, \boldsymbol{\beta}_\mathbf{i})$ is assumed to depend on $\mathbf{Y_i}$ only through $\boldsymbol{\beta}_\mathbf{i}$, i.e., $h(d_i \mid \mathbf{X_i}, \mathbf{Y_i}, \boldsymbol{\beta}_\mathbf{i}) = h(d_i \mid \mathbf{X_i}, \boldsymbol{\beta}_\mathbf{i})$.

These models were first proposed by Wu and Carroll (1988) for modeling nonignorable dropout and have been referred to as random coefficient selection models (Little, 1995). Wu and Carroll (1988) propose their methodology in the setting of a two group longitudinal clinical trial where interest focuses on comparing change over time in the presence of informative dropout. They proposed a random effects model with a random intercept and slope (e.g., a random vector $\boldsymbol{\beta}_\mathbf{i} = (\beta_{1i}, \beta_{2i})'$ for the ith subject). The dropout mechanism was modeled as a multinomial with shared random effects incorporated through a probit link. Specifically, the probability of the ith subject dropping out within the first j intervals is parameterized as $P(d_i \leq \mathrm{j}) = p_{ij} = \phi(\boldsymbol{\alpha}'\boldsymbol{\beta}_\mathbf{i} + \alpha_{0j})$, where $\boldsymbol{\alpha} = (\alpha_1, \alpha_2)$. Large positive values of α_1 or α_2 correspond to the situation where those individuals with large intercept or slopes tend to drop out of the study sooner. They propose jointly estimating the parameters of both probability mechanisms using weighted least squares. Others have proposed shared random effects models of this type. Schluchter (1992) proposed an E-M algorithm for maximum-likelihood estimation for a model where an individual's slope and log survival are assumed multivariate normal. Mori et al. (1994) proposed a model where the slope of continuous repeated data is related to the number of observations on each subject though a shared random effect. Similarly, Follmann and Wu (1995), Ten Have et al. (1998), and Pulkstenis et al. (1998) have proposed shared random effects models for binary longitudinal data subject to missingness. Albert and Follmann (2000) proposed a shared random effects model for repeated count data with informative dropout.

Wu and Bailey (1989) proposed an alternative approach to account for informative dropout which conditions on the dropout times. In this approach, they model the joint distribution of $\mathbf{Y_i}$ and $\boldsymbol{\beta_i}$ given d_i and $\mathbf{X_i}$. Specifically,

$$f(\mathbf{Y_i}, \boldsymbol{\beta_i} \mid d_i, \mathbf{X_i}) = g(\mathbf{Y_i} \mid \boldsymbol{\beta_i}, d_i, \mathbf{X_i},)m(\boldsymbol{\beta_i} \mid d_i, \mathbf{X_i}), \tag{7}$$

where $g(\mathbf{Y_i} \mid \boldsymbol{\beta_i}, d_i, \mathbf{X_i}) = g(\mathbf{Y_i} \mid \boldsymbol{\beta_i}, \mathbf{X_i})$. Little (1995) mentions that this approach fits into the class of models he calls *random coefficient pattern mixture models*. Wu and Bailey (1989) illustrated that the shared random effects model (6) can be well approximated by the conditional models (7). They approximated $\boldsymbol{\beta_i}|d_i$ as normal with constant variance and with mean given as a polynomial expression of d_i, where the variance and polynomial are estimated separately in the two treatment groups. Follmann and Wu (1995) proposed a conditional model for analyzing binary longitudinal data with non-monotonic missing data mechanisms. Albert and Follmann (2000) proposed similar methodology for analyzing repeated count data. They developed three approaches: a full shared random effects model, a likelihood-based, conditional approach, and a GEE-based conditional approach, and applied these approaches for analyzing the epilepsy clinical trial data. Wu and Follmann (1999) discussed a generalization of the conditional model to more closely approximate the shared random effects model when the missing data mechanism is generated through time-dependent shared random effects models.

The shared random effects models are inherently different from the selection models discussed in the previous section. Unlike the selection models in which the missing data mechanism depends on actual (either observed or missed) response values, the missing data mechanism for the shared random effects model depends on an individual's propensity to respond (i.e, an individual's random effect). The choice of model formulation may depend on the scientific problem. Longitudinal data in which missingness is believed to be related to the actual observations (such as the opiate trial in which addicts may miss visits because they took drugs and know that there is a high likelihood that they would test positive) may be more appropriately modeled with a selection model. Longitudinal data in which missingness is believed to be related to an individual's disease process and not a particular realization of this process are better modeled by a shared random effects model. Shared random effects are particularly appropriate for modeling longitudinal data in which the response is highly variable over time. Examples include the epilepsy and the IPPB clinical trials in which dropout and missingness are most likely related to an individual's underlying seizure process or chronic lung disease process, and not to a particular daily seizure count or lung function measurement.

5.4. GEE with Missingness

As discussed previously, GEE is a useful method for analyzing discrete and continuous longitudinal data when the mean response is of primary interest. Unlike likelihood-based methodology, however, GEE produces biased parameter estimates when data are missing at random. Rotnitzky and Wypij (1994) developed expression which can be used to quantify this bias in various settings. Robins et al. (1995) proposed an extension of GEE that allows for unbiased parameter estimation for MAR data. They propose a class of weighted estimating equations which result in consistent estimation of mean structure parameters with a correctly specified missing data mechanism. Their approach reduces to a weighted version of GEE in which each element of the residual vector $(\mathbf{Y}_i - \boldsymbol{\mu}_i)$ is weighted by the inverse of the probability of having a positive response. Paik (1997) discusses alternative GEE based methodology that allows for unbiased parameter estimation for MAR data. She proposes imputation techniques, in which missing observations are imputed in the data set. More recently Rotnitzky, et al. (1998) have proposed GEE estimation for nonignorable missingness.

6. ANALYZING LONGITUDINAL GAUSSIAN DATA WITH MISSINGNESS: IPPB TRIAL

The primary objective in this trial was to compare the rate of change in (FEV_1) over time between standard nebulizer therapy and the experimental IPPB treatment for patients with obstructive pulmonary disease. The trial was designed to test for a change in average slope between the two treatment groups at the end of the study. Analysis was complicated by the large amount of potentially informative dropout (e.g., censoring due to death or loss to follow-up) and intermittently missed observations. The mean number of missed observations is slightly smaller in the IPPB treatment group (3.65 out of 13 in the IPPB group and 4.56 out of 13 in the standard compressor nebulizer therapy group; $P < 0.001$, Wilcoxon rank sun test). In addition, individual estimates of the slope of FEV_1 (rate of change in FEV_1) were positively correlated with the number of missed visits for the IPPB group (Spearman $r = .10$, $p = 0.04$) and essentially uncorrelated for the standard therapy group (Spearman $r = -0.03$,

$p = .53$). We examined the effect of treatment on linear change in FEV_1 with three analyses. First, we fit a linear mixed model (Laird and Ware, 1982) to these data. Second, we compared average individual estimated slopes between the two treatment groups. Third, we fit a conditional model which adjusts for potentially informative missingness.

We model the longitudinal FEV_1 data with the linear mixed model. This approach results in valid inference if missingness is ignorable. The model is

$$Y_{ij} = \beta_0 + \beta_1 t_{ij} + \beta_2 T_i + \beta_3 T_i t_{ij} + \gamma_{i0} + \gamma_{i1} t_{ij} + \varepsilon_{ij} \tag{8}$$

where $\varepsilon_{ij} \sim N(0, \sigma_\varepsilon^2)$ and $\boldsymbol{\gamma}_\mathbf{i} = (\gamma_{i0}, \gamma_{i1})' \sim \text{iid } N(0, \mathbf{D})$, T_i is equal to 1 when the ith subject was randomized to IPPB treatment and equal to 0 when randomized to standard compressor nebulizer therapy, and t_{ij} is the time from randomization for the jth follow-up time on the ith subject. The coefficient β_1 measures change over time, β_2 measures the treatment differences at baseline, and β_3 the treatment differences over time. The two random effects γ_{i0} and γ_{i1} reflect individual departure in baseline FEV_1 measurements and slope, respectively. In addition, the diagonal elements in the random effects covariance matrix D summarize the between subject variation in baseline and slope measurements.

We transformed the outcome variable to the log-scale since the outcome was close to being normally distributed on that scale. We fit this model using the linear mixed models routine in SPLUS (SPLUS version 4.0) The parameter estimates were: $\widehat{\beta}_0 = -.0471$ (SE = .0172), $\widehat{\beta}_1 = -.00331$ (SE = .000355), $\widehat{\beta}_2 = .0203$ (SE = .0241), and $\widehat{\beta}_3$ − .00014 (SE = .00049). The test of whether β_3 is zero provides a test of treatment effect; the Z value was −.28, which suggests that there is no effect of treatment on change in FEV_1 over time.

An alternative to the linear mixed model analysis is a two-stage unweighted analysis in which average individually estimated slopes are compared across treatment arms. Although this approach is valid when missingness is informative (Wu and Bailey, 1989), it can be highly inefficient because all subjects' data are weighted equally (e.g., a subject with only 2 observations gets the same weight in the analysis as a subject with 13 observations). We compared the differences in the slope estimates between the IPPB treatment group and the standard compressor nebulizer therapy group. The difference in average slope by the simple method was computed as −.0000605 (SE = .0010). We compare this value to our estimate of $\widehat{\beta}_3$. Although both approaches result in insignificant effects, the resulting standard error in the simple two-stage approach was twice as large as the standard error obtained with the random effects approach.

In the third approach we condition on the number of missed observations (Wu and Bailey (1989)). Denote m_i as the number of missed observation on the ith subject. We implement the conditional approach by fitting the linear mixed model

$$Y_{ij} = \beta_0 + \beta_1 t_{ij} + \beta_2 T_i + \beta_3 T_i t_{ij} + \beta_4 m_i + \beta_5 T_i m_i + \beta_6 t_{ij} m_i + \beta_7 T_i t_{ij} m_i + \gamma_{i0} + \gamma_{i1} t_{ij} + \varepsilon_{ij} \tag{9}$$

where $\varepsilon_{ij} \sim N(0, \sigma_\varepsilon^2)$ and $\boldsymbol{\gamma}_\mathbf{i} = (\boldsymbol{\gamma}_{i0}, \boldsymbol{\gamma}_{i1})' \sim \text{iid N}(0, \mathbf{D})$. This model was fit using the linear mixed modeling routine in SPLUS. The effect of treatment on average slope can be assessed by comparing slope values averaged over m_i across treatment groups. Specifically, we can assess this effect through the quantity $\beta_3 + [\beta_6 (m_{.1} - m_{.0}) + \beta_7 m_{.1}$ where $m_{.1}$ and $m_{.0}$ are the average number of missed observations in the IPPB and the standard therapy groups, respectively. This was estimated as $-.000640$ and the standard error was estimated by bootstrap as .000677.

Each of the three approaches demonstrates a nonsignificant difference between mean slopes (where the average slope is slightly more negative in the IPPB treatment than in the standard compressor nebulizer therapy group) in the two treatment groups. These results are slightly different from the previously reported results (Intermittent Positive Pressure Trial Group, 1983), where the slopes were estimated as slightly more negative in the standard treatment group than in the IPPB treatment group. This small difference may be due to the fact that the prior comparison was based on analyzing FEV_1 on the original scale and on weighting each individual's slope by the number of observations present.

For our three analyses, the standard error was smallest for the linear mixed model which does not account for potentially informative missingness. The standard error was approximately twice this value for the simple unweighted analysis which adjusts for informative missingness. The conditional model which adjusts for informative missingness is substantially more efficient than the unweighted analysis (i.e., this standard error was 0.68 times that of the unweighted analysis).

7. ANALYZING LONGITUDINAL BINARY DATA WITH MISSINGNESS: OPIATE TRIAL

The opiate clinical trial had substantial amounts of dropout and intermittent missingness and dropout. Over 50% of patients dropped out of the study prematurely. All patients had at least one intermittent missed visit before dropping out or completing the study. We will focus on a key comparison, the comparison of the low-dose methadone (20 mg) group with the experimental buprenorphine treatment group.

Follmann, Wu, and Geller (1994) discuss simple summary measure comparisons for assessing treatment effect in the opiate trial. They show that the estimated proportion of positive tests is correlated with the estimated missing data rate, and that this correlation is greater in the buprenorphine group (r = .51 and .18 in the buprenorphine and methadone group, respectively). The average estimated proportion of positive tests (among nonmissed tests) was .49 and .69 in the buprenorphine and methadone groups, while the average estimated proportion of missed visits was .48 and .58 in these two groups, respectively. All tests of summary measures that involve the comparisons of the proportion of positive responses between the two groups were statistically significant. Z values for (1) a rank tests of average proportion of positive responses, (2) tests of the average proportion of positive response or missing (simple imputation), and (3) O'Brien's rank test (O'Brien, 1984) for the multiple endpoint of proportion of positive responses and proportion of missed visits, were −3.01, −3.48, and −2.70, respectively.

Follmann and Wu (1995) propose a conditional model for for examining treatment effect while adjusting for informative missingness. They fit the generalized linear mixed model

$$\begin{aligned}\text{logit } E(Y_{ij} \mid \mathbf{b_i}, m_i) = \beta_0 + \beta_1 T_i + (1 - T_i)\omega_0 m_i + T_i \omega_1 m_i \\ + (1 - T_i) b_{1i} + T_i b_{2i},\end{aligned} \tag{10}$$

where m_i are the number of missed visits and $\mathbf{b_i}$ is a vector of treatment group specific random effects with mean $\mathbf{0}$ and a diagonal covariance matrix. In addition, the indicator Ti denotes whether a patient is in the buprenophine group. Follmann and Wu (1995) propose parameter estimation assuming a nonparametric mixture for the random effects using methodology described by Follmann and Lambert (1989). More typically, a Gaussian mixture can be assumed and Gaussian quadrature can be used for parameter estimation (e.g., Ten Have et al., 1998). Inference about treatment efficacy can be made by averaging summary statistics over m_i. Follmann and Wu (1995) assess treatment effect using the statistic

$$\frac{1}{n_1} \sum_{T_i = 1} E(Y_{i1} \mid \hat{\mathbf{b}}_\mathbf{i}, m_i) - \frac{1}{n_0} \sum_{T_i = 0} E(Y_{i1} \mid \hat{\mathbf{b}}_\mathbf{i}, m_i), \tag{11}$$

where n_0 and n_1 are the number of patients in group 0 and 1, respectively, and where $\hat{\mathbf{b}}_\mathbf{i}$ are empirical Bayes estimates of the random effects. Standard errors for this statistic were computed using the bootstrap. For the opiate clinical trial data a Z test based on the above statistic divided by its standard error was -3.85, which demonstrates a highly significant treatment effect.

An examination of the opiate trial data suggests that addicts may have periods without opiate-use separated by bouts of opiate-use. Albert (2000) develops a transitional model for binary longitudinal data which allows for nonignorable intermittent missing data and dropout. This is a selection model where the complete data are modeled through a transitional model, and the missing data mechanism is modeled as a first order Markov chain whose parameters depend on the current response value. Unlike the approach of Follmann and Wu, 1995, intermittent missingness is modeled separately from dropout, and the probability of missingness is assumed to depend on the actual value of the response (either observed or missing), and not the propensity to have a positive response. In addition, this model adjusted for day-of-the-week effects. Specifically, the transitional model is

$$\text{logit } P(Y_{it} = 1 \mid Y_{it-1}) = \beta_0 + \beta_1 T_i + \beta_2 \text{Mon}_{it} + \beta_3 \text{Wed}_{it} + \beta_4 Y_{it-1} + \beta_5 T_i Y_{it-1} \tag{12}$$

where Mon_{it} and Wed_{it} are indicator functions which are 1 when the tth visit for the ith subject is a Monday or Wednesday, respectively. The nonignorable missing data mechanism is modeled with a multinomial logit transformation of the probability of changing missing data status over visits. Specifically, we model

$$P(M_{it} = m \mid M_{it-1} = l, Y_{it}) = \frac{\phi(l, m)}{\sum_{m=1}^{3} \phi(l, m)}$$

where $\phi(1, 1)$ is constrained to be 1, $\phi(2, 0) = \phi(2, 1) = 0$, and

$$\phi(l, m) = \exp(\gamma_{0lm} + \gamma_{1lm} T_i + \gamma_{2lm} Y_{it} + \gamma_{3lm} T_i Y_{it}), \tag{13}$$

and where $\mathrm{M}_{it} = 0, 1$, or 2 when the ith subject tth observation is observed, is missing intermittently, or is missing due to dropout, respectively.

Including treatment group T_i by response Y_{it} interactions in (13) allows for different nonignorable missing data mechanisms in the two treatment arms. These interaction terms were highly significant for the opiate data. A global test of treatment effect can be obtained by jointly testing whether β_1 and β_5 are zero. A test of β_5 equal to zero was not significant ($Z = 1.25$) while a test of β_1 was highly significant ($Z = 6.37$). This suggests that the opiate process for patients on buprenophine is significantly different the process when patients are on methadone. The transitional model can then be used to derive summary measures of the opiate-use process that can be compared across treatment groups. Specifically, we estimated the average proportion of positive responses as .61 (SE = .055, obtained with a nonparametric bootstrap) and .34 (SE = .048) for the methadone and buprenorphine groups, respectively. In addition, we estimated the time to the first occurrence of a positive urine test 4 weeks after randomization as 1.75 (SE = .31) and 4.48 (SE = .89) for the methadone and buprenophine groups, respectively. These summary measures demonstrated a large beneficial effect of buprenophine over the standard methadone treatment.

8. ANALYZING LONGITUDINAL COUNT DATA WITH DROPOUT: EPILEPSY CLINICAL TRIAL

Theodore et al. (1995) discussed this trial, which was designed to assess the effect of Felbamate on seizure frequency in patients with intractable partial epilepsy. Patients recruited to this trial had difficulty controlling seizures while on their current antiseizure medications. Patients were taken off their prior medications and randomized to either placebo ($n = 21$) or Felbmate ($n = 19$). Treatment was titrated to full dosage over a 3 day period and patients were followed to monitor daily seizure frequency over an additional 14 day period. A complication of this trial was the large amount of dropout and the large heterogeneity in seizure counts. Time to dropout was earlier in the placebo group, but the difference was not statistically significant ($p = .21$ with a log-rank test). Theodore et al. (1995) discuss various analyses including a rank test to compare the mean daily seizure counts between treatment groups. Albert and Follmann (2000) propose methodology for analyzing repeated count data subject to informative dropout. In particular, a shared random effects model was developed where the repeated count data and the dropout mechanism were jointly modeled by including random effects which are shared between the two probability mechanisms. In addition, conditional likelihood approaches (likelihood and GEE methods) which condition on the dropout times were developed.

We focus here on the likelihood-based conditional model. We fitted the generalized linear mixed model (see Albert and Follmann (2000) for details),

$$\begin{aligned}\log E[Y_{it} \mid \mathbf{b_i}, d_i] = \beta_0 + \beta_1 T_i + \omega_1 \log(d_i)(1 - T_i) \\ + \eta_1 \log(d_i) T_i + (1 - T_i) b_{i1} + T_i b_{i2}\end{aligned} \tag{14}$$

where the choice of a log transformation for the dropout time was made by examining a plot of mean seizure counts by dropout times in each of the two treatment groups. The estimate of ω_1 in (14) was highly significant, while the estimate of η_1 was not significant. This suggests that the informative dropout mechanism is different in the two treatment arms. Treatment effect was assessed using a summary measure which was averaged over the dropout times. Specifically, the test statistic was based on

$$\rho = E_{T_i=1}[\log E(Y_{i1} \mid \mathbf{b_i})] - E_{T_i=0}[\log E(Y_{i1} \mid \mathbf{b_i})]. \tag{15}$$

The treatment effect ρ was estimated by averaging over the dropout times

$$\hat{\rho} = \sum_{T_i=1} \hat{E}[\log E[Y_{i1} \mid d_i, \mathbf{b_i}) \mid \mathbf{b_i}]/n_1 - \sum_{T_i=0} \hat{E}[\log E[Y_{i1} \mid d_i, \mathbf{b_i}] \mid \mathbf{b_i}]/n_0, \tag{16}$$

where

$$\begin{aligned}\hat{E}[\log E[Y_{i1} \mid d_i, \mathbf{b_i}) \mid \mathbf{b_i}] = \hat{\beta}_0 + \hat{\beta}_1 T_i + \hat{\omega}_1 \log(d_i)(1 - T_i) \\ + \hat{\eta}_1 \log(d_i) T_i\end{aligned} \tag{17}$$

and where n_0 and n_1 are the sample sizes in the placebo and treatment groups, respectively ($n_0 = 19$ and $n_1 = 21$). Standard errors were estimated with the bootstrap. The analysis in Albert and Follmann (2000) resulted in a Z statistic of 1.68, which was not statistically significant at the .05 level. Although the rank test suggested a significant effect, based on the analysis with the conditional model, we should be cautious in concluding that Felbamate is effective in this population. More studies are needed to confirm the positive effect of Felbamate.

9. CONCLUSIONS

This chapter discusses recent methodology for analyzing longitudinal data subject to missingness. We reviewed the various types of missing data and discussed how these types of missingness affect various methodologies for analyzing longitudinal data. We also discussed various techniques for analyzing continuous and discrete longitudinal data in clinical trials subject to ignorable and nonignorable missing data.

Data analysis in this paper was done using S-Plus (Version 6.0). S-Plus code for some of the examples in this paper is included in the appendix of Albert (1999). In addition, a general discussion of software for the analysis of longitudinal data is presented in section 7 of Albert (1999).

A major difficulty in analyzing longitudinal data with missingness is that it is difficult to examine the adequacy of models for missingness. Diggle (1989) proposes a test for random dropouts in repeated continuous longitudinal data that can be used to examine whether dropout depends on the past history of the observed process or occurs completely at random. However, it is well recognized that methods that account for nonignorable missing data are very subject to modeling assumptions (Laird, 1988; Little, 1995, and more recently, Scharfstein et al. (1999)). Thus, one approach for analyzing longitudinal clinical trial data with missingness is to model this missingness in various ways and examine the sensitivity of the treatment effect to these modeling assumptions (as we did with the IPPB and opiate clinical trials, for example). Consistent treatment effects under a wide range of missing data models will reassure the investigator that the treatment effect is most probably valid.

REFERENCES

Albert, P. S. (1999). Tutorial in Biostatistics: Longitudinal data analysis (repeated measures) in clinical trials. Statistics in Medicine 18:1707–1732.

Albert, P. S. (2000). A transitional model for longitudinal binary data subject to nonignorable missing data. Biometrics 56:602–608.

Albert, P. S., Follmann, D. A. (2000). Modeling repeated count data subject to informative dropout. Biometrics 56:667–677.

Breslow, N. E., Clayton, D. G. (1993). Approximate inference in generalized linear mixed models. J. Amer. Statist. Assoc. 88:9–25.

Chi, E. M., Reinsel, G. C. (1989). Models for longitudinal data with random effects and AR(1) errors. J. Amer. Statisti. Assoc. 84:452–459.

Conaway, M. R. (1993). Nonignorable nonresponse models for time-ordered categorical variables. Applied Statistics 42:105–115.

Cox, D. R. (1970). The Analysis of Binary Data. London: Chapman and Hall.

Dawson, J. P. (1994). Stratification of summary statistic tests according to missing data patterns. Statistics in Medicine 13:1853–1863.

Dawson, J. D., Lagakos, S. W. (1993). Size and power of two-sample tests of repeated measures data. Biometrics 49:1022–1032.

Diggle, P. J. (1989). Testing for random dropouts in repeated measurement data. Biometrics 45:1255–1258.

Diggle, P., Kenward, M. G. (1994). Informative drop-out in longitudinal data analysis. Applied Statistics 43:49–93.

Diggle, P. J., Liang, K. Y., Zeger, S. L. (1993). Analysis of Longitudinal Data. London: Oxford University Press.

Follmann, D. (1994). Modelling transitional and joint marginal distribution in repeated categorical data. Statistics in Medicine 13:467–477.

Follmann, D. A., Lambert, D. (1989). Generalized logistic regression by nonparametric mixing. J. Amer. Statist. Assoc. 84:295–300.

Follmann, D., Wu, M. (1995). An approximate generalized linear model with random effects for informative missing data. Biometrics 51:151–168.

Follmann, D., Wu, M., Geller, N. L. (1994). Testing treatment efficacy in clinical trials with repeated binary measurements and missing observations. Commun. Statist. Theory Meth. 23:557–574.

Intermittent Positive Pressure Breathing Trial Group (1983). Intermittent positive pressure breathing therapy of chronic obstructive pulmonary disease. Annals of Internal Medicine 99:612–630.

Johnson, R. E., Jaffe, J. H., Fudala, P. J. (1992). A controlled trial of Buprenorphine treatment for opiate dependence. J. Amer. Medical Assoc. 267:2750–2755.

Laird, N. M. (1988). Missing data in longitudinal studies. Statistics in Medicine 7:305–315.

Laird, N. M., Ware, J. H. (1982). Random-effects models for longitudinal data. Biometrics 38:963–974.

Liang, K. Y., Zeger, S. L. (1986). Longitudinal data analyis using generalized linear models. Biometrika 73:12–22.

Lindsey, J. K., Lambert, P. (1997). On the appropriateness of marginal models for repeated measurements in clinical trials. Statistics in Medicine 17:447–469.

Little, R. J. A. (1995). Modeling the drop-out mechanism in repeated-measures studies. J. Amer. Statist. Assoc. 90:1112–1121.

Little, R. J. A., Rubin, D. B. (1987). Statistical Analysis with Missing Data. New York: Wiley.

Little, R. J. A., Wang, Y. (1996). Pattern-mixture models for multivariate incomplete data with covariates. Biometrics 52:98–111.

McCullagh, P., Nelder, J. A. (1989). Generalized Linear Models. London: Chapman and Hall.

Molenberghs, G., Kenward, M. G., Lesaffre, E. (1997). The analysis of longitudinal ordinal data with nonrandom drop-out. Biometrika 84:33–34.

Mori, M., Woolson, R. F., Woodworth, G. G. (1994). Slope estimation in the presence of informative right censoring: modeling the number of observations as a geometric random variable. Biometrics 50:39–50.

Morrison, D. F. (1976). Multivariate Statistical Methods. New York: McGraw-Hill.

O'Brien, P. C. (1984). Procedures for comparing samples with multiple endpoints. Biometrics 40:1079–1087.

Paik, M. C. (1997). The generalized estimating equations approach when data are not missing completely at random. J. Amer. Statist. Assoc. 92:1320–1329.

Pocock, S. J. (1983). Clinical Trials: A Practical Approach. New York: John Wiley and Sons.

Pulkstenis, E. P., Ten Have, T. R., Landis, J. R. (1998). Model for the analysis of binary longitudinal pain data subject to informative dropout through remedication. J. Amer. Statist. Assoc. 93:438–450.

Robins, J. M., Rotnitzky, A., Zhao, L. P. (1995). Analysis of semi-parametric regression models for repeated outcomes in the presence of missing data. J. Amer. Statist. Assoc. 90:106–121.

Rotnitzky, A., Robins, J. M., Scharfstein, D. O. (1998). Semiparametric regression for repeated outcomes with nonignorable nonresponse. J. Amer. Statist. Assoc. 93:1321–1339.

Rotnitzky, A., Wypij, D. (1994). A note on the bias of estimators with missing data. Biometrics 50:1163–1170.

Scharfstein, D. O., Rotnitzky, A., Robins, J. M. (1999) Adjusting for nonignorable dropout using semiparametric nonresponse models (with discussion). J. Amer. Statist. Assoc. 94:1096–1120.

Schluchter, M. D. (1992). Methods for the analysis of informatively censored longitudinal data. Statistics in Medicine 11:1861–1870.

MathSoft, Inc. (2003) S-Plus Version 6.0 User's Guide. Seattle, WA: MathSoft, Inc.

Ten Have, T. R., Kunselman, A. R., Pulkstenis, E. P., Landis, J. R. (1998). Mixed effects logistic regression models for longitudinal binary response data with informative dropout. Biometrics 54:367–383.

Theodore, W. H., Albert, P., Stertz, B., Malow, B., Ko, D., White, S., Flamini, R., Ketter, T. (1995). Felbamate monotherapy: Implications for antiepileptic drug development. Epilepsia 36:1105–1110.

Troxel, A. B., Lipsitz, S. R., Harrington, D. P. (1998). Marginal models for the analysis of longitudinal measurements with nonignorable non-monotone missing data. Biometrika 85:661–672.

Wu, M. C., Bailey, K. R. (1989). Estimation and comparison of changes in the presence of informative right censoring: conditional linear model. Biometrics 45:939–955.

Wu, M. C., Carroll, R. J. (1988). Estimation and comparison of changes in the presence of informative right censoring by modeling the censoring process. Biometrics 44:175–188.

Wu, M. C., Follmann, D. A. (1999). Use of summary measures to adjust for informative missingness in repeated data with random-effects. Biometrics 55:75–84.

Zeger, S. L., Karim, M. R. (1991). Generalized linear models with random effects: A Gibbs' sampling approach. J. Amer. Statist. Assoc. 86:79–95.

Zeger, S. L., Liang, K. Y., Albert, P. S. (1988). Models for longitudinal data: A generalized estimating equations approach. Biometrics 44:1049–1060.

Zeger, S. L., Qaqish, B. (1988). Markov regression models for time-series: A quasi-likelihood approach. Biometrics 44:1019–1031.

12

Statistical Issues Emerging from Clinical Trials in HIV Infection

Abdel G. Babiker and Ann Sarah Walker
Medical Research Council Clinical Trials Unit,
London, England

1. INTRODUCTION

The first randomized trial of antiviral therapy in HIV type 1* infection included 282 patients with AIDS or advanced AIDS-related complex (ARC) and was stopped early in 1986 after an average follow-up of 4 months because of a substantial reduction in mortality in the group who received zidovudine (ZDV) (Fischl et al., 1987). The era of anti-HIV treatment had begun. This chapter will discuss some of the issues faced by clinical trialists and governmental regulatory agencies in the evaluation of therapies for HIV disease over the subsequent years as new anti-HIV drugs have been developed requiring evaluation in clinical trials.

A number of features specific to HIV infection have influenced trial design and interpretation. Even without treatment, the disease has a long asymptomatic phase, on average about 10 years. During this time HIV-infected individuals are essentially well although some laboratory markers, principally the CD4 lymphocyte count and viral load, as measured by HIV RNA in plasma or serum, are indicative of disease progression. As the

---

* Throughout, HIV will be used to denote HIV-1.

disease progresses, individuals become increasingly susceptible to a number of different opportunistic infections and tumors, some of which are life threatening. They may also develop a number of nonspecific symptoms (e.g., fever and weight loss) and hematological and neurological symptoms which may be due to the direct effect of HIV.

It is difficult to find exact parallels between HIV and other diseases. The design of current treatment strategies reflects present ideas about development of drug resistance which have much in common with the chemotherapy of tuberculosis and malignant tumors. However, the need for long-term suppressive therapy, which is likely to be an essential feature of the management of the disease, has much in common with other chronic diseases such as diabetes, hypertension, rheumatoid arthritis, ulcerative colitis, and multiple sclerosis. An additional factor not present in many chronic diseases is the substantial toxicity and burden to the patient of the current effective highly active antiretroviral therapies (HAART). In particular, over the last few years it has become apparent that a substantial proportion of patients taking HAART long term are suffering from metabolic abnormalities and/or significant fat redistribution ("lipodystrophy") that, in combination with other risk factors, may put them at higher risk of cardiovascular disease (Shevitz et al., 2001; Egger et al., 2001). The balance between assessing short-term effects of treatment *regimens* and long-term effects of treatment *strategies* [essentially the difference between testing the direct effect of a treatment regimen under idealized conditions (efficacy) and pragmatic trials of effectiveness which assess the impact of a treatment regimen in clinical practice] has yet to be found.

Many of the issues discussed in other chapters, such as the analysis of failure time and longitudinal data, methods for multiple endpoints and early stopping, and methods for assessing compliance, are highly relevant to clinical trials in HIV infection. HIV trials face several other practical problems which affect their design and analysis and may threaten their successful outcome (Ellenberg et al., 1992; Foulkes, 1998; Albert and Yun, 2001).

As many HIV-infected individuals take large numbers of drugs (both antiretrovirals and prophylaxis), there has been considerable interest in trial designs which maximize the information gained on drugs while minimizing the number of participants involved and the time spent on inferior drug combinations. Factorial designs are attractive to HIV research for two reasons. First, they are the only trial designs that allow investigation of synergistic or antagonistic interactions when these are thought to exist: second, when interactions are assumed to be small, multiple drug effects may be estimated more efficiently in one trial (DeGruttola et al., 1998; Ellenberg et al., 1992; Schoenfeld, in Finkelstein and Schoenfeld, 1995). However, they do have lower power to detect interactions than main treatment effects. When the same endpoint is used to compare more than one treatment regimen, the sample size required to assess one treatment effect must be inflated to incorporate the likely smaller number of events due to both effective treatments. For fixed power, the inflation factor is the ratio of the probability of an event in a nonfactorial trial where there is only one effective treatment to the probability of an event in the factorial trial where both treatments are effective. Therefore in a 2×2 factorial trial, where treatments 1 and 2 have hazard ratios α and β, respectively, compared with placebo, and $1 - \pi$ is the event rate on the double placebo arm on which the sample size is based, the inflation factor can be shown to be

$$\frac{2 \times (2 - \pi - \pi^{\alpha})}{4 - \pi - \pi^{\alpha} - \pi^{\beta} - \pi^{\alpha\beta}}.$$

The inflation factor is only large when event rates are low and treatments moderately efficacious. A practical (rather than statistical) method for reducing patient time spent on inferior drug combinations has been the increasing use of coenrollment in more than one protocol of a clinical trials organization (Larntz et al., 1996). Coenrollment can be more realistic than factorial designs in HIV infection, where the type of interventions to be tested depend on disease stage. However, factorial designs have great potential for trials in HIV infection, in particular in small populations such as children, and also to simultaneously assess different types of treatment strategies, such as testing two regimens of antiretroviral drugs together with two criteria for defining treatment failure and change of treatment.

Regardless of general trial design, the endpoints used to evaluate anti-HIV therapy have changed markedly over the last 15 years. Endpoints used in HIV trials to date include mortality, various measures of morbidity, biological markers of disease progression (surrogate markers), and adverse events. Mortality is the natural choice of endpoint in the definitive evaluation of therapy in a fatal disease such as HIV. It is clearly relevant to patients, it is a unique endpoint, and all trial participants are at risk. However, trials using death as an endpoint need to be much larger and last longer than trials which use earlier endpoints. With the advent of HAART in clinical practice from 1997 [usually consisting of at least two nucleoside analog reverse transcriptase inhibitors (NRTI), with an additional drug which is usually either a nonnucleoside analog reverse transcriptase inhibitor or a protease inhibitor], the use of survival as the primary outcome is likely to be impractical, except in patients with late HIV disease.

As a result, the most commonly used *clinical* outcome measure is time to the first new AIDS-defining event or death. Delaying the onset of the first AIDS event and preventing subsequent new AIDS events is certainly clinically relevant. However, two issues remain: (1) the implications for the size and duration of the trial and (2) the composite nature of this endpoint. Although progression to a new AIDS-defining event or death is more common than mortality, with the advent of HAART this endpoint is likely to be rare enough to still require large numbers of patients to be recruited and followed over a long period, particularly in early HIV disease. However, several international trials with AIDS as a primary clinical endpoint are currently recruiting patients (see, for example, Emery et al., 2002). Some trials in the early 1990s used other (non-AIDS) clinical events (such as AIDS-related complex, ARC) in addition to AIDS or death. These events may provide early evidence of a treatment effect, but their usefulness is questionable because they are largely subjective relatively minor symptoms and are clinically much less important than AIDS. AIDS-defining illnesses, in contrast, are more clinically relevant and can more easily be assessed objectively. However, the current definition of AIDS includes a variety of over 20 different conditions including opportunistic infections and malignancies (Centers for Disease Control, 1992) in addition to a CD4 cell count of less than 200 cells/ml (ignored for the purpose of this discussion). A major issue in using progression to a new AIDS defining event or death is the composite nature of this endpoint, which treats all events equally regardless of their clinical significance. Furthermore, information on second or subsequent AIDS events are ignored (or sometimes not even collected) as is the total number of events experienced by a participant. In the Delta trial (Delta Coordinating Committee, 1996) a total of 1451 AIDS-defining events and 498 deaths were observed in 2765 participants who were AIDS-free at entry. When the relative risks of death associated with different AIDS events were simultaneously estimated from a Cox proportional hazards model using the occurrence of these events as time-dependent covariates, the impact of the different types of AIDS events on mortality ranged between no effect to an increase of about 20-fold. The composite endpoint of progression to AIDS or death utilized 936 (48%) of the total observed events. Thus one clear disadvantage of the composite endpoint of AIDS or death is that more than 50% of all events and the great majority of severe events have not been utilized. Methods for the analysis of multivariate failure time data can be used to include all events in the analysis, and to investigate differences in treatment effects across different AIDS events (see Section 2).

The use of biological markers of disease progression to assess different treatments is attractive because it may provide direct evidence of treatment activity and lead to smaller and shorter trials. Disadvantages in using markers to measure treatment effects include their large within-patient biological variability and problems with quality control. A more relevant criticism is that a biological marker generally measures activity in only one mechanism of action of a drug regimen, be it efficacy or toxicity. Furthermore, the choice of timing of marker measurements and final clinical outcome will clearly affect the degree to which a marker measures the treatment effect on the clinical endpoint. There are a number of examples from other diseases where the inappropriate use of such surrogate markers has led to misleading conclusions and consequently to the inappropriate treatment of many patients, the most notable being the use of anti-arrhythmic drugs (see, for example, Fleming and DeMets, 1996). Candidate markers in HIV include CD4 lymphocyte count and viral load measured by plasma or serum HIV RNA. CD4 lymphocytes are the main target of the HIV virus and a key part of the defence against infection provided by the immune system. Declining numbers of CD4 cells are therefore associated with an increase in susceptibility to infections to which a person would not usually succumb (opportunistic infections). HIV RNA levels in plasma or serum directly measure the number of circulating copies of the virus, and quantitative plasma HIV RNA measurements are now the most commonly used primary outcome measures in phase III trials. Although the prognostic significance of both viral load and CD4 cell count is beyond dispute (Mellors et al., 1997), neither viral load nor CD4 cell counts are particularly strong surrogates for clinical outcome in the evaluation of therapy (HIV Surrogate Marker Collaborative Group, 2000). The assessment of surrogacy of biological markers is discussed in Section 3.1. However, even assuming surrogacy of a marker, a number of issues of analysis remain. If a marker is analyzed as a continuous variable, then repeated measures methods must be employed and informative dropout accounted for (Section 3.2). HIV RNA levels are also often reported as below a limit of assay detectability, so this censoring of continuous data must also be considered. Alternatively, biological markers can be synthesized into failure time data; in this case, methods for interval censored failure time data should be used (Section 3.3).

When drug regimens are taken over the long term, the relative contribution of toxicity and efficacy becomes more important, particularly when endpoints are markers of efficacy only, such as levels of HIV RNA. For example, since 1998 a sizeable proportion of individuals infected with HIV have begun to present with severe disturbances of metabolic parameters and body fat redistribution or "lipodystrophy" (both at levels associated with increased cardiovascular disease risk) (Carr, 1999; Shevitz et al., 2001). The precise relationship between these changes and antiretroviral therapy is currently unclear, although epidemiological studies are ongoing (Friis-Moller, 2002). Toxicity data are a second example of multivariate failure time data with the additional problems of sparse data. The methods described in Section 2 can be used to investigate the effect of treatment on the time to multiple adverse events, but may have little power when there are small numbers of events.

Independently of the choice of endpoint, however, the long asymptomatic phase of HIV infection means that trials which are designed to evaluate the effectiveness of therapy in early disease need to have long-term follow-up. To date more than half of the published phase III trials with clinical endpoints have a median follow-up of 1.5 years or less. Long-term trials are considered undesirable by many clinicians and patient groups because of the urgency of making new treatments available, and the rapid changes in perceptions about therapy. In addition, HIV drugs to date have demonstrated only transient benefit, and so the emphasis has shifted to determining efficacy over short periods of time (particularly in studies sponsored by the pharmaceutical industry for regulatory purposes). This is achieved through trials of relatively short duration using endpoints such as biological markers which occur earlier in the disease and are thus more proximal to randomization. However, there is a clinical need for extra information beyond that required for regulatory purposes: It is precisely because the effect of treatment might be of only very short duration that long-term follow-up is needed to assess durability of the effect as well as the effectiveness of treatment strategies. The transient nature of the benefit of ZDV was only established after the completion of trials with relatively longer duration [the Concorde trial (Concorde Coordinating Committee 1994), and the extended follow-up of the ACTG 019 (Volberding et al., 1994)]. This has been further confirmed by the extended follow-up of the Concorde and Opal trials (Joint Concorde and Opal Coordinating Committee 1998) and the overview of trials of ZDV in asymptomatic and early symptomatic infection (HIV Trialists' Collaborative Group, 1999). The difference between assessing biological efficacy and clinical effectiveness embodied in the difference between explanatory and pragmatic trials (Schwarz and Lellouch, 1967) is central to the arguments for and against longer term follow-up (Schoenfeld, 1996) and the level of agreement expected between short- and long-term results.

The third, and perhaps the most important, reason for short follow-up is the high rate of change from allocated trial therapy (noncompliance or treatment change). In addition to toxicity and tolerability, the reasons for change from allocated treatment include perceived or actual treatment failure, desire to try new but perhaps unproven drugs, or simply the feeling of clinicians and participants that it is "time for a change." Figure 1 shows that the rate of withdrawal from allocated therapy for reasons other than disease progression increases with follow-up but does not appear to depend on the therapy or the size of the trial. The effect of a large number of treatment changes is to reduce the interest of some participants and investigators in the trial because of concerns that the initial treatment

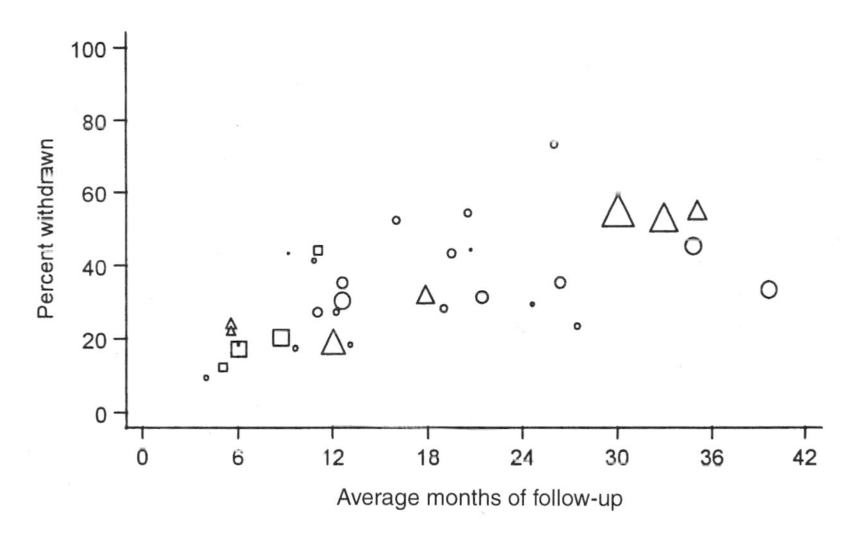

Figure 1 Rate of withdrawal from allocated therapy for reasons other than disease progression by median follow-up in antiretroviral trials with clinical endpoints in HIV infection. ○, monotherapy with NRTIs; △, combination therapy with NRTIs; □, combination therapy including a PI. The size of the symbol is proportional to the size of the trial.

effect might be diluted, the treatment comparison might be confounded and therefore the trial will not provide useful results. That this view is not necessarily correct and should not be used to justify early stopping of a trial of effectiveness is demonstrated by experience in the Delta trial, although there is a clear difference between trials primarily concerned with estimating efficacy rather than effectiveness in the way treatment changes are considered. Delta was a multinational double-blind randomized trial which compared the policy of dual therapy with ZDV plus didanosine (ddl) or zalcitabine (ddC) compared with the policy of monotherapy with ZDV alone (median follow-up 30 months) (Delta Coordinating Committee, 1996). More than 2000 patients had not had anti-HIV therapy prior to entry (Delta 1) and over 1000 had taken ZDV for at least 3 months (Delta 2). There was a high rate of change from allocated treatment in both Delta 1 and Delta 2, with median time from randomization to stopping blinded allocated treatment only about 15 months in Delta 1 (Figure 2).

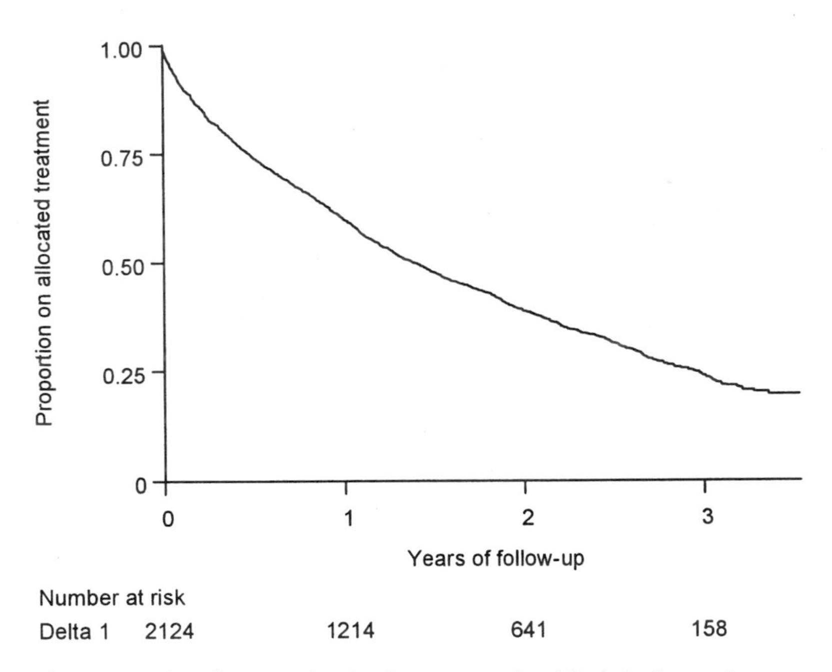

Figure 2 Time from randomization to stopping blinded allocated treatment in Delta 1.

Largely because of this, but also because of "trial fatigue" and of the availability of new drugs [notably lamivudine (3TC)], there was strong pressure to terminate Delta early. The Data and Safety Monitoring Committee (DSMC) finally recommended termination of Delta 3 months before its scheduled completion, not because of the negative impact of the high rate of treatment changes, but because of the clear evidence of the superiority of combination therapy. Table 1 shows that the effect of combination treatment on mortality in Delta 1 became increasingly apparent, and the magnitude of the treatment effect larger, with longer follow-up. Had the trial been stopped on the basis of the high rate of withdrawal from allocated treatment, an important effect would have been missed. This unexpected result (an increasing effect of treatment at least during the first 3 years in spite of a high rate of change from allocated therapy) may be due to the fact that, like Concorde, Delta 1 addressed a generic question on the effectiveness of a treatment policy (namely, initiation of treatment with combination therapy or with monotherapy). Such questions may be more robust to treatment changes of the magnitude observed in Delta, because the treatment changes are part of the policy.

Clearly statistical methods cannot be used to assess rapid changes in therapeutic options. However, transient benefit of anti-HIV therapy can be investigated, at least in the setting of survival data, by either fitting flexible time-dependent treatment effects using natural cubic splines (Hess, 1994), or by considering weighted Schoenfeld residuals (Grambsch and Therneau, 1994). Exploring the impact of treatment changes on the estimated treatment effect in a manner which avoids the introduction of selection bias is considerably complex, and will be considered in detail in Section 4.

Table 1 Relative Risk of Death (RR) in ZDV + ddI and ZDV + ddC Compared to ZDV Alone by Follow-up Time in Delta 1

Years from randomization	Total deaths	ZDV + ddI vs. ZDV		ZDV + ddC vs. ZDV	
		RR	95% CI	RR	95% CI
0–1	49	.77	(.39–1.52)	.78	(.40–1.53)
1–2	151	.60	(.40–.88)	.71	(.49–1.03)
2–3	137	.44	(.29–.67)	.57	(.39–.85)

2. ANALYSIS OF MULTIPLE EVENTS

For the first decade of HIV trials, before the advent of effective therapies, the majority of trials used composite clinical endpoints such as AIDS or death. It soon became clear that analyses of these endpoints were placing undue emphasis on the events that tend to occur earlier in the natural history of the disease. Events in a composite endpoint are likely to be heterogeneous in their effect on subsequent mortality, the physiological system they affect, their response to treatment, and their effect on quality of life. If the majority of early events are less severe events that are more easily treated and have a relatively small impact on patients, then the relevance of the endpoint to clinical practice becomes questionable. In addition, if treatment has a different impact on the different events, comparisons based on the composite endpoint may be misleading. These issues were first considered, in HIV infection at least, by Neaton et al. (1994). On the other hand, large numbers of treatment changes after a first event in the composite endpoint mean that it is only possible to compare treatments in terms of effectiveness not efficacy if events after the first are also included. A number of alternative methods to utilize the available information on all AIDS events have been proposed.

Mocroft et al. (1995) proposed a simple staging system based on a score calculated as a function of the patient's AIDS events and CD4 cell count history up to this time. The proposed score is intuitive, objective, simple to calculate, and can be useful for patient management. However, the use of the score as an outcome measure in clinical trials is likely to give undue emphasis to changes in CD4 count particularly when only a few severe AIDS events are observed. Although moderate changes in CD4 count may be more predictive of mortality than some AIDS events, the predictive ability of CD4 counts may be different in different treatment groups (Sec. 3.1).

Bjorling and Hodges (1997) suggested a rule-based ranking scheme whereby patients are ranked according to their clinical experience throughout follow-up and treatment groups are compared in terms of the ranks. This is intuitively similar to the rank-sum global test proposed by O'Brien for testing multiple endpoints (O'Brien, 1984). Several ranking rules were proposed, based on the total number, severity, and timing of AIDS events. However, this approach can lead to inappropriate conclusions, particularly with heavy censoring, because the method forces a total order in constructing the ranks in a situation where only a partial ordering exists because of the censored observations. For example, in a trial with 10 deaths occurring early among 100 patients in one treatment group and no events in 100 patients in the other group, the ranking method comparing scores with the Wilcoxon rank sum test leads to $p = .36$ while the logrank test gives $p < .005$.

Multivariate failure time data methods can also be used to analyze multiple events in a composite endpoint such as AIDS (Neaton et al., 1994; Finkelstein et al., 1997; Walker et al., 2000). Available techniques include marginal (Wei et al., 1989), frailty (Clayton and Cuzick, 1985; Klein, 1992), and conditional models (Prentice et al., 1981; Kay, 1984), reviewed in Wei and Glidden (1997).

2.1. Marginal Models

Marginal models fully respect the randomization in a clinical trial and are therefore most appropriate for treatment comparisons. In these models, the treatment effect on the hazard of progression to each event (or group of events) is of primary interest, while the correlations between the different events are treated as nuisance parameters. The method of Wei et al. (1989) is based on standard proportional hazards partial likelihood followed by robust adjustment of the covariance matrix of the estimated treatment effect on the marginal hazards [similar to the generalized estimating equations (GEE) of Liang and Zeger (1986)]. For each individual $i = 1, \ldots, I$ the hazard of experiencing an event in group $j = 1, \ldots, J$ is

$$\lambda_{ij}(t) = \lambda_{0j}(t)\ \exp(\beta_j z_i)$$

with z_i the treatment group indicator. A working assumption of independence between events is used to construct a working partial likelihood and large sample martingale arguments are used to derive the variance adjustment. This method can be used to compare the treatment groups with respect to the hazard of progression to different events or groups of events, and is implemented in standard statistical software (SAS, STATA, S+). A summary treatment effect can be calculated from a weighted average of the treatment effect on the separate AIDS events (Wei et al., 1989). The choice of weights is arbitrary, but can depend on clinical considerations. Wei et al. (1989) proposed weighting by the information matrix, while Neaton et al. (1994) proposed using subjective weights elicited from clinicians and patients. Adjustment for multiple testing can be made based on the covariance matrix (see Chapter 6). However, with these marginal multivariate models, Hughes (1997) has shown that the use

Table 2 Cause-Specific Analysis for Progression to a First AIDS-Defining Event or Death in Delta: Relative Risk (RR) for Participants Entering Without AIDS

		ZDV + ddl vs. ZDV		ZDV + ddC vs. ZDV	
Event	Total events	log(RR)	(se)	log(RR)	(se)
AIDS I	756	−.277	(.091)	−.109	(.088)
AIDS II	96	−.617	(.256)	−.362	(.239)
Death	84	.082	(.266)	−.016	(.275)
First	936	−.279	(.081)	−.132	(.078)

of events after the first may lead to loss in power in estimating event-specific treatment effects in some situations when a substantial number of participants change their allocated treatment after the first event.

Based on the relative risk of mortality associated with the occurrence of AIDS events, the AIDS events in Delta can be divided into two categories, where AIDS II are events of poorer prognosis (relative risk of death greater than 5: namely multifocal leukoencephalopathy, non-Hodgkin's and cerebral lymphomas, indeterminate cerebral lesions, HIV encephalopathy, and HIV wasting syndrome) and AIDS I consists of the remaining less severe events. The vast majority (81%) of first events were AIDS I. The effect of randomized group on the cause-specific hazards for progression to AIDS I, AIDS II, and death are shown in Table 2, together with the composite endpoint analysis. Table 3 gives the parameter

Table 3 Marginal Analysis of Multiple Endpoints for the ZDV + ddl Versus ZDV Alone Comparison in Delta (for Participants Entering Without AIDS)

		ZDV + ddl vs. ZDV			
				Correlations	
	Total events	log (RR)	(se)	AIDS I	AIDS II
AIDS I	525	−.307	(.088)		
AIDS II	116	−.500	(.191)	.21	
Death	342	−.346	(.109)	.52	.45
Any	983	−.343	(.085)	—	
First	624	−.281	(.081)	—	—

estimates (log relative risk) for the ZDV + ddI versus ZDV comparison in Delta from the multivariate marginal model, together with the correlation matrix. The closed testing procedure of Marcus et al. (1976) applied to the estimates in Table 3 shows that ZDV + ddI significantly reduces the marginal hazard to AIDS I, AIDS II, and death ($p < .02$).

2.2. Frailty Models

Frailty models represent the association between events experienced by the same individual as the effect of a single unobservable covariate (frailty w_i), conditional upon which the times to the different events are assumed independent. For each individual $i = 1, \ldots, I$ the hazard of experiencing an event in group $j = 1, \ldots,$ J is now

$$\lambda_{ij}(t) = \lambda_{0j}(t) \exp(\beta_j z_i) w_i.$$

Semiparametric inference for multivariate failure time data was developed for gamma-distributed frailties (Klein, 1992), although inverse Gaussian and positive stable frailties can also be used (Wang et al., 1995, Klein et al. 1992). Parameter estimation proceeds via the EM algorithm (Dempster et al., 1977). A profile likelihood estimate is constructed for the baseline hazard, resulting in a likelihood for the effect of factors and the frailty parameters similar to the partial likelihood. However, complex (numerical) maximization routines are required to estimate the parameters of the continuous frailty distributions. Further, standard errors should be adjusted for the use of the profile likelihood estimate for the nonparametric baseline hazard (Andersen et al., 1997).

Currently, a SAS macro is available for implementing the gamma frailty model (Klein and Moeschberger, 1997), but only with a common nonparametric baseline hazard across event groups [$\lambda_{0j}(t) = \lambda_0(t) \forall j$]. This is clearly inappropriate for a composite endpoint such as AIDS or death when the underlying rates vary substantially across the individual events making up the composite endpoint. A simpler semiparametric method of estimation assumes the frailties come from a finite number of frailty subpopulations, with the simplest form a binary frailty similar to that proposed for multivariate binary data by Babiker and Cuzick (1994). Now the frailty $w_i = \exp(\gamma U_i)$, where $U_i \in \{0, 1\}$ with $P(U_i = 1) = \theta$. This model is estimable using standard software for Poisson regression (Walker, 1999). Table 4 gives the parameter estimates (log relative risk) for the ZDV + ddI versus ZDV comparison in Delta from the multivariate semiparametric binary frailty model, together with the correlation matrix. Models with

Table 4 Binary Frailty Analysis of Multiple Endpoints for the ZDV + ddl Versus ZDV Alone Comparison in Delta (for Participants Entering Without AIDS)

		ZDV + ddl vs. ZDV			
				Correlations	
	Total events	log (RR)	(se)	AIDS I	AIDS II
AIDS I	525	−.264	(.938)		
AIDS II	116	−.500	(.166)	.274	
Death	342	−.395	(.111)	.415	.283
Any	983	−.329	(.083)	—	—

Note: Estimated proportion of frail individuals was .22, and the relative risk associated with being frail was 32.26.

parametric hazards are considerably easier to fit (Pickles and Crouchley, 1995), but at the expense of potential model misspecification.

Whether parametric or nonparametric hazards are used, parameter estimates from any frailty model are conditional on the frailty and must be interpreted as such. Ratios of hazards averaged over the frailty distribution can be constructed for comparison with the hazard ratio from the corresponding marginal model, but these depend on the (profile) baseline hazard and thus vary over time. In addition, in the setting of clinical trials, although the randomization ensures that the unobservable frailty covariates are on average identically distributed in the different treatment groups, it does not ensure that the effect of the frailty of the hazard is independent of treatment group: that is, there may be frailty-treatment group interactions.

2.3. Conditional and Multistate Models

Conditional and multistate models extend the concept of frailty models further by conditioning treatment effects on more of an individuals' covariate history than the value of a single unobserved covariate. Prentice et al. (1981) propose a conditional model which can be used to investigate recurrent events of the same kind, based on proportional hazards models and conditional on the history of the event and covariate processes [denoted $\Delta(t)$ and $X(t)$, respectively]. One choice is to condition on the previous number of events experienced by the individual. The hazard for the jth event in individual i is then

$$\lambda_{ij}\{t \mid \Delta(t), X(t)\} = \lambda_{0j}(t) \exp(\beta_j z_i).$$

Time can either be measured from randomization, or from the previous event. This type of recurrence model can be fitted in any standard software which allows data to be input in the counting process formulation for failure time data and simultaneously allows stratification of the baseline hazard (such as SAS, STATA, and S+).

Multistate models (Kay, 1984) extend these conditional models further to include conditioning information on the type rather than merely the number of previous events. Separate proportional hazards models are specified for transitions between any pair of events or group of events. All estimated treatment effects must now be interpreted conditionally on the entire covariate history. Table 5 gives the parameter estimates (log relative risk) for the ZDV + ddI versus ZDV comparison in Delta from the multistate model. The effect of combination therapy on the overall rate of progression to AIDS II events is much less clear from this model.

A distinction has to be drawn between accurately modelling disease processes and covariate effects, and presenting the likely effects of treatment in a manner which is easily understood by clinicians and patients, and applied to clinical practice. For the latter marginal models remain the most appropriate for use in clinical trials, while for the former the simple frailty models present an alternative which is easy to interpret. Conditional and frailty models provide a richer alternative for hypothesis generating.

Table 5 Multistate Analysis of Multiple Endpoints for the ZDV + ddI Versus ZDV Alone Comparison in Delta (for Participants Entering Without AIDS)

Transition			ZDV + ddI vs. ZDV	
From	To	Total events	Log (RR)	(se)
Entry	AIDS I	759	−.281	(.090)
Entry	AIDS II	98	−.662	(.254)
Entry	Death	79	.216	(.281)
AIDS I	AIDS II[a]	67	−.155	(.293)
AIDS I	Death[a]	284	−.311	(.147)
AIDS II	Death[a]	135	−.122	(.213)

[a] Timescale measured from previous event.

3. BIOLOGICAL MARKERS OF DISEASE PROGRESSION

Without a doubt, the greatest change in the design of HIV trials over the last 15 years has been the move from clinical endpoints to the use of endpoints based on biological markers of disease progression. The 1990s saw substantial statistical interest in the validation of these markers as surrogates for clinical outcome. Eventually, however, the FDA and other regulatory authorities decided to licence anti-HIV drugs on the basis of their effects on these markers rather than on clinical outcome. Plasma HIV RNA measurements are now the most commonly used primary outcome measures in Phase III trials.

3.1. Surrogacy

A perfect surrogate for clinical outcome should satisfy the condition that a test of the null hypothesis of no treatment effect on the marker should also be a valid test of the null hypothesis based on clinical outcome (Prentice 1989). This requires that

1. The ability of the marker to predict clinical outcome should be independent of treatment.
2. The marker should capture any relationship, positive or negative, between the treatment and clinical outcome.

In the Concorde trial (Concorde Coordinating Committee, 1994), immediate treatment with ZDV induced significant increases in CD4 count, which remained on average more than 30 cells/μL higher than in the deferred treatment group for at least 3 years. Yet clinical outcome up to 3 years showed no significant difference between the two treatment groups in mortality or progression to AIDS or death, and with longer follow-up there was a significant excess of deaths in the immediate group. Thus CD4 does not seem to satisfy conditions 1 and 2. Neither of the Prentice conditions for surrogacy, condition 2 in particular, appear to be adequately satisfied by HIV RNA viral load. In the Delta trial, plasma and/or serum was available for viral load assessment in about 40% of the participants. Compared to ZDV alone, the unadjusted relative risk (95% confidence interval, CI) of disease progression or death (after week 8) was 0.60 (0.46 to 0.78) for ZDV + ddl and .66 (.51 – .85) for ZDV + ddC. After adjustment for viral load at baseline and week 8, disease-free survival was substantially worse in the two combination groups relative to ZDV monotherapy: the adjusted relative risks were 1.31 (1.00 to 1.71) and 1.52 (1.15 to 2.02) respectively (Delta, 1999).

In practice a single marker that captures all of the treatment effect is unlikely to exist. A more realistic goal is to require that, in addition to the lack of interaction between treatment and marker in their effect on clinical outcome (1), the marker captures a substantial proportion of the treatment effect on the clinical endpoint. The statistical properties of the proportion of treatment effect explained by the marker (PTE) were investigated by Freedman et al. (1992) and Lin et al. (1997) in the contexts of logistic regression and Cox proportional hazards regression, respectively. The marginal methods for the analysis of multivariate failure time data described in Section 2 can be used to simultaneously model

$$\lambda_i(t \mid z_i) = \lambda_{01}(t) \exp(\alpha z_i) \tag{1}$$

$$\lambda_i(t \mid z_i, X) = \lambda_{02}(t) \exp\{\beta z_i + \gamma \quad X(t)\} \tag{2}$$

where z_i is the treatment group indicator and $X(t)$ represents the possibly time-dependent history of the marker. Models (1) and (2) cannot strictly hold simultaneously, but the first model, which is not conditional on the marker process, is assumed to correspond approximately to the integrated second model. This will hold provided either $\gamma\ E\{X(t)\}$ or $\Lambda_{02}(t) - \int_0^t \lambda_{02}\ (u)\ du$ is small. Under these conditions the PTE is defined by PTE $= 1-\beta/\alpha$. Confidence intervals for the PTE can be obtained using the Delta method or Fieller's theorem (Fieller, 1940). Using the Delta method, the variance of the PTE can be estimated by

$$\sigma^2 = \frac{V_\alpha}{\hat{\alpha}^2}\left[\frac{V_\beta}{V_\alpha} + \left(\frac{\hat{\beta}}{\hat{\alpha}}\right)^2 - 2 \times \frac{\hat{\beta}}{\hat{\alpha}} \times \frac{V_{\alpha\beta}}{V_\alpha}\right]$$

where V_α, V_β, and $V_{\alpha\beta}$ are the elements of the robust variance matrix. Logrank based methods for estimating PTE have also been developed based on the difference between logrank observed and expected events stratified by marker levels (DeMasi and Babiker 1998), avoiding the assumption of proportional hazards.

The PTE by serial CD4 cell counts for AIDS or death has been estimated by Choi et al. (1993) and Lin et al. (1993) as −.01, .31, and −.13 from three trials of ZDV (Volberding et al., 1990; Fischl et al., 1987; and Fischl et al., 1990, respectively). The PTE by CD4 at weeks 16 and 8 for AIDS or death after this time point in the second two trials has also been estimated at .46 (95% Cl −.14 to .08) and .28 (95% Cl .06 to .51) respectively (Choi et al., 1993; Lin et al., 1997). CD4 cell counts over time and at fixed time points therefore appear to be only an incomplete surrogate for clinical outcome.

Estimates of PTE clearly tend to be imprecise, and can even lie outside the range of zero to one because PTE is related to the *net* effect of treatment. A surrogate marker might be considered important if the lower confidence limit for the PTE exceeded a level such as .75 (since a perfect surrogate has PTE = 1). Lin et al. (1997) showed that the power of detecting the lower confidence limit greater than .75 remained low, at only 50% even when the treatment effect was about 8 standard deviations in size. Therefore, reasonably precise estimation of the PTE is likely to require that the effect of treatment on a clinical outcome be assessed much more precisely (with a smaller standard error) than needed to show a significant result on the clinical event itself. Such a trial would be likely to be stopped early before such significant evidence accumulated in any case. More importantly, even if PTE is estimated to be near 1 with a high degree of confidence, this by itself does not guarantee that the marker is a good surrogate (DeGruttola et al., 1997). The reason is that if the treatment has a negative impact on clinical outcome through processes not mediated via the marker, a poor surrogate can have PTE close to 1. Thus, while these methods may lead to the identification of poor surrogates, they cannot validate surrogacy, which requires a more general understanding of mechanisms of disease and drug action.

Rather than considering the PTE, Buyse and Molenberghs (1998) propose assessing the surrogacy of an endpoint (rather than a marker process) via the relative effect defined by RE $= \alpha/\gamma$, where γ is the effect of treatment on the surrogate endpoint,

$$\lambda_i(x \mid z_i) = \lambda_{03}(x) \exp(\gamma z_i).$$

However, similarly to PTE, validating surrogate endpoints using the RE requires large numbers of observations.

Daniels and Hughes (1997) explored the issue of surrogacy by a Bayesian meta-analysis of the correlation between treatment-induced changes in biological markers and treatment effect on clinical outcome. This is a more promising approach, although it may be limited by the amount and nature of data available from the trials. The estimated treatment difference on the clinical outcome $\hat{\theta}_k$ and the marker response $\hat{\gamma}_k$ in each trial, $k = 1, \ldots, I$ are assumed to follow a joint normal distribution,

$$\begin{pmatrix} \hat{\theta}_k \\ \hat{\gamma}_k \end{pmatrix} \sim N\left\{ \begin{pmatrix} \theta_k \\ \gamma_k \end{pmatrix}, \begin{pmatrix} \sigma_k^2 & \rho_k \sigma_k \nu_k \\ \rho_k \sigma_k \nu_k & \nu_k^2 \end{pmatrix} \right\}$$

where sampling variation is represented by σ_k and ν_k. θ_k is assumed to be related to γ_k through a simple linear fixed effects model, $\theta_k|\gamma_k \sim N(\alpha + \beta\gamma_k, \tau^2)$, leading to

$$\begin{pmatrix} \hat{\theta}_k \\ \hat{\gamma}_k \end{pmatrix} \sim N\left\{ \begin{pmatrix} \alpha + \beta\gamma_k \\ \gamma_k \end{pmatrix}, \begin{pmatrix} \sigma_k^2 + \tau^2 & \rho_k\sigma_k\nu_k \\ \rho_k\sigma_k\nu_k & \nu_k^2 \end{pmatrix} \right\}.$$

If the marker is a perfect surrogate, then we expect $\alpha = 0$, $\beta \neq 0$, and $\tau^2 = 0$. Noninformative priors are placed on the regression coefficients (α, β, γ_k), a positive prior is placed on τ^2, and (σ_k^2, ν_k^2, ρ_k) are replaced by their within trial (empirical Bayes) estimates. Gibbs sampling is used for estimation (Gilks et al., 1996). This method allows for the fact that both clinical outcome and marker outcome are measured with error. Using this technique to assess mean change and AUC (area under the curve) in CD4 and RNA as surrogates for progression to AIDS or death, CD4 and RNA were concluded to be jointly important as prognostic factors, but only partial surrogates, for clinical outcome (HIV Surrogate Marker Collaborative Group, 2000). At 24 weeks change in CD4 alone accounted for 0.34 (95% Cl .16–.53) of the observed treatment effect, change in RNA accounted for 0.45 (95% Cl .24–.67), and changes in both RNA and CD4 jointly accounted for 0.57 (95% Cl .31–.84) of the treatment effect on AIDS or death to 2 years.

3.2. Analysis of Biological Markers as Continuous Variables

The majority of clinical trials in HIV disease now have biological markers as outcome measures, notably viral load as measured by HIV RNA, and thus (in the absence of sufficient information on surrogacy) evaluate the effect of treatment on the markers of anti-HIV efficacy only. When markers are treated as continuous outcome measures, methods for the analysis of longitudinal data must be used as in Chapter 11. Treatment groups are compared in terms of the trajectory of the marker or a summary of such a trajectory. Possible summaries include

1. Level or change at a fixed time point
2. Average level as measured by the area under the curve (AUC)
3. Average slope of marker trajectory
4. Time to achieve a given threshold level

However, participants are not followed beyond the end of the trial therapy in many HIV trials and so intention to treat has been more rarely used. The rationale is that biological markers measure efficacy and that no efficacy is expected after withdrawal from the trial regimen. This excludes either continuing benefit from continuation of other therapy, or more importantly leads to bias if one group with superior marker response stop therapy more quickly due to toxicity. Data will often be incomplete due to dropouts from toxicity or personal withdrawal and dropout will commonly be informative (Touloumi et al., 2002). In the analysis of biological markers as continuous variables in the medical literature, dropout is generally handled either by basing analysis only on those with complete data, or by using the last observation carried forward (LOCF). Mean values at various time points after randomization can then be compared using pointwise tests. Clearly, more advanced methods of analysis of incomplete data are possible including GEE and multilevel models in standard software such as SAS, Stata, and S+, as well as Bayesian methods (Raab and Parpia, 2001). However, none of the above methods addresses the issue of informative dropout. More recently, longitudinal models which explicitly include information on the dropout process have been developed (see, for example, Diggle and Kenward, 1994; Touloumi, 1999; Hogan and Laird, 1997a, b). All these models for longitudinal data can be used with the intention-to-treat principle, assessing the effect on the marker of efficacy of the policy of giving the treatment regimens.

When comparing treatment groups in terms of change in HIV RNA from baseline, it is also important to recognize that the continuous data itself is often censored (Hughes, 2000). In general, at any time point after randomization a number of HIV RNA measurements will be reported as less than the level of detectability of the assay, for example, RNA < 400 or RNA < 50. Often this left censoring is ignored, assuming that RNA $<$ 400 is equivalent to RNA $= 400$. A number of appropriate statistical methods for parametric and nonparametric analysis of this type of measurements are available (Hughes, 2000; Journot et al., 2001). For example, normal interval regression can be used, where the likelihood contribution for the interval censored data is the probability that the true value lies within the known interval, rather than the probability that it equals some fixed value (Long, 1997). Parametric or nonparametric failure time methods can be used to incorporate the left censoring with the dependent variable RNA rather than time, and compare treatment groups or calculate medians (Flandre et al., 2002). Gehan's modification of the Wilcoxon test (Gehan, 1965) can also be used as a nonparametric rank test. Mixed models can be used to model longitudinal data incorporating this left censoring and informative dropouts (Lyles et al., 2000). More complicated mixture models allowing for highly skewed data with extra probability mass below the limit of detection of the assay have also been developed but do not currently take informative dropout into account (Moulton et al., 2002).

3.3. Analysis of Biological Markers as Failure Time Data

Rather than comparing levels of biological markers over time or at arbitrarily chosen time points, biological markers can also be used to define time-to-event endpoints, for example, time to achieve either a prespecified fixed level, or percentage change from baseline. For example, a successful outcome can be defined as time to reach a threshold such as <50 copies of HIV RNA per milliliter (or undetectable viral load on the assays), or a treatment failure can be defined as time to a rebound above baseline after initial reduction. An endpoint such as RNA rebound or failure of viral suppression needs to take into account the likely trajectories of viral load decline in response to therapy: generally a window of 16–24 weeks has been considered an appropriate period for viral load to drop to undetectable levels (DeGruttola et al., 1998). How to account for unsuccessful or slow initial response to treatment must also be considered (Gilbert et al., 2000). There is still a measure of arbitrariness in the definition of these endpoints since they are likely to depend on factors which may have no clinical significance, such as the lower limit of quantification of the RNA assay chosen or a convenient round number.

In clinical trials RNA is generally only measured at specific time points post baseline (clinic visits) so that the exact time of occurrence of a marker defined endpoint is never known. A rigorous approach to the analysis of time to virological failure therefore requires the use of interval censored failure data techniques. This is particularly important when data are sparse, or the intervals between successive marker measurements are wide, since it is then that the most bias is likely to occur in approximations such as taking the failure time as the midpoint between visits or the first visit at which the event is observed to have already happened.

Suppose T_i denotes the unobserved marker event time, such as the time that viral load first drops to undetectable levels. The observed interval-censored data consists of an interval (L_i, R_i) where L_i is the time of the last clinic visit with detectable viral load and R_i is the time viral load was first observed to be undetectable. If T_i could be observed exactly, then $L_i = R_i$, when T_i is left censored, $L_i = 0$, and when T_i is right censored, $R_i = \infty$. Both semiparametric and parametric approaches have been developed to estimate the effects of covariates such as treatment group on the failure times T_i.

A (semiparametric) extension to Cox's proportional hazards model for interval censored data was originally proposed by Finkelstein (1986) by parameterizing the cumulative baseline hazard in a sufficiently fine manner. Suppose that now s_k denote times from trial entry such that all L_i and R_i are contained in the set of s_k. Then the failure data log-likelihood can be expressed as

$$\sum_i \log \sum_k c_{ik} \left[\exp\{-\exp(\beta z_i + \gamma_{k-1})\} - \exp\{-\exp(\beta z_i + \gamma_k)\}\right]$$

where

$$c_{ik} = I\{(s_{k-1}, s_k] \subset (L_i, R_i]\}, \quad \text{and}$$
$$\gamma_k = \log[-\log\{\Pr(T > s_k \mid X = 0)\}]$$

represents the cumulative baseline hazard. Newton-Raphson can be used to maximize the log likelihood to simultaneously estimate β and γ. The major disadvantage with this method is that the number of parameters to be estimated (γ) increases with the number of individuals unless the visit times are fixed for all individuals. Rank-based methods and methods based on multiple imputation are also available but are considerably more complex computationally.

By imposing the relatively weak assumption of constant hazards across predefined time intervals a parametric model with a fixed number of parameters can be fitted without imposing strong assumptions about the required failure time distribution. Generalized linear model approaches to estimation in this model have been developed (Carsenten, 1996; Farringdon, 1996; Smith et al., 1997), extending the logistic model for right censored data of Efron (1988). Suppose the time axis is divided into intervals $I_1, \ldots, I_m$ with $I_j = [t_{j-1}, t_j]$ and with hazard a constant λ_j within each interval. Then the failure data likelihood is

$$\prod_i \exp\left(-\sum_j a_{ij}\lambda_j\right) \times \left\{1 - \exp\left(-\sum_j b_{ij}\lambda_j\right)\right\}$$

where a_{ij} is the time in I_j in which patient i is known to not have had the event, and b_{ij} is the time in I_j during which the event could have occurred. The hazards λ_j are therefore the parameters of a generalized linear model with a log link and Bernoulli error. However, estimation using generalized linear models requires that the linear predictor is constrained to be positive throughout the iterations. Sparse data or inappropriate intervals can produce negative hazards. An alternative is to estimate the λ_j using the EM algorithm (Lindsey and Ryan, 1998), where the complete data is the exact (unobserved) failure times for those who experienced the event and the censoring times for those right censored. The complete data log likelihood is therefore

$$\sum_j (D_j \ln \lambda_j - \lambda_j Y_j)$$

where D_j is the number of events in I_j and Y_j is the person-time at risk in I_j. Poisson regression can therefore be used to estimate λ_j using D_j as response and log Y_j as offset. The conditional probability of a patient's event occurring in an interval I_j and the conditional expected time at risk in I_j given current λ_j can be calculated by considering the location of (L_i, R_i) with respect to I_j. These quantities can then be used in the Poisson regression. Standard errors can be estimated using methods such as Louis (1982) or Meng and Rubin (1991).

Finally, fully parametric failure time data models provide greater stability when event data are sparse or intervals are wide (Lindsey, 1998; Lindsey and Ryan, 1998). However, this stability comes at the expense of potential model misspecification. Both nonparametric and parametric methods have been recently extended to multivariate data (Betensky and Finkelstein, 1999; Goggins and Finkelstein, 2000).

An alternative to interval-censored failure time data analysis is to group the data and use a discrete survival model; for example failure time observations R_i could be grouped by weeks from randomization (indexed by k below). A logistic model for the regression analysis of discrete failure time data has been proposed by Sun (1997), relating the hazard of failure at discrete time point s_k to covariates via

$$\frac{\lambda_k}{1 - \lambda_k} = \exp(w_k \beta z + \gamma_k)$$

where w_k is a prespecified weight used to construct tests. Under this model the failure data log–likelihood function is

$$\sum_i \log \sum_k c_{ik} \left[\prod_{l=1}^{k-1} \{1 + \exp(w_l \beta z_i + \gamma_l)\}^{-1} \right] \left\{ \frac{\exp(w_k \beta z_i + \gamma_k)}{1 + \exp(w_k \beta z_i + \gamma_k)} \right\}$$

with $c_{ik} = I\{(s_{k-1}, s_k) \subset (L_i, R_i)\}$ as before. β and γ can be estimated using Newton-Raphson maximization of the log likelihood, with standard errors estimated from the Hessian. Interval-censored and discrete models for the analysis of virologic endpoints have not been widely used so far. Instead, the time of the assay has been used as the true time of the event.

In the medical literature, analyses of virologic endpoints after randomization have often been based on comparison of proportions experiencing the endpoint by a fixed time T_0, *excluding* participants who change treatment or are lost to follow-up before T_0 (standard on treatment analysis). More recently, a "noncompleter equals failure" analysis (NC = F) has been proposed as an attempt to include all participants in a simple manner. Under NC = F, patients who change treatment are included in the analysis and assumed to have failed at the time of dropout. This method is also likely to lead to biased estimates of the treatment effect if the reasons for dropout are different in the two treatment groups. Assuming that either none or all (NC = F) of those who change treatment or are lost to follow-up have events are extreme case analyses (although the most conservative extreme case approach would be to define noncompleter equals failure in the experimental treatment arm, and noncompleter equals success in the standard arm). A similar approach has recently been described as a sensitivity method for assessing the effect of missing data (Molenberghs et al., 2001). If the number of noncompleters is substantial there may be large differences between the methods in the absolute proportions experiencing the event as well as in the differences between randomized groups. If treatment changes are the reason for noncompletion, then some methods have been proposed to adjust for the treatment changes while retaining unbiased estimation of treatment differences.

4. ADJUSTING FOR CHANGES FROM ALLOCATED TREATMENT

Analysis by the intent-to-treat (ITT) principle is generally accepted as the most appropriate for randomized controlled trials. All follow-up from all eligible patients are included in the analysis in the treatment group to which they were originally assigned. In contrast, "on treatment" analyses are restricted to patients on allocated therapy at the time of analysis (so follow-up is censored at the time of change from allocated therapy in survival analysis). Clearly focusing on events that occur during the allocated treatment period or shortly after can lead to misleading results. Many trials in HIV infection only collect information until participants stop allocated trial therapy, and therefore the only analysis possible is an on-treatment analysis. It is important to note that only the intent-to-treat (ITT) analysis is unbiased under the null hypothesis of no treatment difference and that on treatment analyses can produce significantly biased estimates of treatment effect for a variety of reasons, the most common being that participants with worse prognosis are more likely to change treatment in *both* treatment groups. Direct comparison of patients according to treatment actually received therefore incurs major selection bias. However, several methods are available to adjust the ITT estimate of treatment effect for the treatment changes that occurred in a manner which preserves the randomization. Thus the direct efficacy of the treatment regimens can be compared as intended, in addition to the effectiveness of the policy of applying the treatment regimens in practice (ITT).

Randomization-based methods for adjusting for treatment changes are also described in Chapter 10. Methods for adjusting for treatment changes at randomization have been proposed by Sommer and Zeger (1991) and Cuzick et al. (1997) for binary treatment outcomes, and by Newcombe (1988) for continuous outcomes. The difference in outcome adjusting for treatment changes essentially equals the intention-to-treat difference divided by the difference between the two treatment groups in the proportion receiving the treatment as allocated. For treatment changes which can occur at any time, rather than only at randomization, a variety of randomization-based methods using causal modelling have been developed by Robins and coworkers (Robins and Tsiatis, 1991; Robins and Greenland, 1994; Mark and Robins, 1993; White and Goetghebeur, 1998). These models make no assumptions about the relationship between treatment changes and prognosis. A Stata macro is available for the simplest model, described below (White et al., 2002).

Only randomization-based methods for survival data will be considered here. In brief, for a participant who experiences an event at time T_i, the treatment history, represented by time dependent covariate $\mathbf{z}_i(t)$, is assumed to modify the true unobserved underlying lifetime U_i, in the absence of treatment via the causal accelerated life model

$$U_i = \int_0^{T_i} \exp\{\beta^T \mathbf{z}_i(u)\}\ du.$$

The underlying lifetime is independent of treatment group, and therefore β can be estimated using a logrank test for U_i. The point estimate is the value of β at which the logrank test for a difference between the treatment groups in U_i is 0, and the 95% confidence interval for β the range of values for which the logrank test is not significant at the 5% level. The test of $\beta = 0$ is the intention-to-treat logrank test, and therefore the p value is unchanged by the adjustment for treatment changes.

When not all patients experience the event of interest, censoring of the failure times by withdrawal or end of study depends on the treatment actually received, and is therefore informative on the U scale. This is easy to see by considering individuals with detrimental treatment history ($|\beta^T z_i(t)| >> 0$): Individuals experiencing events just before their censoring time C_i would not have had these events observed if their treatment history had been more favorable. Recensoring is one procedure for dealing with this informative censoring: Each U_i is "recensored" by the minimum censoring time over all time-dependent values of $\mathbf{z}(t)$ that were possible within the ith patient's randomized treatment group. Thus for a patient censored at C_i,

$$U_i = \min\left[\left[\int_0^{T_i} \exp\{\beta^T \mathbf{z}_i(u)\} du, \quad \min_{\mathbf{z}(u) \text{ in ith group}} \left[\int_0^{C_i} \exp\{\beta^T \mathbf{z}(u)\} du\right]\right]\right].$$

Although such randomization-based methods are appealing in that they do not introduce bias into the comparison of the treatment groups, the effect of treatment from the accelerated failure time model β represents a ratio by which time to event is extended in one treatment group. For example, with two treatment groups and without censoring, if $\mathbf{z}(t)$ indicates whether a patient is taking the experimental treatment at time t, then $U_i = T_i^0 + e^{\beta} T_i^1$ where T_i^0 is the total time patient i spent on the standard treatment and T_i^1 is the total time patient i spent on the experimental treatment. Then $e^{-\beta}$ is the factor by which time to event is multiplied if a patient receives the experimental treatment continuously compared with continuously receiving the standard treatment. However, this is unfamiliar to many clinicians and statisticians who are more used to expressing the treatment effect as a hazard ratio. The estimated time ratio in the accelerated life model can be used to "correct" the observed event times T_i to those which would have been observed under the scenario represented by the treatment variable $\mathbf{z}(t)$, denoted T_i^*. For example, with $\mathbf{z}(t)$ as above and ignoring treatment changes in the experimental group, $T_i^* = T_i$ in the experimental treatment group, whereas in the standard group

$$T_i^* = T_i + (e^{-\beta} - 1)T_i^{01} + (e^{\beta} - 1)T_i^{10}$$

where T_i^{mn} is the time on the T scale that the treatment received was m but would have been n under the scenario represented by $\mathbf{z}(t)$. T^* is recensored in a similar manner to U, and then a "corrected" hazard ratio can be estimated using standard methods on T^* for comparison with the standard intention-to-treat hazard ratios.

Example. In the Concorde trial participants were randomized to immediate ZDV or ZDV deferred until the onset of symptoms (ARC or AIDS). Many participants started open label ZDV before clinical disease progression, mainly on the basis of persistently low CD4 counts after a protocol amendment one year into the trial. The effect of these treatment changes is to make the two treatment arms more similar, that is, to move the estimate of the treatment effect toward the null. Methods not based on the randomization (such as proportional hazards modelling with "on treatment" covariates) are subject to particularly large bias in Concorde, because in both groups by far the strongest predictor of starting ZDV is prognosis. Therefore comparing patients by whether or not they had taken ZDV is a comparison of prognosis, not the treatment arms themselves (White et al., 1997). Using the accelerated failure time model above, there are several choices for the treatment history covariate $\mathbf{z}(t)$:

$z_{\mathrm{ITT}}(t)$ = 1 for immediate, 0 for deferred ZDV

$z_{\mathrm{NOW}}(t)$ = indicator of being on ZDV at time t

$z_{\mathrm{EVR}}(t)$ = indicator of being assigned to receive ZDV before time t (that is, 1 for immediate or after open ZDV in deferred)

$z_{\mathrm{EVP}}(t)$ = indicator of being assigned to receive ZDV before time t, other than at or after the onset of ARC or AIDS (that is, 1 for immediate, or after open ZDV in deferred if open ZDV before ARC or AIDS)

The concept of transient treatment effect can also be incorporated into these models by restricting the effect of ZDV to only a limited period, for example, by defining

$z_{\mathrm{EVR1}}(t)$ = indicator of being assigned to receive ZDV within the previous year at time t

and similarly for $z_{\mathrm{EVP1}}(t)$. However, these treatment covariates do not correspond to the difference between the two treatment arms under any scenario of treatment changes.

Table 6 shows the log time ratios for progression to the three major clinical endpoints in Concorde adjusted for the various scenarios described above (White et al., 1998, 1999). Correcting for treatment

Table 6 Semiparametric Adjustment for Changes from Allocated Trial Therapy in Concorde

	ARC, AIDS, or death		Endpoint AIDS or death		Death	
Scenario	β	95% CI	β	95% CI	β	95% CI
ITT	−.101	(−.245, .041)	.004	(−.140, .137)	.093	(−.028, .227)
NOW	−.262	(−.517, .061)	.006	(−.308, .383)	.414	(−.104, 2.082)
EVR	−.178	(−.377, .041)	.004	(−.274, .217)	.172	(−.102, .858)
EVP			.004	(−.230, .178)	.132	(−.078, .344)
EVR1	−.870	(. , .134)	.013	(. , .710)	.750	(. , 1.260)
EVP1			.013	(−1.857, .554)	.435	(−.534, .746)

Note: β is a log time ratio from the accelerated failure time model. Lower confidence limit is missing when the logrank test statistic is greater than −1.96 at β = −3. For progression to ARC, AIDS, or death, EVP is an identical scenario to EVR.

changes increased the estimated benefit of immediate ZDV in delaying progression to ARC, AIDS, or death and the estimated disadvantage of immediate ZDV in accelerating death. Correspondingly, the confidence intervals became wider, reflecting the increased uncertainty because of the treatment changes and indicating the maximum effect that might have been missed in the trial. The necessity of some form of recensoring can be shown by considering proportional hazards models using treatment history as covariates. Treatment history strongly predicts events on the T scale, the U scale, and the recensored U scale, but only predicts end of follow-up on the nonrecensored U scale, showing that censoring is informative on the U scale. Simulations show that in Concorde, failing to recensor incurs a small bias, but has little effect on the overall error in the estimation because the standard deviations of the recensored estimator are larger.

5. CONCLUSIONS

Clinical trials in HIV over the first decade of antiretroviral therapy were mainly set up to evaluate two classes of anti-HIV drugs, the reverse transcriptase and protease inhibitors. The second decade of HIV clinical trials is seeing a wider diversity as further classes of anti-HIV drugs become available (such as fusion inhibitors and immune modulators), strategy trials are designed to investigate order and length of administration of drug combinations, salvage trials are developed for patients failing on HAART, and trials move into areas of nondrug interventions such as genotypic and phenotypic resistance testing. As individuals take HAART for increasing periods of time, toxicity data are likely to play a more important role, particularly with the advent of reported metabolic dysfunction and lipodystrophy. Methods which incorporate both efficacy and safety into treatment comparisons may become more widely used (Tubert-Bitter et al., 1995; Thall and Cheng, 1999). It is also likely that the use of biological markers in making treatment decisions will be further refined, and that measures of drug resistance will become trial endpoints. However, issues discussed in this chapter such as choice of trial design and endpoints, the analysis of biological markers and their interpretation, and compliance will continue to be important and present new statistical challenges.

REFERENCES

Albert, J. M., Yun, H. (2001). Statistical advances in AIDS therapy trials. Statistical Methods in Medical Research 10:85–100.

Andersen, P. K., Klein, J. P., Knudsen, K. M., Tabanera y Palacios, R. (1997). Estimation of variance in Cox's regression model with shared gamma frailties. Biometrics 53:1475–1484.

Babiker, A. G., Cuzick, J. (1994). A simple frailty model for family studies with covariates. Statistics in Medicine 13:1679–1692.

Betensky, R. A., Finkelstein, D. M. (1999). A non-parametric maximum likelihood estimator for bivariate interval censored data. Statistics in Medicine 18: 3089–3100.

Bjorling, L. E., Hodges, J. S. (1997). Rule-based ranking schemes for antiretroviral trials. Statistics in Medicine 16:1175–1191.

Buyse, M., Molenberghs, G. (1998). Criteria for the validation of surrogate endpoints in randomized experiments. Biometrics 54:1014–1029.

Carr, A., Samaras, K., Thorisdottir, A., Kaufmann, G. R., Chisholm, D. J., Cooper, D. A. (1999). Diagnosis, prediction, and natural course of HIV-1 protease-inhibitor-associated lipodystrophy, hyperlipidaemia, and diabetes mellitus: a cohort study. Lancet 353:2093–2099.

Carsenten, B. (1996). Regression models for interval censored survival data: application to HIV infection in Danish homosexual men. Statistics in Medicine 15:2177–2189.

Centers for Disease Control (1992). 1993 revised classification system for HIV infection and expanded surveillance case definition for AIDS among adolescents and adults. Mortality and Morbidity Weekly Report 41:1–19.

Choi, S., Lagakos, S. W., Schooley, R. T., Volberding, P. A. (1993). CD4 Lymphocytes are an incomplete surrogate marker for clinical progression in persons with asymptomatic HIV infection taking zidovudine. Annals of Internal Medicine 118:674–680.

Clayton, D., Cuzick, J. (1985). Multivariate generalizations of the proportional hazards model. Journal of the Royal Statistical Society A 148:82–117.

Concorde Coordinating Committee (1994). Concorde: MRC/ANRS randomised double-blind controlled trial of immediate and deferred zidovudine in symptom-free HIV infection. Lancet 343:871–882.

Cuzick, J., Edwards, R., Segnan, N. (1997). Adjusting for non-compliance and contamination in randomized controlled trials. Statistics in Medicine 16: 1017–1029.

Daniels, M. J., Hughes, M. D. (1997). Meta analysis for the evaluation of potential surrogate markers. Statistics in Medicine 16:1965–1982.

DeGruttola, V., Fleming, T. R., Lin, D. Y., Coombs, R. (1997). Validating surrogate markers - are we being naive? Journal of Infectious Diseases 175: 237–246.

DeGruttola, V., Hughes, M. D., Gilbert, P., Phillips, A. (1998). Trial design in the era of highly effective antiviral drug combinations for HIV infection. *AIDS* 12(suppl A):S149–S156.

Delta Coordinating Committee (1996). Delta: a randomised double-blind controlled trial comparing combinations of zidovudine plus didanosine or zalcitabine with zidovudine alone in HIV-infected individuals. Lancet 348: 283–291.

Delta Coordinating Committee and Virology Group (1999). An evaluation of HIV RNA and CD4 cell count as surrogates for clinical outcome. AIDS 13: 565–573.

DeMasi, R. A., Babiker, A. G. (1998). Nonparametric estimation of the proportion of treatment effect explained by a surrogate marker. Presented at the 1998 ENAR conference, April 1, 1998.

Dempster, A. P., Laird, N. M., Rubin, D. R. (1977). Maximum likelihood from incomplete data via the EM algorithm. Journal of the Royal Statistical Society B 39:1–38.

Diggle, P., Kenward, M. G. (1994). Informative drop-out in longitudinal analysis (with discussion). Journal of the Royal Statistical Society C 43:49–93.

Efron, B. (1988). Logistic regression, survival analysis and the Kaplan Meier curve. Journal of the American Statistical Association 83:414–425.

Egger, M., Junghans, C., Friis-Moller, N., Lundgren, J. D. (2001). Highly active antiretroviral therapy and coronary heart disease: the need for perspective. AIDS 15(Suppl. 5):S193–S201.

Ellenberg, S. S., Finkelstein, D. M., Schoenfeld, D. A. (1992). Statistical issues arising in AIDS clinical trials (with discussion). Journal of the American Statistical Association 87:562–583.

Emery, S., Abrams, D. I., Cooper, D. A., Darbyshire, J. H., Lane, H. C., Lundgren, J. D., Neaton, J. D. (2002). The evaluation of subcutaneous Proleukin (R) (interleukin-2) in a randomized international trial: rationale, design, and methods of ESPRIT. Controlled Clinical Trials 23:198–220.

Farringdon, C. P. (1996). Interval censored survival data: a generalised linear model approach. Statistics in Medicine 15:283–292.

Fieller, E. C. (1940). The biological standardisation of insulin. Journal of the Royal Statistical Society 7:S1–S15.

Finkelstein, D. M. (1986). A proportional hazards model for interval-censored failure time data. Biometrics 42:845–854.

Finkelstein, D. M., Schoenfeld, D. A., Stamenovic, E. (1997). Analysis of multivariate failure time data from an AIDS clinical trial. Statistics in Medicine 16:951–961.

Fischl, M. A., Richman, D. D., Grieco, M. H., Gottlieb, M. S., Volberding, P. A., Laskin, O. L., Leedom, J. M., Groopman, J. E., Mildvan, D., Schooley, R. T., Jackson, G. G., Durack, D. T., King, D., the ZDV Collaborative Working Group. (1987). The efficacy of azidothymidine (ZDV) in the treatment of patients with AIDS and AIDS-related complex: A double-blind, placebo-controlled trial. New England Journal of Medicine 317:185–191.

Fischl, M. A., Richman, D. D., Hansen, N., Collier, A. C., Carey, J. T., et al. (1990). The safety and efficacy of zidovudine (AZT) in the treatment of subjects with mildly symptomatic human immunodeficiency virus type 1 (HIV) infection. Annals of Internal Medicine 112:727–737.

Flandre, P., Durier, C., Descamps, D., Launay, O., Joly, V. (2002). On the use of magnitude of reduction in HIV-1 RNA in clinical trials: Statistical analysis and potential biases. *Journal of Acquired Immune Deficiency Syndromes* 30:59–64.

Fleming, T. R., DeMets, D. L. (1996). Surrogate endpoints in clinical trials: Are we being misled? Annals of Internal Medicine 125:605–613.

Foulkes, M. A. (1998). Advances in HIV/AIDS statistical methodology over the past decade. Statistics in Medicine 17:1–25.

Freedman, L. S., Graubard, B. I., Schatzkin, A. (1992). Statistical validation of intermediate endpoints for chronic diseases. Statistics in Medicine 11:167–178.

Friis-Moller, N., Weber, R., Reiss, P., Thiébaut, R., et al., for the DAD Study Group. (2003) Cardiovascular disease risk factors in HIV patients—association with antiretroviral therapy. Results from the DAD Study. AIDS 17:1179–1193.

Gehan, E. A. (1965). A generalized two-sample Wilcoxon test for doubly censored data. Biometrika 52:620–653.

Gilbert, P. B., Ribaudo, H. J., Greenberg, L., Yu, G., Bosch, R. J., Tierney, C., Kuritzkes, D. R. (2000). Considerations in choosing a primary endpoint that measures durability of virological suppression in an antiretroviral trial. AIDS 14:1961–1972.

Gilks, W. R., Richardson, S., Spiegelhalter, D. J. (1996). Markov Chain Monte Carlo in practice. London: Chapman and Hall.

Goggins, W. B., Finkelstein, D. M. (2000). A proportional hazards model for multivariate interval-censored failure time data. Biometrics 56:940–943.

Grambsch, P. M., Therneau, T. M. (1994). Proportional hazards tests and diagnostics based on weighted residuals. Biometrika 81:515–526.

Hess, K. R. (1994). Assessing time-by-covariate interactions in proportional hazards regression models using cubic spline functions. Statistics in Medicine 13:1045–1062.

HIV Surrogate Marker Collaborative Group (2000). Human Immunodeficiency virus type 1 RNA level and CD4 count as prognostic markers and surrogate endpoints: a meta-analysis. AIDS Research and Human Retroviruses 16: 1123–1133.

HIV Trialists' Collaborative Group (1999). Zidovudine, didanosine and zalcitabine in the treatment of HIV infection: meta-analyses of the randomised evidence. Lancet 353:2014–2025.

Hogan, J. W., Laird, N. M. (1997a). Mixture models for the joint distribution of repeated measures and event times. Statistics in Medicine 16:239–257.

Hogan, J. W., Laird, N. M. (1997b). Model-based approaches to analysing incomplete longitudinal and failure time data. Statistics in Medicine 16:259–272.

Hughes, M. D. (1997). Power considerations for clinical trials using multivariate time-to-event data. Statistics in Medicine 16:865–882.

Hughes, M. D. (2000). Analysis and design issues for studies using censored biomarker measurements with an example of viral load measurements in HIV clinical trials. Statistics in Medicine 19:3171–3191.

Joint Concorde and Opal Coordinating Committee (1998). Long-term follow-up of randomized trials of immediate versus deferred zidovudine in symptom-free HIV infection. AIDS 12:1259–1265.

Journot, V., Chêne, G., Joly, P., Savès, M., Jacqmin-Gadda, H., Molina, J.-M., Salamon, R., the ALBI Study Group (2001). Viral load as a primary outcome in Human Immunodeficiency Virus trials: a review of statistical analysis methods. Controlled Clinical Trials 22:639–658.

Kay, R. (1984). Multistate survival analysis: An application in breast cancer. Methods of Information in Medicine 23:157–162.

Klein, J. P. (1992). Semiparametric estimation of random effects using the Cox model based on the EM algorithm. Biometrics 48:795–806.

Klein, J. P., Moeschberger, M., Li, Y. H., Wang, S. T. (1992). Estimating random effects in the Framingham Heart Study. In: Goel, P. K., Klein, J. P., eds. Survival Analysis: State of the Art. Boston: Kluwer Academic Publishers, pp. 99–120.

Klein, J. P., Moeschberger, M. L. (1997). Survival analysis: techniques for censored and truncated data. New York: Springer-Verlag.

Larntz, K., Neaton, J. D., Wentworth, D. N., Yurik, T. (1996). Data analysis issues for protocols with overlapping enrollment. Statistics in Medicine 15: 2445–2453.

Liang, K-Y., Zeger, S. L. (1986). Longitudinal data analysis using generalized linear models. Biometrika 73:13–22.

Lin, D. Y., Fischl, M. A., Schoenfeld, D. A. (1993). Evaluating the role of CD4-lymphocyte counts as surrogate endpoints in HIV clinical trials. Statistics in Medicine 12:835–842.

Lin, D. Y., Fleming, T. R., De Gruttola, V. (1997). Estimating the proportion of treatment effect explained by a surrogate marker. Statistics in Medicine 16:1515–1527.

Lindsey, J. C., Ryan, L. M. (1998). Methods for interval-censored data. Statistics in Medicine 17:219–238.

Lindsey, J. K. (1998). A study of interval censoring in parametric regression models. Lifetime Data Analysis 4:329–354.

Long, J. S. (1997). Regression Models for Categorical and Limited Dependent Variables. Thousand Oaks, CA: Sage Publications.

Louis, T. A. (1982). Finding the observed information matrix when using the EM algorithm. Journal of the Royal Statistical Society B 44:226–233.

Lyles, R. H., Lyles, C. M., Taylor, D. J. (2000). Random regression models for human immunodeficiency virus ribonucleic acid data subject to left censoring and informative dropouts. Applied Statistics 49:485–497.

Marcus, R., Peritz, E., Gabriel, K. R. (1976). On closed testing procedures with special reference to ordered analysis of variance. Biometrika 63:655–660.

Mark, S. D., Robins, J. M. (1993). A method for the analysis of randomized trials with compliance information: An application to the multiple risk factor intervention trial. Controlled Clinical Trials 14:79–97.

Mellors, J. W., Muñoz, A., Giorgi, J. V., Margolick, J. B., Tassoni, C. J., Gupta, P., Kingsley, L. A., Todd, J. A., Saah, A. J., Detels, R., Phair, J. P. (1997). Plasma viral load and CD4 + lymphocytes as prognostic markers of HIV-1 infection. Annals of Internal Medicine 126:946–954.

Meng, X. L., Rubin, D. B. (1991). Using EM to obtain asymptotic variance-covariance matrices: the SEM algorithm. Journal of the American Statistical Association 86:899–909.

Mocroft, A. J., Johnson, M. A., Sabin, C. A., Lipman, M., Elford, J., Emery, V., Morcinek, J., Youle, M., Janossy, G., Lee, C. A., Phillips, A. N. for the Royal Free/Chelsea and Westminster Hospitals Collaborative Group. (1995). Staging System for clinical AIDS patients. Lancet 346:12–17.

Molenberghs, G., Kenward, M. G., Goetghebeur, E. (2001). Sensitivity analysis for incomplete contingency tables: The Slovenian plebiscite case. Applied Statistics 50:15–29.

Moulton, L. H., Curriero, F. C., Barroso, P. F. (2002). Mixture models for quantitative HIV RNA data. Statistical Methods in Medical Research 11:317–325.

Neaton, J. D., Wentworth, D. N., Rhame, F., Hogan, C., Abrams, D. I., Deyton, L. (1994). Considerations in choice of a clinical endpoint for AIDS clinical trials. Statistics in Medicine 13:2107–2125.

Newcombe, R. G. (1988). Explanatory and pragmatic estimates of the treatment effect when deviations from allocated treatment occur. Statistics in Medicine 7:1179–1186.

O'Brien, P. C. (1984). Procedures for comparing samples with multiple endpoints. Biometrics 40:1079–1087.

Pickles, A., Crouchley, R. (1995). A comparison of frailty models for multivariate survival data. Statistics in Medicine 14:1447–1461.

Prentice, R. L., Williams, B. J., Peterson, A. V. (1981). On the regression analysis of multivariate failure time data. Biometrika 68:373–379.

Prentice, R. L. (1989). Surrogate endpoints in clinical trials: Definition and operational criteria. Statistics in Medicine 8:431–440.

Raab, G. M., Parpia, T. (2001). Random effects models for HIV marker data: Practical approaches with currently available software. Statistical Methods in Medical Research 10:101–116.

Robins, J. M., Tsiatis, A. A. (1991). Correcting for non-compliance in randomized trials using rank preserving structural failure time models. Communications in Statistics—Theory and Methods 20:2609–2631.

Robins, J. M., Greenland, S. (1994). Adjusting for differential rates of prophylaxis therapy for PCP in high-dose versus low-dose AZT treatment arms in an AIDS randomized trial. Journal of the American Statistical Association 89:737–749.

Schoenfeld, D. A. (1995). Issues in the testing of drug combinations. In: Finkelstein, D. M., Schoenfeld, D. A., eds. AIDS Clinical Trials: Guidelines for Design and Analysis. New York: Wiley.

Schoenfeld, D. A. (1996). Long-term follow-up in AIDS clinical trials. Statistics in Medicine 15:2366–2539.

Schwartz, D., Lellouch, J. (1967). Explanatory and pragmatic attitudes in therapeutic trials. Journal of Chronic Disease 20:637–648.

Shevitz, A., Wanke, C. A., Falutz, J., Kotler, D. P. (2001). Clinical perspectives on HIV-associated lipodystrophy syndrome: an update. AIDS 15:1917–1930.

Smith, P. J., Thompson, T. J., Jereb, J. A. (1997). A model for interval-censored tuberculosis outbreak data. Statistics in Medicine 16:485–496.

Sommer, A., Zeger, S. L. (1991). On estimating efficacy from clinical trials. Statistics in Medicine 10:45–52.

Sun, J. (1997). Regression analysis of interval-censored failure time data. Statistics in Medicine 16:497–504.

Thall, P. F., Cheng, S. C. (1999). Treatment comparisons based on two-dimensional safety and efficacy alternatives in oncology. Biometrics 55:746–753.

Touloumi, G., Pocock, S. J., Babiker, A. G., Darbyshire, J. H. (1999). Estimation and comparison of rates of change in longitudinal studies with informative drop-outs. Statistics in Medicine 18:1215–1233.

Touloumi, G., Pocock, S. J., Babiker, A. G., Darbyshire, J. H. (2002). Impact of missing data due to selective drop-outs in cohort studies and clinical trials. Epidemiology 13:347–355.

Tubert-Bitter, P., Bloch, D. A., Raynauld, J. P. (1995). Comparing the bivariate effects of toxicity and efficacy of treatments. Statistics in Medicine 14:1129–1141.

Volberding, P. A., Lagakos, S. W., Koch, M. A., Pettinelli, C. B., et al. (1990). Zidovudine in asymptomatic HIV infection: a controlled trial in persons with fewer than 500 CD4-positive cells per cubic millimeter. New England Journal of Medicine 322:941–949.

Volberding, P. A., Lagakos, S. W., Grimes, J. M., Stein, D. S., Balfour, H. H., Reichman, R. C., Bartlett, J. A., Hirsch, M. S., Phair, J. P., Mitsuyasu, R. T., Fischl, M. A., Soeiro, R., the AIDS Clinical Trials Group of the National Institute of Allergy and Infectious Diseases (1994). The duration of zidovudine benefit in persons with asymptomatic HIV infection. Journal of the American Medical Association 272:437–442.

Walker, A. S. (1999).The analysis of multivariate failure time data with application to multiple endpoints in trials in HIV infection. Unpublished PhD thesis, University College, London.

Walker, A. S., Babiker, A. G., Darbyshire, J. H. (2000). Analysis of multivariate failure-time data from HIV clinical trials. Controlled Clinical Trials 21:75–93.

Wang, S. T., Klein, J. P., Moeschberger, M. L. (1995). Semi-parametric estimation of covariate effects using the positive stable frailty model. Applied Stochastic Models and Data Analysis 11:121–133.

Wei, L. J., Lin, D. Y., Weissfeld, L. (1989). Regression analysis of multivariate incomplete failure time data by modelling marginal distributions. Journal of the American Statistical Association 84:1065–1073.

Wei, L. J., Glidden, D. V. (1997). An overview of statistical methods for multiple failure time data in clinical trials. Statistics in Medicine 16:833–839.

White, I. P., Walker, A. S., Babiker, A. G., Darbyshire, J. H. (1997). Impact of treatment changes on the interpretation of the Concorde trial. AIDS 11:999–1006.

White, I. R., Goetghebeur, E. J. T. (1998). Clinical trials comparing two treatment policies: which aspect of the treatment policies make a difference? Statistic in Medicine 17:319–339.

White, I. R., Babiker, A. G., Walker, A. S., Darbyshire, J. H. (1999). Randomization-based methods for correcting for treatment changes: examples from the Concorde trial. Statistics in Medicine 18:2617–2634.

White, I. R., Walker, A. S., Babiker, A. G., Darbyshire, J. H. (2002). Strbee: Randomization-based efficacy estimator. The Stata Journal 2:140–150.

Index of Abbreviations*

*The page reference gives the first use of an abbreviation in a chapter.

Index of Clinical Trials Used as Examples

Subject Index